SURGERY - PROCEDURES, COMPLICATIONS, AND RESULTS

CURRENT UNDERSTANDING AND NEW TECHNIQUES IN REFRACTIVE SURGERY

Surgery - Procedures, Complications, and Results

Additional books in this series can be found on Nova's website under the Series tab.

Additional e-books in this series can be found on Nova's website under the e-book tab.

Eye and Vision Research Developments

Additional books in this series can be found on Nova's website under the Series tab.

Additional e-books in this series can be found on Nova's website under the e-book tab.

SURGERY - PROCEDURES, COMPLICATIONS, AND RESULTS

CURRENT UNDERSTANDING AND NEW TECHNIQUES IN REFRACTIVE SURGERY

MICHAEL O'KEEFE
EDITOR

NOVA BIOMEDICAL

New York

For permission to use material from this book please contact us:
Telephone 631-231-7269; Fax 631-231-8175
Web Site: http://www.novapublishers.com

NOTICE TO THE READER

Library of Congress Cataloging-in-Publication Data

ISBN: 978-1-62808-748-2

Library of Congress Control Number: 2013945712

Published by Nova Science Publishers, Inc. † New York

Contents

Preface vii

Acknowledgments ix

Chapter 1 LASEK Complications **1**
David P. S. O'Brart

Chapter 2 LASIK Complications **25**
Marco Tavolato and Lucio Buratto

Chapter 3 Dry Eyes in Patients Undergoing Refractive Surgery **35**
Ian John Dooley

Chapter 4 Corneal Ectasia **55**
Gerard N. Kervick

Chapter 5 Refractive Surgery in Patients with Strabismus **73**
Gillian O'Mullane and Caitriona Kirwan

Chapter 6 Pediatric Refractive Surgery **91**
William F. Astle, Santa Heede, Peter T. Huang and Emi Sanders

Chapter 7 Intraocular Lens Power Calculations Post Refractive Surgery **115**
Grainne Brosnan

Chapter 8 High Order Aberrations **127**
Caitriona Kirwan

Chapter 9 Medical Legal Issues **145**
Marc B. Guerin

Chapter 10 Long-Term Refractive Changes after Refractive Surgery **155**
Andrea Ryan and Michael O'Keefe

Chapter 11 Corneal Topography **187**
Arthur Cummings

Chapter 12 Phakic Intraocular Lens Implants **201**
Sarah Moran

Chapter 13 Supracor **219**
Andrea Ryan and Michael O'Keefe

Chapter 14 Corneal Inlays **231**
Caroline Baily and Michael O'Keefe

Chapter 15 Management of Keratoconus **245**
Edward Loane and William J. Power

Chapter 16 Femtosecond Laser Cataract Surgery **269**
Sheraz M. Daya and Marcela Espinosa-Lagana

Chapter 17 Corneal Grafting **281**
Tim Fulcher

About the Editor **295**

Index **297**

Preface

Refractive surgery has radically changed the boundaries of ophthalmology. It has opened up new frontiers, stimulated new techniques and new technology. More important it has improved the quality of life for millions of people.

It has resulted in numerous publications with many books written and thousands of peer publications published in many journals. A minority of patients are unhappy due to complications or poor outcome. The challenge remains to find ways of helping these patients and reducing their numbers. The other challenge is to open up new frontiers in presbyopia. In this book we cannot address everything but our main aim is to bring greater clarity to some of the current techniques and to outline some of the future techniques.

Acknowledgments

I would like to thank all the Irish and foreign contributors for their time and efforts. I am indebted to Helen Murphy for her organizational and secretarial skills.

In: Current Understanding and New Techniques … ISBN: 978-1-62808-748-2
Editor: Michael O'Keefe

Chapter 1

LASEK Complications

David P. S. O'Brart *
Guy's and St. Thomas' NHS Foundation Trust,
London, England

Introduction

It has been over a decade since the technique of Laser Epithelial Keratomileusis (LASEK) was described separately by Camellin [1], Azar [2], and Shah [3]. Unlike PRK, where the central epithelium is wholly debrided by blades or brushes, in the classically described LASEK technique an epithelial flap with a superior hinge is created by means of a peri-operative application of a dilute solution of alcohol, which creates a cleavage plane between the lamina lucida and the lamina densa of the epithelial basement membrane [4]. Following Excimer laser treatment, the intact epithelial sheet is typically re-positioned over the ablated corneal stroma and to keep it in place a bandage contact lens is applied during the first few days post-operatively. The reported purpose of replacing the epithelial sheet is to reduce post-operative pain, speed visual recovery and decrease the risk of iatrogenic haze occasionally seen after PRK by diminishing the early epithelial-stromal wound-healing interactions [1-3]. Such epithelial flaps, unlike the deeper partial-thickness stromal flaps created in LASIK, are not associated with intra-lamellar flap complications such as diffuse lamellar keratitis, permanent wrinkling, flap melt, epithelial in-growth, etc, which can, albeit rarely, severely limit visual performance following LASIK [5].

Whilst LASIK offers clear advantages in terms of rapidity of post-operative recovery, multiple comparative studies using modern laser platforms have demonstrated similar medium and long-term visual and refractive outcomes between LASEK and LASIK for low-hyperopic and low-, moderate- and even high-myopic corrections [6-15]. Indeed, a recent study by Kirwan and O'Keefe demonstrated less induction of higher order aberrations in LASEK compared to LASIK-treated eyes [14]. A finding which has also been reported in two

* David P.S. O'Brart MD FRCS FRCOphth - Consultant Ophthalmic Surgeon. Guy's and St. Thomas' NHS Foundation Trust, London SE1 7EH, England. Email: davidobrart@aol.com.

recent published prospective studies by Wallau and Campos and Moshirfar et al. comparing PRK and LASIK, with less induction of higher order aberrations in PRK-treated eyes [16-17].

Comparative studies of LASEK and PRK have demonstrated no consistent significant differences in clinical outcomes. In terms of early postoperative recovery, whilst Leccisotti et al. [18] demonstrated no differences, Autrata and Rehurek [19] and Lee et al. [20] in prospective bilateral studies found less pain and faster visual recovery after LASEK. In contrast, Litwak et al. [21] found more pain and slower epithelial healing after LASEK, although they exposed the epithelium to 20% alcohol for 45 seconds, which would result in the death of virtually all cells in the flap [22]. In the only reported comparative study of hyperopic corrections, Autrata and Rehurek [23] reported less pain, faster visual recovery, and quicker refractive stability with LASEK compared with PRK. A more recent randomized, bilateral clinical study by Einollahi et al. utilizing confocal microscopy comparing mechanical versus alcohol-assisted epithelial debridement with PRK reported retarded epithelial healing time and decreased retro-ablation stromal keratocyte density with mechanical debridement [24].

In terms of visual and refractive outcomes, recently published meta-analyses by Zhao et al. and Cui et al. of clinical outcomes of LASEK and PRK in myopia, whilst in demonstrating less sub-epithelial haze at one and three months after surgery with LASEK failed to demonstrate any differences in primary outcome (UCVA, manifest refractive spherical equivalent) or secondary outcome (epithelial healing, pain, haze) measures after these time points [25-26]. Similarly, Ghoreishi et al. in a randomized controlled trial comparing alcohol-assisted versus mechanical epithelium removal in PRK in 1250 eyes found entirely comparable results between the two techniques [27].

With regards to other methods of surface Excimer laser ablation, whilst Teus et al. in a randomized prospective trial comparing LASEK and Epi-LASEK demonstrated faster visual rehabilitation and better safety and efficacy after LASEK for low to moderate myopic corrections [28], Hondur et al. in a prospective, bilateral study of Epi-LASIK and LASEK for myopia found comparable results between the two methods at 1 year [29] and Reilly in a retrospective chart review reported less pain and a trend towards less haze with Epi-LASIK [30].Similarly, whilst Aslanides et al. in a randomized, bilateral prospective study comparing trans-epithelial to alcohol-assisted PRK reported lower pain scores, faster epithelial healing and less haze at six months with the all laser technique [31], Luger et al. in a randomized, bilateral study demonstrated no differences in efficacy or safety between the two techniques [32].

Published outcomes of LASEK procedures over the past decade are very encouraging [6-33]. In a review article by Teneri et al. , the cumulative reported safety index of 11 peer-reviewed papers was 1.0, with only a single eye of nearly 1,500 studied, losing two or more lines of BSCVA due to a macular cyst unrelated to the LASEK procedure [33]. Reported predictability was excellent with 83% of eyes within +0.50 D of the intended correction at 6 months, with an efficacy index of 0.947 [33]. Similarly, the author's own experience with this technique has been very positive with excellent efficacy and safety not only for low and moderate myopia but also for high myopia (-6.00 to -12.00 diopters) and hyperopic corrections [34-35].

Such results are the product of two decades of increasing knowledge of laser tissue interactions and corneal wound-healing responses, the development and access to advanced technologies, and meticulous attention to detail with regards to preoperative patient education and counselling, preoperative evaluation, operative procedures, and postoperative care. A detailed knowledge of possible complications both sight threatening and non-sight threatening, their avoidance and management is absolutely essential in order to minimize adverse events postoperatively and optimize visual and refractive outcomes and patient satisfaction. This is especially important taking into consideration the elective nature of keratorefractive procedures and the associated high patient expectations.

Intra-Operative Complications

Alcohol Escape and Peri-Operative Pain

The LASEK procedure is relatively easy to perform and takes only a few minutes to undertake. It is normally painless. However, if alcohol escapes from underneath the LASEK well onto the bulbar conjunctival surface, then significant ocular pain and discomfort can result. Alcohol escape should be avoided not only to facilitate a painless surgical procedure but also as it might cause limbal epithelial stem cell damage, which may delay epithelial healing, and conjunctival epithelial damage, which will increase post-operative discomfort and inflammation. To avoid this complication, patients should receive adequate topical anaesthesia with 2-3 drops of topical Tetracaine 1% (which also helps facilitate the alcohol epithelial removal). They should be fully informed of the need to stay still during alcohol application and told that they will experience a pressure sensation when the well is placed on the globe and loss of visual clarity as it is filled with alcohol. Firm, but not excessive, pressure should be used when holding the LASEK well on the ocular surface. Should alcohol escape occur, the ocular surface should be immediately irrigated with balanced saline solution, the conjunctival and corneal surface dried and the well re-applied for the remainder of the application time.

Poor Epithelial Flap

With application of 15-20% alcohol for 25-40 seconds, the fashioning of an intact epithelial flap with an adequate superior hinge is usually straightforward [1-3, 22-23, 33-35]. However, in a few cases, the epithelium may be especially adherent. In the author's experience, this tends to occur in individuals who have undertaken excessive long-term contact lens wear. This has been similarly noted by Claringbold, who also identified young men and postmenopausal women as having more adherent epithelium [36]. In such eyes the author increases alcohol exposure time to 30 seconds instead of 25. Camellin, in his series, reported difficulty in obtaining an intact epithelial flap in 12% of eyes [1. 37]. The author reported adherent and incomplete epithelial flaps in 4% of high myopic [34] and 6% of hyperopic eyes [35].

If adherence is encountered, replacing the flap and applying alcohol for 10 more seconds usually facilitates improved flap creation. However, if it is not possible to obtain a complete epithelial flap, then the procedure can be simply converted to a PRK technique by mechanically debriding the epithelium with the knowledge that although the patient may [20,

23-24] or may not [21] experience more postoperative pain and a slightly slower visual recovery, the long-term clinical outcomes are the same [25-27].

Free Flap

It is the author's observation that, the corneal epithelium is often less adherent superiorly than inferiorly, which helps facilitate superior hinge formation. However, it may be occasionally difficult to fashion an adequate epithelial hinge and a free epithelial flap can occasionally occur.

This tends to be more common in the treatment of hyperopic eyes where much larger (9.00 to 10.00 millimetre (mm)) flaps need to be fashioned. In such cases the flap can still be repositioned over the ablated stromal surface, although care should be taken to ensure the flap is placed basal epithelial-side down. Following replacement of a free flap a few minutes drying time should be allowed and a bandage contact lens can then be carefully inserted in the usual manner to keep the epithelium in place. Post-operative care can then continue in the usual manner.

It should be noted, however, that for many surgeons it is their usual practice to discard the epithelial flap before contact lens placement. Liu et al. reported less post-operative pain and faster visual recovery with a flap removal technique in a series of 582 patients [38], whilst Taneri et al. in a comparative case series demonstrated no difference in terms of pain, epithelial closure time and haze development in eyes treated with flap retention or removal [39]. Similarly, Kalyvainaki et al. in a double-masked, bilateral randomized study of epi-LASIK found no differences with discarding or keeping the epithelium. It is therefore not unreasonable to simply discard the epithelium in cases of free or poor flaps as the ultimate refractive and visual outcome should still be very satisfactory.

Early Postoperative Complications (Hours/Days)

Pain

While some comparative studies have shown no differences [18], others have reported less postoperative pain after LASEK compared with PRK [19-20]. Camellin reported that over 60% of his patients experienced little/no pain following LASEK [37]. However, it is the author's experience [34-35] that the majority of individuals do experience pain/discomfort during the first 1-24 hours after LASEK and a number of individuals may report considerable pain.

Most surgeons prescribe oral analgesics for 2-3 days after the procedure, both opiate and non-opiate. Topical non-steroidal anti-inflammatory agents have been shown to be efficacious in reducing pain following LASEK and other ocular surface ablation procedures [41-43]. A number of different agents have been utilized with efficacy being demonstrated with topical Indomethacin 0.1%, Diclofenac 0.5%, Nepfenac 0.1% and Ketolorac 0.4% [41-43]. Care must be exercised, however, with administration of these agents as corneal melting has been reported very rarely with their usage [44-46]. They should only be used for a few days following surgery, in limited dosage and patients must be carefully counselled regarding their correct usage and dosage.

Considerable pain relief without any detrimental effects on visual and refractive recovery has also been demonstrated by Verma et al. with the use of limited and supervised topical anaesthetic administration after PRK [47-48]. In the author's practice great benefit has been found, with no detrimental effects, with the use of topical preservative free anaesthetic drops (Benoxinate 0.4%) in a limited dosage, with a maximum of 1 drop every 2 hours for the first 18 hours following surgery (maximum of 10 drops in total) for acute pain control after LASEK [34, 35].

Patents must, however, must be very carefully counselled as to the importance regarding the correct dosage of such agents as keratatopathy after LASEK with their excessive use has been reported [49].

Delayed Epithelial Healing

In the author's experience, epithelial closure is usually present in myopic LASEK corrections within 3-4 days [34] and hyperopic corrections, which have larger overall ablation diameters, within 3-7 days following surgery [35]. Kornilovsky reported epithelial closure at 4 days [50], Camellin et al. 4-5 days [1, 37], and Lee et al. 3.68+0.69 days [20] in myopic LASEK corrections. Taneri et al. in a review article reported a closure rate of 78% at 3 days and 99% at one week [33].

Most surgeons remove bandage contact lenses between 3 and 5 days or when epithelial closure is complete. Late epithelial closure beyond 5-7 days is unusual. Such patients need to be carefully examined and monitored because of the risks of underlying stromal melt, the ongoing risk of infection, and the possible development of late corneal haze and scarring. Any signs of stromal infiltration should alert the practitioner to the possibility of potential sight-threatening complications such as an infection or melt. Conditions predisposing to delayed epithelial closure include dry eye problems, preservative toxicity, drug allergy (topical antibiotics), topical drug abuse and over-usage (non-steroidal anti-inflammatory and anaesthetic drops) and limbal stem cell anomalies.

Prior to surgery, it is vital to eliminate patients with dry eye problems, as this may exacerbate epithelial healing problems following surgery. Patients with overt dry eye problems do not make good candidates for laser refractive surgery and are contraindicated. Those with mild dry eye symptoms and signs can be treated prior to surgery with ocular lubricants, punctal plugs, aggressive treatment of concurrent lid disease and Omega-3 oral supplementation [51-52]. If satisfactory resolution occurs, then keratorefractive surgery may be possible provided there is no associated manifest connective tissue problem. Whilst surface laser ablation is generally associated with less induction of post-operative dry eye problems [53], if delayed epithelial healing occurs in the presence of dry eye, ocular lubricants, punctal plugging and Omega-3 supplementation should be implemented immediately [51-52].

Toxicity to preservatives and drug allergy should be suspected in cases of retarded epithelial healing and in the presence of a history of previous intolerance to contact lens solutions, continuing conjunctival injection and punctate epithelial erosions. In eyes where epithelial closure is delayed beyond 4-5 days, the use of preservative free-medications is advisable.

Patients with conjunctival cicatrizing conditions and limbal stem cell deficiencies are not candidates for keratorefractive surgery and should be excluded preoperatively by careful slit-lamp biomicroscopic examination.

Slow Visual Recovery

Immediately after LASEK, provided an intact epithelial flap has been created and successfully replaced, patients typically notice an immediate improvement in unaided postoperative visual performance. It is not uncommon for patients to then experience a reduction in visual acuity after the first 12-24 hours, as epithelial cells within the flap damaged by alcohol swell and die [22] or occasionally if the flap sloughs off. Patients should be warned before surgery, that although ocular pain redness and swelling improve after 12-24 hours, early visual impairment is not unusual and will not influence the ultimate final outcome. Vision begins to improve after a few days following epithelial closure and even in high myopic corrections (greater than -6.0D) 90% of eyes have an UCVA of 20/40 or better and 70% of 20/30 or better by one week [34]. For low myopic corrections and in younger patients, visual recovery is much faster. With hyperopic LASEK corrections, visual recovery is typically more protracted [35]. Less than 50% of such patients achieve an UCVA of 20/40 or better by one week, as epithelial regeneration is slower in the presence of larger flap diameters and older patients and myopic over-correction during the first few weeks and months after surgery is usual [35]. Hyperopic LASEK patients need to counselled pre-operatively that although functional unaided near vision may be achieved during the first few weeks, satisfactory levels of unaided distance visual acuity may take several weeks and even months [35].

Protracted visual recovery in the early post-operative period, beyond that considered above, is typically the result of delayed or irregular epithelial healing. As discussed above, predisposing causes include dry eye, preservative toxicity, drop allergy, anaesthetic and non-steroidal eye drop abuse, infection and pre-existing ocular surface anomalies. Prevention is always better than cure and it is obligatory that all patients have a complete pre-operative ophthalmic consultation and examination by a suitably experienced practitioner with a thorough knowledge of anterior segment disease so that pre-existing conditions are adequately treated prior to surgery and unsuitable patients with untreatable and/or extensive ocular surface disorders are excluded. In the presence of delayed epithelial healing, infectious and non-infectious keratitis must be excluded, investigated and appropriately managed, the tear film optimized [51-52] and correct compliance with topical medication ensured [44-46, 49].

Sterile Infiltrates

Punctate sterile epithelial infiltrates without stromal infiltration may develop during the first few weeks after LASEK. They may occasionally be the result of dry eye and/or preservative toxicity/drug allergy. They can be treated by optimizing the pre-corneal tear film and frequent preservative-free topical corticosteroid administration.

Occasionally, anterior stromal infiltration may occur. In these cases infectious keratitis needs to be excluded and eyes with an associated overlying epithelial defect must be assumed infected and investigated and treated appropriately. Where the overlying epithelium is closed and the anterior chamber quite, such eyes may be treated by increasing the frequency of topical corticosteroid medication, while maintaining antibiotic cover until the infiltrates have resolved [54]. However, the patient must be kept under very careful observation and a high degree of suspicion for infective keratitis be maintained and if in any doubt appropriate microbiological specimens must be taken.

Early Infectious Keratitis

Infectious keratitis is a very rare event after LASEK and other surface laser ablation procedures with a reported incidence in one multicentre study of 18,651 eyes of 0.2% [55]. It has been postulated, that as the infectious process commences at the epithelial level in LASEK/PRK and not intrastromally as in LASIK, it might be easier to manage in terms of the taking of microbiological specimens and antimicrobial penetration [56]. Because of its serious sight-threatening potential, Surgeons need to maintain a high level of suspicion with regards to its occurrence. In suspected cases immediate and aggressive management is imperative, with the taking of appropriate microbiological specimens and targeted intensive topical antimicrobial therapy. With such management, good visual acuity is usually restored [55, 57-58]. In de Rojas's multicentre study of surface ablation procedures including LASEK, 72% of cases presented within 7 days, cultures were positive in about 50%, Staphylococcus was the most frequently isolated organism and over 90% retained a corrected distance acuity of 20/40 or better [55].

In order to minimize the potential occurrence of infective keratitis, patients must be examined preoperatively for signs of active lid margin disease, which must be treated appropriately with lid hygiene and if indicated systemic tetracyclines before considering laser refractive procedures. Following laser refractive surgery, practitioners typically advocate the use of a broad spectrum prophylactic topical antibiotic regimen until epithelial closure is complete. Common therapies include the use of an aminoglycoside, such as tobramycin, which covers gram-negative organisms including Pseudomonas, and/or a Fluoroquinolone, which cover both gram-positive and gram-negative species. Preferred agents include Ofloxacin and fourth-generation fluoroquinolones such as gatifloxacin, and moxifloxacin.

Early Postoperative Complications (Days/Weeks)

Slow Visual Recovery

At 1 month over 80% of myopic eyes after LASEK achieve an UCVA of 20/20 or better [6-9, 11-15, 18-21, 23, 25-26, 28-39]. Occasionally, however, visual recovery may take longer, up to 3-4 months. As well as residual refractive error, this can be due to epithelial irregularity because of delayed epithelial healing (as discussed above). Such patients need to be carefully examined to exclude the presence of sight-threatening complications such as late infective keratitis, non-infective keratitis/melt, and steroid-induced raised intraocular pressure.

In hyperopic LASEK corrections, visual recovery is generally slower, with less than 40% of eyes achieving an UCVA of 20/20 or better at 1 month due to myopic overcorrection that may take several months to settle, especially in high-order corrections greater than +3.00 D [35].

Intraocular Steroid Pressure Response

Although randomized clinical studies have indicated little benefit from topical corticosteroid administration following surface Excimer laser procedures [59], the vast majority of Surgeons still prescribe topical steroids during the first few weeks after LASEK/PRK to minimize the development of corneal haze. Fluorometholone 0.1% (FML) is often the preferred agent, as its reduced ocular penetration reduces the risk of associated intra-ocular complications such as increased intraocular pressure, enhanced risk of infective keratitis and cataract formation [59-61]. When prescribing such medications, it is essential to monitor patients for an intraocular pressure response if they are used for longer than 10 days. Idealy patients should have intraocular pressure measurements every 2 weeks while they are administering such medications [62]. With FML usage, steroid-induced ocular hypertension has been reported in up to 3% of cases [60]. Should an elevated intraocular response occur, the steroid medication should, if possible, be terminated. Topical anti-glaucomatous medications, in the first instance preservative-free Timoptol 0.25% twice daily (unless contraindicated), may be prescribed. Preservative-free Aproclonidine 1% three times a day is useful if the pressure is greater than 30mmHg. Systemic Acetazolamide is rarely required. The intraocular pressure usually returns to normal levels a 1-2 weeks after stopping the steroid drops. The use of new steroid agents, designed to produce less intraocular pressure problems, such as Loteprednol etabonate 0.5% in laser refractive surgery is as yet to be evaluated.

Recurrent Corneal Erosion Syndrome

Fifteen to 20% of patients undergoing LASEK and PRK report "dryness" and discomfort on first opening their eyes when waking in the morning or in the middle of the night [63]. Such symptoms are indicative of mild recurrent corneal erosion syndrome. They occur during the first few post-operative few months post-operatively and then typically resolve. In persistent cases or when symptoms become frequent and problematic the use of topical lubricant ointments such as Lacrilube and Simple at night for 8-10 weeks is often successful in alleviating and resolving such problems. In cases with pre-existing lid disease, systemic tetracyclines are a useful adjunctive treatment, possibly due to inhibition of metalloproteinase-9 [64]. Optimization of the tear film with ocular lubricants, punctal plugging and Omega-3 supplementation is often beneficial [51-52].

After 9-12 months, in persistent cases that have not responded to medical therapy, it may be necessary perform a peripheral anterior stromal puncture procedure. This can be performed as a quick outpatient procedure under topical anaesthesia with a 25G needle. The stromal punctures are directed to the 360-degree, 3.0mm para-central/peripheral corneal area outside the central optical zone, both to avoid scar formation across the visual axis and as the epithelium overlying the area of ablation is typically firmly adherent to the underlying stroma (Figure 1).

In the author's experience of 12 years of performing LASEK, anterior stromal puncture has been necessary in 10 eyes of six patients (<0.5%) when symptoms have persisted after 9 months. In all cases, it has resulted in improvement/resolution of symptoms, with only one case requiring a repeat procedure.

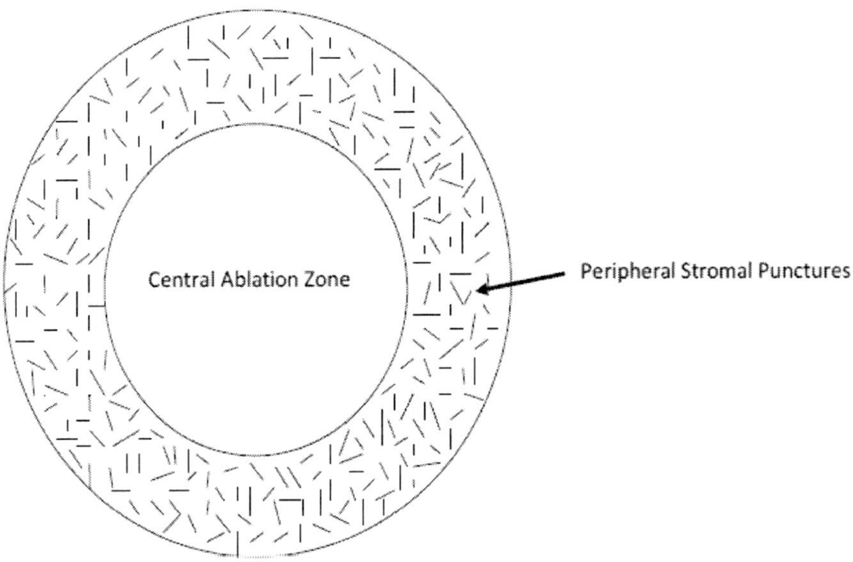

Figure 1. The stromal punctures are directed to the 360-degree, 3.0mm para-central/peripheral corneal area outside the central optical zone.

Symptoms of recurrent erosion syndrome are more common after surface ablation procedures than LASIK [65]. In the author's experience it is more common with low order myopic corrections (typically less than -4.00 D) and in myopic rather than hyperopic corrections due to the width of the stromal ablation. Patients should be counselled and warned preoperatively about the occurrence of such symptoms as they can have a significantly adverse effect on patient satisfaction [65].

Prior to alcohol administration, it is can be useful to test the adherence of the epithelium with a LASIK sponge. If the epithelium moves and wrinkles it likely that there is an underlying epithelial basement membrane dystrophy and then the procedure can be performed without alcohol administration and early medical therapy, with topical lubricants before sleeping, instigated immediately post-operatively. In eyes with signs of epithelial basement membrane dystrophy pre-operatively (epithelial cysts and whorls seen on slit lamp examination), it is the author's practice not only to warn the patient prior to surgery of the increased risks of recurrent erosion syndrome but to combine the LASEK procedure with a peripheral anterior stromal puncture technique (figure 1).

Corneal Melt

Corneal melting after LASEK/PRK is an extremely rare occurrence. Cases have been reported in the presence of collagen vascular diseases such as systemic lupus erythematosus (SLE) [66]. It is important to exclude such patients preoperatively. Some practitioners regard collagen vascular diseases as only a relative contraindication to refractive laser surgery with surgery being considered possible in cases of completely controlled systemic disease with no ocular manifestations and no clinical signs or history of dry-eye symptoms [67]. However, the presence of active systemic disease with past ocular involvement and dry eye is an absolute contraindication.

As well as collagen vascular diseases other predisposing causes for corneal melting after LASEK include dry eye, anaesthetic [49] and non-steroidal eye drop abuse [44-46], infection and pre-existing ocular surface anomalies. It has been particularly associated with the use of non-steroidal drops, which have been shown to induce the production of collagenases and matrix metalloproteinases [44-46]. It is for this reason that the author prefers not to prescribe these medications after keratorefractive surgery and prefers limited topical anaesthesia application for the first 18 hours after surgery.

If corneal melting should occur, then associated dry eye problems must be immediately and aggressively treated and infectious keratitis excluded. If being administered, topical anaesthetic and non-steroidal drops should be stopped. Expert sub-specialist ophthalmic medical management is required with intensive topical preservative-free corticosteroid and systemic immunosuppressive therapy. Further surgical interventions such as amniotic membrane grafting and keratoplasty may be necessary [44-46, 49, 67].

Herpes Simplex Keratitis

Patients with recurrent herpes simplex keratitis are not candidates for routine keratorefractive surgery. Phototherapeutic keratectomy (PTK) can be useful in selected cases, but reactivation may occur [68], and such eyes require prophylactic systemic antivirals (Acyclovir 400mg bd starting for two weeks prior to surgery and for 6 months following surgery). Any eye with an unexplained corneal scar preoperatively must be regarded as suspicious and a full history must be taken. In patients that develop labial herpes simplex during the early/medium postoperative period, it is recommended that they are prescribed systemic prophylactic acyclovir.

Late Infectious Keratitis

Late infectious keratitis is a rare event after LASEK. As discussed above the incidence of infectious keratitis after surface laser ablation procedures is 0.2% with the majority of cases occurring within the first week after surgery [55]. Infection presenting after the first week in similarity to those cases after LASIK tend occur in the presence of atypical organisms such as mycobacterium species [69] and fungi [70-71].

Surgeons must be aware of the occurrence of such late infections so they can be adequately managed. Patients should be informed that they must return promptly with any symptoms of pain, redness, and sudden visual loss occurring in the first couple of months after surgery.

In such patients especially where there are signs of corneal infiltration/melting there should be a high suspicion of late infectious keratitis. Microbiological specimens should be taken, particularly for atypical organisms, and appropriate antimicrobial therapy instigated. In the presence of worsening signs and symptoms and negative cultures, corneal biopsy and even therapeutic keratoplasty may be required. The role of corneal cross-linking in such cases is as yet undetermined and requires further evaluation but may perhaps be of benefit [72].

Medium-Term Postoperative Complications (Weeks/Months)

Overcorrection/Undercorrection

For corrections between +4.00 and -8.00 D and up to -5.00 DC published studies of LASEK indicate that 80-90% of eyes achieve refractive outcomes within +0.50 D of that intended [6-9, 11-15, 18-21, 23, 25-26, 28-39], with refractive stability being achieved by 1-3 months in myopic [34] and 3-6 months in hyperopic corrections [35]. Uncommonly, over- and under-correction may occur especially in high-order corrections [34-35]. Reported re-treatment rates vary between 0 and 7% [6-9, 11-15, 18-21, 23, 25-26, 28-39]. In cases of early regression especially in the presence of sub-epithelial haze some practitioners advocate the use of topical corticosteroids [61, 73] although not all such cases respond and re-treatment may be necessary.

The optimum timing of re-treatment is as yet undetermined. It should not be undertaken before at least two stable refractive measurements have been obtained at least 3 months apart. It is advisable not to consider re-treatment in cases of myopic surface Excimer laser ablation before 6-9 months, and for hyperopic cases before 12 months, due to the risk of precipitating an aggressive healing response. In such eyes which have undergone previous corneal surgery, the use of intra-operative Mitomycin-C (MMC) is advisable to reduce post-operative haze formation [74]. Careful pre-operative evaluation with corneal topography and tomography is essential to ensure that any regression, especially in myopic cases and where there has been an increase in cylindrical refractive error, is not due to an ectatic process.

Haze

As Excimer laser refractive surgery is undertaken on healthy eyes any deterioration in postoperative corneal transparency and hence visual performance is of great concern. In PRK, sub-epithelial haze can arise within the ablated area 3-4 weeks following surgery, with maximal disturbances at 3-6 months. Haze development is associated with increasing depths of stromal ablation and small optical zone treatments [75-78]. In LASEK, it has been postulated that the formation of an intact epithelial layer to cover the lasered area might reduce epithelial-stromal cytokine cross-talk during the initial phases of postoperative wound healing and induce less haze [1-3]. With regards to haze, prospective bilateral comparative studies of LASEK versus PRK have demonstrated contradictory results. Hashemi et al. reported no differences [79], while Autrata and Rehurek [19] and Lee et al. [20] found less haze in eyes undergoing LASEK. In the author's own published series, with modern laser platforms and large optical zone diameters of 6.50mm or greater, visually significant haze formation is an infrequent event even in high myopic and hyperopic corrections, with 90% of corneas being completely clear or showing only the merest trace of haze at 6-12 months post-operatively [34-35]. Because of the increased risks of visually-significant haze development with high corrections, small ablation diameters, and increasing depths of stromal ablation, it is the author's protocol to only treat eyes with LASEK (without adjunctive MMC) for corrections between +2mm and -6.00 D and up to -2.5 DC, to only use optical zones of 6.5mm for myopia and 7.0mm for hyperopia and to limit the maximum depth of stromal ablation to less than 100μm.

For surface ablation procedures including LASEK and especially for high order corrections, many surgeons advocate the adjunctive use of MCC. MMC is a DNA alkylating agent, derived from Streptomyces Caepitosus. It inhibits DNA/RNA replication especially in rapidly dividing cells such as fibroblasts and thereby suppresses wound healing. Its use as an adjunctive medication applied intra-operatively immediately after laser ablation in PRK was first suggested by Talamo over two decades ago [80]. Re-interest in surface ablation over the past decade led to resurgence in its usage and now routine implementation, especially in high corrections and eyes at risk for the development of haze such as those which have undergone previous corneal surgery. Leccisotti in a prospective, randomized, double-masked, paired eye study of PRK corrections between -6.5 and -10 diopters (D) reported statistically less haze in eyes treated with MMC 0.2mg/ml for 45 seconds albeit with a reported over-correction of 6% [81]. Similarly, Wallau and Campos as well as demonstrating better outcomes for PRK with MMC compared to LASIK, reported no haze after PRK with the use of MMC [82]. A recent meta-analysis of clinical outcomes comparing surface ablation with and without 0.02% MMC showed that it indeed reduces haze in PRK, although the results of MMC in conjunction with laser assisted sub-epithelial keratomileuis (LASEK) were less certain [83].

There is, however, some controversy concerning the use of MMC in keratorefractive surgery. Corneal and sclera melting both early (within months) and late (after many years) has been reported following its peri-operative application in pterygium surgery [83]. Certainly there are concerns regarding its potential unknown long-term complications after laser refractive surgery, with reported delays in epithelial wound healing [84], although other investigators have not found such changes [85]. In relation to possible endothelial damage, in a recently published review article Roh and Funderburgh identified five clinical studies in the peer-reviewed literature, three of which reported no change in corneal endothelial density, while two found statistically significant cell loss following MMC application after surface ablation [86]. A more recent prospective study with 0.02% MMC applied for 40 seconds showed no change in central endothelial counts at 6 months after surgery [87]. Similarly, Gambato et al. in a randomized bilateral study using in vivo confocal microscopy with five year follow-up found no changes in endothelial cell counts, epithelial thickness, keratocyte density, number of corneal nerve fibres, nerve beadings, nerve branching and tortuosity with the intraoperative use of MMC 0.02% [88,89].

Whilst these studies afford support for the use of peri-operative MMC, large series, longer follow-up studies are required to determine the precise influence many decades after LASEK/PRK of intra-operative MMC on the health and functioning of the cornea and its endothelium. In the meantime, pre-operatively patients should be informed and consented concerning the possibility of rare and as yet undetermined possible long-term complications associated with MMC usage. It is the author's personal preference to reserve the adjunctive use of MMC in LASEK to eyes undergoing myopic corrections >-6.0D, hyperopic corrections >+2D, astigmatic corrections >2.5DC and in eyes with previous corneal surgery such as keratoplasty, radial keratotomy (RK) and previous surface ablations.

Although there is evidence to suggest that topical corticosteroids merely delay rather than prevent haze formation [59], in eyes where haze greater than grade I (easily visible with the slit lamp) develops during the first 3 months, it is recommended that topical corticosteroids are prescribed (preservative-free Dexamethasone 0.1%) possibly in conjunction with preservative-free topical Timoptol 0.25% twice daily (providing there is no contraindication to its usage) to negate steroid intraocular pressure responses [61]. The topical steroid medication should be tapered over a 6 to 12 week period, with careful bi-weekly monitoring of the intraocular pressure. It is important to note that with or without the use of topical steroids, long-term studies indicate that with time haze however dense will clear in the vast majority of eyes with return of any associated loss of BSCVA [90, 91].

In eyes with persistent and significant haze (>grade 2 beyond 9-12 months post-surgery) steroid medication will only have a limited effect [59]. Although haze does very gradually clear with time [90, 91], further surgical intervention may be necessary depending on any associated loss of BSCVA, regression of correction and patient preference. A number of surgical options for persistent post-PRK/-LASEK haze are available. Vigo et al. reported a series of 35 eyes of 30 patients with severe haze and regression after PRK, that underwent 6-12 months after surgery epithelial debridement and scraping of the stromal surface with topical application of MMC 0.02% applied for 30-45 s. All eyes had significant improvements in corneal transparency and refractive error and only 2 required a further debridement treatment [92]. Porges et al. presented a series of 8 eyes 7 patients with severe haze following PRK who were treated with phototherapeutic keratectomy (PTK) to remove the haze layer augmented with intraoperative MMC 0.02% [93]. All eyes had an improvement in visual performance [93]. It is the author's preferred practice to use a corneal wavefront topography-assisted excimer laser ablation augmented with intraoperative MMC 0.02% to treat such eyes [94]. This is best performed when the refractive status and corneal appearance has been stable for at least 6 months and should not ideally be performed until 12 months after the original procedure. A transepithelial approach is most beneficial with the laser being used to remove the epithelium, as epithelial hyper/hypoplasia smooths much of the underlying irregularities caused by the haze formation, and the epithelium is typically very adherent overlying areas of aggressive haze. When using MMC, it is necessary to under-correct the spherical and cylindrical component of the intended refractive correction by about 10%. Very rarely, cases of severe haze cannot be managed with excimer laser re-treatment and may require deep anterior lamellar corneal grafting procedures.

Night Vision Disturbances/Halos

In the early days of excimer laser keratorefractive procedures, night vision disturbances and halo phenomena in mesopic and scotopic conditions were not infrequent with the use of small (4-6 millimeter) diameter optical zone treatments [75, 78, 95]. This was due to this mismatch between the optical zone size and mesopic/scotopic pupil diameter and the spherical profile of the corrections. Such phenomena were associated with considerable patient dissatisfaction and in some cases have persisted with over 12 years of reported follow-up [91, 95]. With a greater understanding of the need to evaluate the preoperative pupil diameter, the use of larger optical zone treatments (>6mm), the advent of wavefront technology the development of aspheric ablation profiles to reduce the induction of fourth-order spherical aberration postoperatively, the incidents of such problems have reduced dramatically [34, 96].

Patients, especially professional drivers, must be counselled preoperatively as to the rare occurrence of night vision disturbances that may preclude driving on unlit roads such as motorways [97]. Careful pre-operative evaluation of mesopic/scotopic pupil diameter is mandatory [97]. Matching the optical zone to the pupil diameter should be attempted and the use of aspheric ablations profiles, (wavefront-optimized or total wave-front) is mandatory in modern keratorefractive surgery especially with myopic corrections and in patients with mesopic/scotopic pupil diameters greater than 6.5mm [96, 97].

If night vision disturbances should occur, some benefit may be derived from the use of Brimondine tartrate 0.2% or Pilocarpine 1% eye drops to induce miosis, taken half an hour before driving on unlit roads [97, 98]. Wavefront-guided re-treatments with optical zone enlargements may be useful in problematic cases [97].

Recurrent Erosion

Continuing symptoms 9-12 months after LASEK may be treated with a 360° peripheral anterior stromal puncture procedure, as described above (figure 1). In the author's experience of 10 cases over the past 12 years, this has resulted in improvement/resolution of symptoms, with only one case requiring a repeat procedure If, however, anterior stromal puncture does not alleviate the problem, then it may be necessary to perform an epithelial debridement and 15-20μm ablation depth, 10mm diameter PTK procedure, which has been shown to be efficacious for the management of recurrent corneal erosion syndrome [99].

Late Postoperative Complications (Months/Years)

Overcorrection/Undercorrection

See above.

Haze

See above.

Recurrent Corneal Erosion Syndrome

See above.

Ectasia

Whilst ectasia occurs less often after PRK/LASEK than after LASIK [100], because of the greater degradation of corneal biomecahnics in LASIK due to its inherent flap creation [101], ectasia has been reported after PRK even with low myopic corrections [100, 102]. Such cases typically occur in eyes with abnormal topography indicative of forme fruste or early keratoconus [100, 102], and whilst there are case series of successful and stable outcomes of PRK in eyes with mild keratoconus [103-104], surface ablation is controversial and not recommended in such eyes because of the risk of post-operative ectasia.

Careful preoperative corneal topographic, wavefront and tomographic evaluation is necessary in all eyes to identify abnormal patterns, and most devices now have statistical packages that identify high-risk cases, which should not be treated. Preoperative corneal pachymetric measurements are essential prior to surface ablative procedures and any eyes with central pachymetric measurements of less than 500μm although in many cases suitable for surgery [105], should be regarded with some suspicion. It is also recommended to leave all eyes with a residual minimal central corneal thickness of 400μm as a precaution against problems with long-term corneal biomechanical instability and to perform corneal collagen cross-linking if it becomes necessary should ectasia develop.

Eyes with ectasia after keratorefractive surgery typically present with myopic and especially oblique/against the rule astigmatic regression/induction. They show features of irregular astigmatism and usually inferior steepening on corneal topography and anterior and posterior protrusion on corneal tomography. Should ectasia occur, topical anti-glaucomatous medications may slow/reverse progression and treatment should be initiated [107]. Riboflavin (Vitamin B2)/UV-A (370nn) light corneal collagen cross-linkage CXL appears to halt the progression of ectasia and should certainly be considered in eyes with central corneal thicknesses of at least 400μm or greater [107, 108]. In terms of visual rehabilitation, rigid contact lens fitting is the mainstay of treatment. Intra-stromal corneal ring (Intacs) insertion has been shown to be of benefit in mild-to-moderate cases, improving both UCVA, BSCVA, and contact lens fitting [109] and is such cases it is the author's preference to generally use single inferior Intacs insertion [109] (figure 2). In eyes with advanced ectasia intolerant to contact lenses, deep anterior lamellar keratoplasty may be the only option.

Over recent years, CXL has been used in combination with other procedures such as topography-guided PRK to optimize visual and refractive outcomes in keratoconus and even in post-LASIK ectasia [110-112]. Combined CXL and limited topography-guided PRK, with ablation depths less than 50 micrometers (μm), in eyes with moderate keratoconus and post-LASIK ectasia has been shown to be effective with significant improvements in visual, refractive and topographic parameters and stabilization of the ectatic process in the vast majority of eyes [110-112]. Labiris et al. demonstrated that such combined procedures are associated with significant improvements in quality of life scores [113]. Follow-up of these combined PRK CXL treatments in what are chronic progressive conditions, however, is limited to only 1-3 years so that long-term biomechanical stability has not really been fully elucidated.

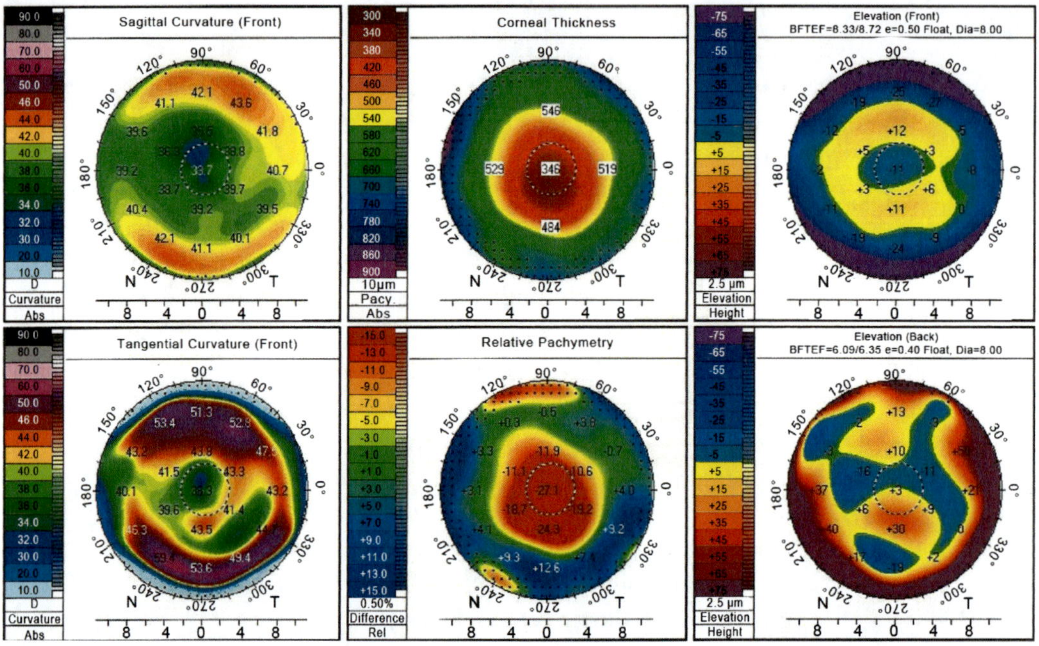

Figure 2. Tomography scan of an eye that developed ectasia 2 years after LASEK, which has been completely stable for 8 years following 250um inferior Intacs insertion and CXL and which retains a visual acuity of 20/20 unaided.

It is known that PRK itself reduces the biomechanical strength of the cornea [102] and progression of ectasia after PRK with CXL has been reported [110] as well as the occasional occurrence of visually significant corneal haze/scarring [114]. Despite these unknowns in carefully selected cases with contact lens intolerance, limited ablation depths, adequate corneal thickness and low grade ectasia, with adequate counselling and fully informed consent as to the risk of progression combined CXL and topographic-PRK treatments might on the basis of the recent published literature be considered.

References

[1] Ciberle M. LASEK may offer the advantages of both LASIK and PRK. *Ocular Surgery News*, International edition, 28 March 1999.

[2] Azar DET, Ang RT, Lee JB, Kato T, Chen CC, Jain S, Gabison E, Abad JC. Laser subepithelial keratomileusis: electron microscopy and visual outcomes of flap photorefractive keratectomy. *Curr. Opin. Ophthalmol.* 2001; 12:323-328.

[3] Shah S, Sebai Sarhan AR, Doyle SJ, Pillia CT, Dua HS. The epithelial flap for photorefractive keratectomy. *BR. J. Ophthalmol.* 2001; 85: 393-396.

[4] Espana EM, Grueterich M, Mateo A, Romano AC, Yee SB, Yee RW, Tseng SC. Cleavage of corneal basement membrane components by ethanol exposure in laser-assisted subepithelial keratectomy. *J. Cataract Refract. Surg.* 2003 Jun; 29(6): 1192-7.

[5] Melki SA, Azar DT. LASIK complications: etiology, management and prevention. *Surv. Ophthalmol.* 2001; 46: 95-116.

[6] Scerrati E. Laser in situ keratomileusis vs. laser epithelial keratomileusis (LASIK vs. LASEK). *J. Refract. Surg.* 2001; 17: S219-S21.

[7] Kaya V, Oncel B, Sivrikaya H, Yilmaz OF. Prospective paired comparison of laser in situ keratomileusis and laser epithelial keratomileusis for myopia less than -6.00 diopters. *J. refract. Surg.* 2004; 20(3): 233-8.

[8] Tobaigy FM, Ghanem RC, Sayegh RR, Hallak JA, Azar DT. A control-match comparison of laser epithelial keratomileuis and laser in situ keratomileusis for low to moderate myopia. *Am. J. Ophthalmol.* 2006; 142(6): 901-8.

[9] Huang P, Liu J., Xia YJ, Zhong YY, Chen YG. Comparison of laser in situ keratomileusis and laser-assisted subepithelial keratomy for myopia more than -10.00 diopters. *Beijing Da Xue Xue Bao* 2007; 39(5): 498-502.

[10] Ghadhfan F, Al-Rajhi A, Wagoner MD. Laser in situ keratomileusis versus surface ablation: visual outcomes and complications, *J. Cataract Refract. Surg.* 2007; 33(12): 2041-8.

[11] Teus MA, de Bentio-Llopis L, Sanchez-Pina JM. LASEK versus LASIK for the correction of moderate myopia. *Optom. Vis. Sci.* 2007; 84(7): 605-10.

[12] Tietjen A. Muller C, Sekundo W. A prospective individual comparison between laser in situ keratomileusis and laser subepithelial keratectomy for myopia. 1-year follow-up results. *Ophthalmologe* 2008; 105(10): 921-6.

[13] de Benito-Llopis L, Teus MA, Sanchez-Pina JM. Comparison between LASEK with mitomycin C and LASIK for the correction of myopia of -7.00 to -13.75. *J. Refract. Surg.* 2008; 24(5): 516-23.

[14] Kirwan C, O'Keefe M. Comparative study of higher-order aberrations after conventional laser in situ keratomileusis and laser epithelial keratomileusis for myopia using the technolas 217z laser platform *Am. J. Ophthalmol.* 2009; 147: 910:77-83.

[15] Townley D, Kirwan C, O'Keefe M. One year follow-up of contrast sensitivity following conventional laser in situ keratomileusis and laser epithelial keratomileusis. *Acta Ophthalmol.* 2012; 90(1):81-5.

[16] Wallau AD, Campos M. One-year outcomes of a bilateral randomised prospective clinical trial comparing PRK with mitomycin C and LASIK. *Br. J. Ophthalmol.* 2009 Dec; 93(12): 1634-8.

[17] Moshirfar M, Schliesser JA, Chang JC, Oberg TJ, Mifflin MD, Townley R, Livingston MK, Kurz CJ. Visual outcomes after wavefront-guided photorefractive keratectomy and wavefront-guided laser in situ keratomileusis: Prospective comparison. *J. Cataract Refract. Surg.* 2010 Aug; 36(8): 1336-43.

[18] Leccisotti A. Laser-assisted subepithelial keratectomy (LASEK) without alcohol versus photorefractive keratectomy (PRK). *Eur. J. Ophthalmol.* 2003; 13: 676-680.

[19] Autrata R, Rehurek J. Laser-assisted subepithelial keratectomy for myopia: two-year follow-up. *J. Cat. Refract. Surg.* 2003; 29: 661-668.

[20] Lee JB, Seong GJ, Lee JH, Seo KY, Lee YG, Kim EK. Comparison of laser epithelial keratomileusis and photorefractive keratectomy for low to moderate myopia. *J. Cataract Refract. Surg.* 2001; 27: 565-570.

[21] Litwak S, Zadok D, Garcia-de Quevedo V, Robledo N, Chayet AS. Laser-assisted subepithelial keratectomy versus photorefractive keratectomy for the correction of myopia. A prospective comparative study. *J. Cataract Refract. Surg.* 2002; 28: 1330-1333.

[22] Gabler B, Winkler von Mohrenfels C, Dreiss AK, Marshall J, Lohmann CP. Vitality of epithelial cells after alcohol exposure during laser-assisted subepithelial keratectomy flap preparation. *J. Cataract Refract. Surg.* 2002; 28: 1841-1846.

[23] Autrata R, Rehurek J. Laser-assisted subepithelial keratectomy for the correction of hyperopia: results of a 2-year follow-up. *J. Cataract Refract. Surg.* 2003; 29: 2105-2114.

[24] Einollahi B, Baradaran-Rafii A, Rezaei-Kanavi M, Eslani M, Parchegani MR, Zare M, Feizi S, Karimian F. Mechanical versus alcohol-assisted epithelial debridement during photorefractive keratectomy: a confocal microscopic clinical trial. *J. Refract. Surg.* 2011 Dec; 27(12): 887-93.

[25] Zhao LQ, Wei RL, Cheng JW, Li Y, Cai JP, Ma XY. Meta-analysis: clinical outcomes of laser-assisted subepithelial keratectomy and photorefractive keratectomy in myopia. *Ophthalmology.* 2010 Oct; 117(10): 1912-22.

[26] Cui M, Chen XM, Lu P. Comparison of laser epithelial keratomileusis and photorefractive keratectomy for the correction of myopia: a meta-analysis. *Chin. Med. J.* (Engl.) 2008; 121(22): 2331-5.

[27] Ghoreishi M, Attarzadeh H, Tavakoli M, Moini HA, Zandi A, Masjedi A, Rismanchian A. Alcohol-assisted versus Mechanical Epithelium Removal in Photorefractive Keratectomy. *J. Ophthalmic Vis. Res.* 2010 Oct; 5(4): 223-7.

[28] Teus MA, de Benito-Llopis L, García-González M. Comparison of visual results between laser-assisted subepithelial keratectomy and epipolis laser in situ keratomileusis to correct myopia and myopic astigmatism. *Am. J. Ophthalmol.* 2008 Sep; 146(3): 357-362.

[29] Hondur A, Bilgihan K, Hasanreisoglu B. A prospective bilateral comparison of epi-LASIK and LASEK for myopia. *J. Refract. Surg.* 2008 Nov; 24(9): 928-34.

[30] Reilly CD, Panday V, Lazos V, Mittlestaedt BR. PRK vs LASEK vs Epi-LASIK: A comparison of corneal haze, poastoperative pain and visual recovery in moderate to high myopia. *Nepal J. Ophthalmol.* 2010 Jul; 2(4): 97-104.

[31] Aslanides IM, Padroni S, Arba Mosquera S, Ioannides A, Mukherjee A. Comparison of single-step reverse transepithelial all-surface laser ablation (ASLA) to alcohol-assisted photorefractive keratectomy. *Clin. Ophthalmol.* 2012; 6:973-80.

[32] Luger MH, Ewering T, Arba-Mosquera S. Consecutive myopia correction with transepithelial versus alcohol-assisted photorefractive keratectomy in contralateral eyes: one-year results. *J. Cataract Refract. Surg.* 2012 Aug; 38(8): 1414-23.

[33] Taneri S, Zieske JD, Azar DT. Evolution techniques, clinical outcomes and pathophysiology of LASEK: review of literature. *Survey of Ophthalmology* 2004; 49: 576-602.

[34] O'Brart DPS, Attar M, Hussien B, Marshall J. Laser epithelial keratomileusis (LASEK) for the correction of high myopia with the Schwind ESIRIS flying-spot laser. *J. Refract. Surg.* 2006 Mar; 22(3): 253-62.

[35] O'Brart DP, Mellington F, Jones S, Marshall J. Laser epithelial keratomileusis for the correction of hyperopia using a 7.0-mm optical zone with the Schwind ESIRIS laser. *J. Refract. Surg.* 2007; 23: 343-54.

[36] Claringbold TV 2nd. Laser-assisted subepithelial keratectomy for the correction of myopia. *J. Cataract Refract. Surg.* 2002 Jan; 28(1): 18-22.

[37] Camellin M. Laser epithelial keratomileusis for myopia. *J. Refract. Surg.* 2003 Nov-Dec; 19(6): 666-70.

[38] Liu XQ, Xu L, Yi CJ. Flap removal or flap preservation during LASEK surgery. *Cell Biochem. Biophys.* 2010 May; 57(1): 45-8. .

[39] Taneri S, Oehler S, Koch J, Azar D. Effect of repositioning or discarding the epithelial flap in laser-assisted subepithelial keratectomy and epithelial laser in situ keratomileusis. *J. Cataract Refract. Surg.* 2011 Oct; 37(10): 1832-46.

[40] Kalyvianaki MI, Kymionis GD, Kounis GA, Panagopoulou SI, Grentzelos MA, Pallikaris IG. Comparison of Epi-LASIK and off-flap Epi-LASIK for the treatment of low and moderate myopia. *Ophthalmology.* 2008 Dec; 115(12): 2174-80.

[41] Badala F, Fioretto M, Macri A. Effect of topical 0.1% indomethocin solution versus 0.1% fluorometholone acetate on the ocular surface and pain control following laser subepithelial keratomileusis (LASEK). *Cornea* 2004; 23: 550-443.

[42] Caldwell M, Reilly C. Effects of topical nepafenac on corneal epithelial healing time and postoperative pain after PRK: a bilateral, prospective, randomized, masked trial. *J. Refract. Surg.* 2008 Apr; 24(4): 377-82.

[43] Solomon KD, Donnenfeld ED, Raizman M, Sandoval HP, Stern K, VanDenburgh A, Cheetham JK, Schiffman R; Ketorolac Reformulation Study Groups 1 and 2. Safety and efficacy of ketorolac tromethamine 0.4% ophthalmic solution in post-photorefractive keratectomy patients. *J. Cataract Refract. Surg.* 2004 Aug; 30(8): 1653-60.

[44] Zanini M, Savini G, Barboni P. Corneal melting associated with topical diclofenac use after laser-assisted subepithelial keratectomy. *J. Cataract Refract. Surg.* 2006 Sep; 32(9): 1570-2.

[45] Mian SI, Gupta A, Pineda R 2nd. Corneal ulceration and perforation with ketorolac tromethamine (Acular) use after PRK. *Cornea.* 2006 Feb; 25(2): 232-4.

[46] Guidera AC, Luchs JI, Udell IJ. Keratitis, ulceration, and perforation associated with topical nonsteroidal anti-inflammatory drugs. *Ophthalmology.* 2001 May; 108(5): 936-44.

[47] Verma S, Corbett MC, Marshall J. A prospective, randomized, double-masked trial to evaluate the role of topical anesthetics in controlling pain after photorefractive keratectomy. *Ophthalmology.* 1995 Dec; 102(12): 1918-24.

[48] Verma S, Corbett MC, Heacock G, Patmore A, Marshall J. A comparative study of the duration and efficacy of Tetracaine 1% and bupivacaine 0.75% in controlling pain following photorefractive keratectomy (PRK). *Eur. J. Ophthalmol.* 1997; 7:327-333.

[49] Rao SK, Wong VW, Cheng AC, Lam PT, Lam DS. Topical anaesthesia-induced keratopathy after laser-assisted subepithelial keratectomy. *J. Cataract Refract. Surg.* 2007; 33(8): 1482-4.

[50] Komilovsky IM. Clinical results after subepithelial photorefractive keratectomy (LASEK). *J. Refract Surg.* 2001; 17: S222-S223.

[51] Albietz JM, McLennan SG, Lenton LM. Ocular surface management of photorefractive keratectomy and laser in situ keratomileusis. *J. Refract. Surg.* 2003 Nov-Dec; 19(6): 636-44.

[52] Ong NH, Purcell TL, Roch-Levecq AC, Wang D, Isidro MA, Bottos KM, Heichel CW, Schanzlin DJ. Epithelial Healing and Visual Outcomes of Patients Using Omega-3 Oral Nutritional Supplements Before and After Photorefractive Keratectomy: A Pilot Study. *Cornea.* 2012 Nov 5. [Epub ahead of print]

[53] Lee JB, Ryu CH, Kim J, Kim EK, Kim HB. Comparison of tear secretion and tear film instability after photorefractive keratectomy and laser in situ keratomileusis. *J. Cataract Refract. Surg.* 2000 Sep; 26(9): 1326-31.

[54] Lifshitz T, Levy J, Mahler O, Levinger S. Peripheral sterile corneal infiltrates after refractive surgery. *J. Cataract Refract. Surg.* 2005; 31; 31(7): 1392-5.

[55] De Rojas V, Llovet F, Martinez M, Cobo-Soriano R, Orteega-Usobiaga J, Beltran J, Baviera J. Infectious keratitis in 18,651 laser surface ablation procedures. *J. Cataract Refract. Surg.* 2011; 37(10): 1822-31.

[56] Rouweyha RM, Chuang AZ, Mitra S, Phillips CB, Yee RW. Laser epithelial keratomileusis for myopia with the autonomous laser. *J. Refract. Surg.* 2002; 18: 217-224.

[57] Laplace O, Bolurcier T, Chaumeil C, Cardine S, Nordmann JP (2004) Early bacterial keratitis after laser-assisted subepithelial keratectomy. *J. Cataract Refract. Surg.* 30: 2638-2640.

[58] Parthasarathy A, Theng J, Ti SE, Tan DT. Infectious keratitis after laser epithelial keratomileusis. *J. Refarct. Surg.* 2007; 23(8): 832-5.

[59] O'Brart DPS, Lohmann CP, Klonos G, Corbett MC, Pollock WST, Kerr Muir MG, Marshall J. The effects of topical corticosteroids and plasmin inhibitors on refractive outcome, haze and visual performance after excimer laser photorefractive keratectomy: a prospective, randomised, observer-masked study. *Ophthalmology* 1994; 101: 1565-1574.

[60] Li C, Zhang J, Huang C. The clinical analysis of corticosteroid ocular hypertension and corticosteroid glaucoma after photorefractive keratectomy. *Zhonghua Yan Ke Za Zhi* 1999; 35: 179-182.

[61] Arshinoff SA, Opalinski Y. The pharmacotherapy of photorefractive keratectomy. *Comp. Ophthalmol. Update* 2003; 4:225-233.

[62] Nagy ZZ, Szabó A, Krueger RR, Süveges I. Treatment of intraocular pressure elevation after photorefractive keratectomy. *J. Cataract Refract. Surg.* 2001 Jul; 27(7): 1018-24.

[63] Hovanesian JA, Shah SS, Maloney RK. Symptoms of dry eye and recurrent erosion syndrome after refractive surgery. *J. Cataract Refract. Surg.* 2001; 27: 577-584.

[64] Dursun D, Kim MC, Solomom A, Pflugfelder SC. Treatment of recalcitrant recurrent erosions with inhibitors of matrix metalloproteinases-9, Doxycycline and corticosteroids. *Am. J. Ophthalmol.* 2001; 132: 8-13.

[65] Hovanesian JA, Shah SS, Maloney RK. Symptoms of dry eye and recurrent erosion syndrome after refractive surgery. *J. Cataract Refract. Surg.* 2001; 27(4): 577-84.

[66] Seiler T, Wollensak J. Complications of laser keratomileusis with the excimer laser. *Klin. Monatsbl. Augenheilkd.* 1991; 200: 648-563.

[67] Simpson RG, Moshirfar M, Edmonds JN, Christiansen SM, Behunin N. Laser in situ keratomileusis in patients with collagen vascular disease: a review of the literature. *Clin. Ophthalmol.* 2012; 6: 1827-37.

[68] Fagerholm P, Ohman L, Orndahl M. Phototherapeutic keratectomy in herpes simplex: clinical results in 20 patients. *Acta Ophthalmol.* 2004; 72: 457-460.

[69] Rodriquez B, Holzinger KA, Le LH, Winkle RK, Allen RD. Mycobacterium chelonae keratitis after laser-assisted subepithelial keratectomy. *J. Cataract Refract. Surg.* 2006; 32: 1059-1061.

[70] Maverick KJ, Conners MS. Aureobasidium pullulans fungal keratitis following LASEK. *J. refract. Surg.* 2007; 23(70:727-9.

[71] Jung SW, Kwon YA, Lee MK, Song SW. Epidermophyton fungal keratitis following laser-assisted subepithelial keratectomy. *J. cataract Refract. Surg.* 2009; 35(12): 2157-60.

[72] Iseli HP, Thiel MA, Hafezi F, Kampmeier J, Seiler T. Ultraviolet A/riboflavin corneal cross-linking for infectious keratitis associated with corneal melts. *Cornea.* 2008 Jun; 27(5): 590-4.

[73] Lee RW, Lee SB. Update on laser subepithelial keratectomy (LASEK). *Curr. Opin. Ophthalmol.* 2004; 15: 333-341.

[74] Chen SH, Feng YF, Stojanovic A, Wang QM. Meta-analysis of clinical outcomes comparing surface ablation for correction of myopia with and without 0.02% mitomycin C. *J. Refract. Surg.* 2011 Jul; 27(7): 530-41.

[75] Garty DS, Kerr, Muir MG, Marshall J. Photorefractive keratectomy with an argon fluoride excimer laser: a clinical study. *Refract. Corneal. Surg.* 1991; 7:420-435.

[76] Salz JJ, Maguen E, Nesburn AB et al. A two-year experience with excimer laser photorefractive keratectomy for myopia. *Ophthalmology* 1993; 100: 873-882.

[77] Lohmann CP, Patmore A, O'Brart DPS, Reischl U, Winkler von Mohrenfels C, Marshall J. Regression and wound healing after excimer laser PRK: a histopathological study on human corneas. *Eur. J. Ophthalmol.* 1997; 7: 130-138.

[78] O'Brart DPS, Corbett MC, Lohmann CP, Kerr Muir MG, Marshall J. The effects of the ablation diameter on the outcome of photorefractive keratectomy: a prospective, randomised, double-blind study. *Arch. Ophthaolmol.* 1995; 113: 438-443.

[79] Hashemi H, Fotouhi A, Foudazi H, Sadeghi N, Payvar S. Prospective, randomized, paired comparison of laser epithelial keratomileusis and photorefractive keratectomy for myopia less than -6.50 diopters. *J. Refract. Surg.* 2004 May-Jun; 20(3): 217-22.

[80] Talamo JH, Gollamudi S, Green WR, De La Cruz Z, Filatov V, Stark WJ. Modulation of corneal wound healing after excimer laser keratomileusis using topical mitomycin C and steroids. *Arch. Ophthalmol.* 1991 Aug; 109(8): 1141-6.

[81] Leccisotti A. Mitomycin C in photorefractive keratectomy: effect on epithelialization and predictability. *Cornea.* 2008 Apr; 27(3): 288-91.

[82] Wallau AD, Campos M. One-year outcomes of a bilateral randomised prospective clinical trial comparing PRK with mitomycin C and LASIK. *Br. J. Ophthalmol.* 2009 Dec; 93(12): 1634-8.

[83] Chen SH, Feng YF, Stojanovic A, Wang QM. Meta-analysis of clinical outcomes comparing surface ablation for correction of myopia with and without 0.02% mitomycin C. *J. Refract. Surg.* 2011 Jul; 27(7): 530-41.

[84] Ti SE, Tan DT. Tectonic corneal lamellar grafting for severe scleral melting after pterygium surgery. *Ophthalmology.* 2003 Jun; 110(6): 1126-36.

[85] Kremer I, Ehrenberg M, Levinger S. Delayed epithelial healing following photorefractive keratectomy with mitomycin C treatment. *Acta Ophthalmol.* 2012 May; 90(3): 271-6.

[86] Roh DS, Funderburgh JL. Impact on the corneal endothelium of mitomycin C during photorefractive keratectomy. *J. Refract. Surg.* 2009 Oct; 25(10): 894-7.

[87] Zare M, Jafarinasab MR, Feizi S, Zamani M. The effect of mitomycin-C on corneal endothelial cells after photorefractive keratectomy. *J. Ophthalmic Vis. Res.* 2011 Jan; 6(1): 8-12.

[88] Gambato C, Miotto S, Cortese M, Ghirlando A, Lazzarini D, Midena E. Mitomycin C-assisted photorefractive keratectomy in high myopia: a long-term safety study. *Cornea.* 2011 Jun;30(6):641

[89] Midena E, Gambato C, Miotto S, Cortese M, Salvi R, Ghirlando A. Long-term effects on corneal keratocytes of mitomycin C during photorefractive keratectomy: a randomized contralateral eye confocal microscopy study. *J. Refract. Surg.* 2007 Nov; 23(9 Suppl): S1011-4.

[90] O'Brart DPS, Patsoura E, Jaycock PD, Raan MS, Marshall J. Excimer laser photorefractive keratectomy for hyperopia: 7.5 year follow-up. *J. Cat. Ref. Surg.* 2005; 31: 1104-1113.

[91] Rajan M, Jaycock P, O'Brart DPS, Marshall J. A long-term study of photorefractive keratectomy: 12 year follow-up. *Ophthalmology* 2004; 111: 1813-1824.

[92] Vigo L, Scandola E, Carones F. Scraping and Mitomycin C to treat haze and regression after photorefractive keratectomy for myopia. *J. Refract. Surg.* 2003; 19:449-454.

[93] Proges Y, Ben-Haim O, Hirsh A, Levinger S. Phototherapeutic keratectomy with Mitomycin C for corneal haze following photorefractive keratectomy for myopia. *J. Refract. Surg.* 2003; 19:40-43.

[94] Rajan M, O'Brart DPS, Parel P, Falcon M, Marshall J. Topography-guided customized laser-assisted subepithelial keratectomy for the treatment of postkeratoplasty astigmatism. *J. Cataract Refract. Surg.* 2006; 32: 949-957.

[95] Rajan M, O'Brart DPS, Jaycock P, Marshall J. Effects of ablation diameter on long-term refractive stability and corneal transparency after photorefractive keratectomy. *Ophthalmology* 2006; 113: 1798-1806.

[96] Mastropasqua L, Toto L, Zuppardi E, Nubile M, Carpineto P, Di Nicola M, Ballone E. Photorefractive keratectomy with aspheric profile of ablation versus conventional photorefractive keratectomy for myopia correction: six-month controlled clinical trial. *J. Cataract Refract. Surg.* 2006 Jan; 32(1): 109-16.

[97] Salz JJ, Trattler W. Pupil size and corneal laser surgery. *Curr. Opin. Ophthalmol.* 2006; 17: 373-379.

[98] Kesler A, Shemesh G, Rothkoff L, Lazar M. Effect of brimonidine tartrate 0.2% ophthalmic solution on pupil size. *J. Cataract Refract. Surg.* 2004; 30: 1707-1710.

[99] O'Brart DPS, Kerr Muir MG, Marshall J. Excimer laser phototherapeutic keratectomy for recurrent erosions. *Eye* 1994; 8:378-83.

[100] Randleman JB, Woodward M, Lynn MJ, Stulting RD. Risk assessment for ectasia after corneal refractive surgery. *Ophthalmology.* 2008 Jan; 115(1): 37-50.

[101] Kamiya K, Shimizu K, Ohmoto F. Comparison of the changes in corneal biomechanical properties after photorefractive keratectomy and laser in situ keratomileusis. *Cornea.* 2009 Aug; 28(7): 765-9.

[102] Reznik J, Salz JJ, Klimava A. Development of unilateral corneal ectasia after PRK with ipsilateral preoperative forme fruste keratoconus. *J. Refract. Surg.* 2008 Oct; 24(8): 843-7.

[103] Cennamo G, Intravaja A, Boccuzzi D, Marotta G, Cennamo G. Treatment of keratoconus by topography-guided customized photorefractive keratectomy: two-year follow-up study. *J. Refract. Surg.* 2008 Feb; 24(2):145-9.
[104] Koller T, Iseli HP, Donitzky C, Ing D, Papadopoulos N, Seiler T. Topography-guided surface ablation for forme fruste keratoconus. *Ophthalmology.* 2006 Dec; 113(12): 2198-202.
[105] de Benito-Llopis L, Teus MA, Sánchez-Pina JM, Fuentes I. Stability of laser epithelial keratomileusis with and without mitomycin C performed to correct myopia in thin corneas: a 15-month follow-up. *Am. J. Ophthalmol.* 2008 May; 145(5): 807-12.
[106] Hiatt JA, Wachler BS, Grant C. Reversal of laser in situ keratomileusis-induced ectasia with intraocular pressure reduction. *J. Cataract Refract. Surg.* 2005; 31: 1652-1655.
[107] Wollensak G, Spörl E, Seiler T (2003) Riboflavin/ultraviolet-A-induced collagen cross linking for the treatment of Keratoconus. *Am. J. Ophthalmol.* 135: 620-627.
[108] Hafezi F, Kanellopoulos J, Wiltfang R, Seiler T. Corneal collagen crosslinking with riboflavin and ultraviolet A to treat induced keratectasia after laser in situ keratomileusis. *J. Cataract Refract. Surg.* 2007 Dec; 33(12): 2035-40.
[109] Sharma M, Boxer Wachler BS. Comparison of single segment and double segment Intacs for Keratoconus and post-LASIK ectasia. *Am. J. Ophthalmol.* 2006; 141: 891-895.
[110] Kanellopoulos AJ, Binder PS. Management of corneal ectasia after LASIK with combined, same-day, topography-guided partial transepithelial PRK and collagen cross-linking: the athens protocol. *J. Refract. Surg.* 2011 May; 27(5): 323-31.
[111] Kymionis GD, Portaliou DM, Kounis GA, Limnopoulou AN, Kontadakis GA, Grentzelos MA. Simultaneous topography-guided photorefractive keratectomy followed by corneal collagen cross-linking for keratoconus. *Am. J. Ophthalmol.* 2011 Nov; 152(5): 748-55.
[112] Tuwairqi WS, Sinjab MM. Safety and efficacy of simultaneous corneal collagen cross-linking with topography-guided PRK in managing low-grade keratoconus: 1-year follow-up. *J. Refract. Surg.* 2012 May; 28(5): 341-5.
[113] Labiris G, Giarmoukakis A, Sideroudi H, Gkika M, Fanariotis M, Kozobolis V. Impact of Keratoconus, Cross-Linking and Cross-Linking Combined With Photorefractive Keratectomy on Self-Reported Quality of Life. *Cornea.* 2012 Jan 10.
[114] Kymionis GD, Portaliou DM, Diakonis VF, Kontadakis GA, Krasia MS, Papadiamantis AG, Coskunseven E, Pallikaris AI. Posterior linear stromal haze formation after simultaneous photorefractive keratectomy followed by corneal collagen cross-linking. *Invest. Ophthalmol. Vis. Sci.* 2010 Oct; 51(10): 5030-3.

In: Current Understanding and New Techniques …
Editor: Michael O'Keefe
ISBN: 978-1-62808-748-2

Chapter 2

LASIK Complications

***Marco Tavolato*[1*] *and Lucio Buratto*[2]**
[1]Centro Oculistico San Paolo, Padova, Italy
[2]Centro Ambrosiano Oftalmico, Milano, Italy

Abstract

The expectations of patients facing refractive surgery are often highly exaggerated, so even a simple hypocorrection can be experienced as a complication. Plus, since all refractive operations are rarely mandatory, any real complications are perceived by patients as extremely serious.

Theoretically every LASIK complication can be avoided, or at least minimized, by paying attention to all the surgical technique details and performing an accurate pre-op evaluation of the patient. It is fundamental to exclude subjects from treatment who have significant contraindications and use all precautions to minimize any complications.

The surgeon's experience is a very important factor, but equally so is the use of modern, perfectly operational equipment, with a constant maintenance service.

Complications of the Lamellar Cut with Femtosecond Lasers

Intraoperative

- Vertical Gas Breakthrough: rare complication characterized by the appearance of air bubbles between the epithelium (due to its rupture) and the applanation cone. It is more frequent in procedures with very thin flaps or in the presence of corneal scarring. If this complication presents during the creation of the flap, the procedure should be interrupted and flap creation postponed for a few months increasing the cut

* Email: salvatore.ferrandes@buratto.com.

depth (evaluating whether to use a microkeratome) or by modifying the surgical technique (PRK with the use of Mitomycin C or implanting a phakic IOL).

- Anterior Chamber Bubble: appearance of bubbles in the anterior chamber while using a femtolaser. This seems to be caused by the passage of plasma bubbles in the anterior chamber, through the Schlemm's canal. This complication is more frequent with an imperfect centering of the flap with very peripheral pocket. The presence of these bubbles does not preclude performance of the treatment with excimer laser, except for possible interference with the eye-tracking system. The bubbles reabsorb spontaneously in a few hours.
- Opaque Bubble Layer: collection of gas bubbles created during a cut with femtosecond laser in the intrastromal cornea lamellas above and below the cutting plane. If they present in the early cutting phase (Early Opaque Bubble Layer) they are due to a lack of evacuation space for the gas bubbles produced during the cut. The creation of a peripheral intrastromal pocket at the beginning of the cut for the gas bubbles to escape decreases the incidence of this phenomenon. If they appear in the already cut corneal flap area (Late Opaque Bubble Layer) they are due to incomplete separation of the corneal tissue, thus lifting of the flap could be more difficult and the eye-tracking system may not work correctly.

Postoperative

- Post Op - Transient Light Sensitivity Syndrome: the symptom is a significant photophobia with preserved visual acuity and absence of other disorders; it presents 6 to 12 weeks after surgery. Treatment involves the use of topical steroids with symptoms disappearing in 2-3 weeks. The pathogenesis seems to be correlated to an activation of intrastromal keratocytes following femtolaser treatment. This complication has almost disappeared with the decrease in the energy values needed to create the flap.
- Post OP - Rainbow glare: very rare complication where patients report the perception of a glare of colored lights in their peripheral vision field, primarily observing a source of punctiform light on a dark background. The objective exam is negative and visual acuity is preserved. It decreases spontaneously over time. It may be due to the diffractive effect of the surface of the cut created with the femtosecond laser. Modern femtolasers make it possible to create a very uniform cut surface, with decrease of the incidence of this complication.

Intraoperative Flap Complications

These types of complications were more frequent with the use of microkeratomes; today with the use of femtosecond lasers they are much rarer.

- Incomplete cut: the main cause for this complication is a loss of suction when performing the cut. Other causes may be an electrical or mechanical blocking of the instrument. For this reason the microkeratome or femtolaser must be connected to an uninterruptible power supply, in order to prevent problems related to black outs. Prevention of this complication requires correct exposure of the eye bulb so that too much force does not have to be exerted on the bulb with the suction ring or with the microkeratome which must be able to move freely. The instruments must always be inspected and tested before starting an operation.

- o Incomplete cut with femtolaser: if the loss of suction occurs outside the visual axis (i.e. an optic zone of at least 4.5-5 mm) it is possible, after having waited for the plasma bubbles to reabsorb, to reposition the suction ring; then using the same applanation cone, to continue with the cut at the same depth; generally, however, it is preferable to postpone the operation. If the loss is near the visual axis the procedure needs to be stopped without lifting the flap and a new cut after a few months at a greater depth set up or a surface ablation.
- o Incomplete cut with microkeratome: if there is a block in advancing it is important to invert the movement direction and remove the suction ring. In the event of a total block the suction is stopped and the ring and microkeratome are removed in a single maneuver moving them in the opposite direction from the hinge site. If the cut area permits a refractive ablation with an adequate optic zone the treatment is continued, vice versa the flap is stretched again and the operation postponed. It can be performed 3-6 months later, with a deeper cut than the first, or by converting the procedure into a surface technique.

- Flap buttonhole: the flap may be perforated with very thin cuts. This complication no longer occurs with the use of femtolaser. The following causes may be linked to the microkeratome: incorrect selection of the plane, an insufficient suction, too dry cornea, edema of the epithelium, poor microkeratome and blade quality. Anatomical causes include: very curved corneas or strong irregular astigmatism. To prevent this complication it is essential to use modern microkeratomes, avoid excessive administration of anesthetic eye drops to prevent epithelium swelling and always change the blade after each cut. It is necessary to reposition the flap very carefully; normally, after a centrally perforated flap, patients return to the pre-op situation in terms of functional and refractive vision. In more unfortunate cases, there may also be interface epitelization and possible melting due to penetration of the epithelial cells, not just from the edge of the flap but also from the buttonhole, so it becomes practically impossible to clean the flap interface. At this point the flap has to be removed and the epithelium allowed to regrow like in a PRK. A long-term approach to these eyes may be through retreatment with LASIK with a deeper cut (after 3-6 months) or with a transepithelial PRK (for irregular surfaces or minor central and paracentral opacities).
- Free cap: complication where the vertical cut involves all 360°, without creation of a hinge. A predisposing factor for this is a very wide (greater than 14.5 mm) or flat (average keratometric value less than 41.00 D) cornea. A cornea of this type protrudes relatively less compared to a normal cornea in the suction ring and thus presents a portion of cornea with a smaller diameter for the microkeratome blade. The following non-anatomical but mechanical problems can cause "free cap": poor

microkeratome assembly, use of a ring which does not allow sufficient cornea exposure, inadequate suction. The use of femtolaser eliminates all of the free cap causes listed to here. However, even using this instrument it is possible, if creating very thin flaps (90μm), to tear the flap with the microspatula during the lifting maneuver. For these reasons it is fundamental to always make the appropriate corneal markings. In the presence of "free cap" the flap is positioned with the epithelial surface facing down in the anti-desiccation chamber adding one or two drops of BSS (no fluid must be placed above the stromal surface of the flap) and the laser treatment is performed. Once the laser ablation is completed it may be useful to put a drop of BSS directly on the center of the corneal bed: the surface tension of the fluid helps placement of the flap on the stromal bed. At this point the flap is reapplied to the corneal bed being careful to position it exactly in its original site, aligning the preoperative markings. At the end of the operation a therapeutic contact should be applied. If it is not possible to obtain correct flap alignment and stretching it is possible to convert the technique into a PRK by sacrificing the flap and applying a contact lens which lets the epithelium regrow.

Intraoperative Excimer Laser Complications

Complications linked to excimer laser can be almost completely avoided by using modern instruments which are periodically tested and which are placed in dedicated rooms (constant temperature and humidity). The laser must have a centered beam, correct level of energy, a uniform qualitative beam, thus the surgeon must never perform a treatment without first having performed a fluence test.

Postoperative Complications

Flap displacement: movement of the flap in the immediate postoperative period or the first 24 hours. The main causes are an incomplete adhesion of the flap to the stromal bed, excessive eye dryness, rubbing movements by the patients or an accidental trauma to the flap during postoperative instillation therapy. For this reason it is very important to assess patients with a slit lamp before discharging them to check correct flap alignment, instruct them on how to apply postoperative drops, recommend that they not rub their eyes in the initial postoperative days and ask them to use sunglasses during the day and protective transparent cups when sleeping.

Treatment involves relifting and repositioning the flap; in these cases it is advisable to wait a few minutes before removing the blepharostat to allow good flap adhesion and possibly use a contact lens for 24 hours.

Diffuse Lamellar Keratitis (DLK): keratitis of toxic genesis which present in the immediate postoperative period (2nd-4th day). It is characterized by infiltration of inflammatory cells in the interface.

Pathogenic hypotheses include: contamination of the interface, significant epithelial defects, hypersensitivity to bacterial proteins denatured by the sterilization procedures, contamination by the meibomian glands and povidone iodine toxicity.

It is divided into 4 stages:

- Stage 1: presence of whitish granular cells in the interface in the periphery of the flap, no effect on visual axis. This is found fairly frequently on the first postoperative day (2-4%). Normally it is self-limiting; frequent topical steroid treatment is recommended.
- Stage 2: presence of whitish granular cells in the interface with involvement of the visual axis. Presentation is on the second-third day after surgery with an incidence of 0.5%. The patient needs to be monitored closely to prevent progression to more advanced stages. It is essential to start a very frequent topical steroid treatment (1 drop of Prednilosone every hour during the day and if possible every 2-3 hours at night).
- Stage 3: presence of significant whitish cell aggregates in the center of the visual axis, with transparent corneal periphery. Presentation is on the third-fourth postoperative day (0.2%); the patient may report a slightly cloudy vision with decrease in visus, but it may be completely asymptomatic. In these cases the flap should be relifted with interface irrigation with BSS and interface cleaning with a soaked Merocel sponge. This should be associated with a very frequent topical steroid treatment (1 drop of Prednilosone every hour during the day and if possible every 2-3 hours at night).
- Stage 4: central corneal melting in the interface caused by collagenase released from the aggregated inflammatory cells (0.02%). The patient reports a significant decrease in vision with hypermetric shift. The flap should not be lifted due to possible additional stromal tissue loss while manipulating. Often central corneal scarring remains. The treatment for this phase is prevention with periodic check ups which show early stages of DLK. Once the repair process is completed an anterior lamellar keratoplastic procedure can be performed if the cornea surface or stroma have significant repercussions on vision.

Flap folds (micro and macro striae): Striae are parallel lines which form on the flap surface in the immediate postoperative period. The most commons causes are: thin flap (less than 100 microns), incorrect positioning of the flap at the end of surgery (marking before lifting the flap is always recommended), high refraction defects, dehydration of the flap stromal surface from excessive exposure time, flap edema from excessive interface irrigation, pre-op use of vasoconstrictors such as phenyleprine or brimonidine to minimize subconjunctival hemorrhages caused by the suction ring, dislocation of the flap during post-op instillation of eye drops or due to patient rubbing.

Treatment needs to be as early as possible: striae are present in the first hour after surgery and they are easy to remove if done immediately. The more time passes the more difficult they are to remove.

- Very thin striae (microstriae): they are found fairly frequently after LASIK operations and are caused by wrinkling of the Bowman membrane; they rarely result in vision disorders or loss thus no intervention is needed.
- Larger striae (macrostriae): they can reduce the patient's visual acuity due to the onset of irregular astigmatisms and opacity of the folds with significant disturbances such as haloes and starbursts. If they are found on the first day after surgery, they require immediate treatment by relifting the flap, washing the interface and repositioning. Ironing the flap with a Merocel sponge soaked with BBS perpendicularly to the direction of the striae is recommended. The blepharostat needs to be removed after a few minutes so that the flap adheres correctly to the stromal bed. In these cases a contact lens should be applied.

Striae which are not diagnosed early become permanent because the epithelium fills the spaces created by the flap folds and the collagen fibers tend to contract. In this situation it becomes necessary to soak the flap by distilled water instillation on the cornea surface for a few minutes. This procedure is used to swell the epithelium and break the cell bonds to make removal easier. At this point the epithelium is removed with a PRK spatula, and a few more drops of distilled water are instilled on the surface to obtain further flap swelling and relaxation of the striae. Then the flap is lifted, irrigating the interface with BSS (do not use distilled water which would swell the stroma bed!) and the flap repositioned. An ironing maneuver can be performed using blunt spatulas. A contact lens needs to be applied at the end of the procedure. If these procedures are not enough and the striae are still present the next day, instillation of a drop of instilled water every hour for a day can be prescribed (with the contact lens in place). For persistent cases some Authors propose a PTK on the epithelial and stromal surfaces or suturing the flap perpendicular to the striae.

Infections: this is a very rare, but potentially devastating complication. The most frequent pathogens include: gram positive bacteria (*Staphilococcus aureus*) in early infections (within a week), atypical mycobacteria (*Mycobacterium chelone*) in later infections (2-3 weeks). Fungal infections (*Candida, Fusarium*) are very rare and often have a late onset. Predisposing causes for an infection include: intraoperative infection due to lack of sterilization during the operation, patient non-compliance with postoperative antibiotic treatment, predisposing palpebral situations (e.g. chronic blepharitis) and patient non-compliance with hygiene rules and behaviors in post-op period.

The clinical picture is characterized by a decrease in vision, conjunctival hyperemia, sensation of a foreign body and photophobia. Examination with a slit lamp shows cornea infiltration which can be localized at all levels: flap, interface or stroma. They can be associated with corneal ulcer, anterior chamber reaction, epithelial deficit and interface epithelial growth.

The main differential diagnosis is with a DLK, however in infections the eye is often more inflamed and does not respond to steroid treatment. In addition, onset is often one week from treatment, while in DLK onset is earlier. Other clinical pictures which can imitate an infection include: the presence of a peripheral sterile infiltrate, an interface epithelial growth and the presence of interface impurities.

Treatment includes:

- For infiltrates located in the interface, early flap lifting is required with removal of all infective foci in order to perform microbiological cultures and an antibiogram, abundant washing of the interface with Vancocin 50mg/ml for early infections or amikacin 35mg/ml for later forms.
- For superficial infiltrates the flap does not need to be lifted
- Treatment with topical broad spectrum antibiotics: in early forms fourth generation fluoroquinolones (gatifloxacin 0.3% or moxifloxacin 0.5%) every 30 minutes, alternating with 50mg/ml fortified cefazolin eye drops. In late forms fourth generation fluoroquinolones (gatifloxacin 0.3% or moxifloxacin 0.5%) every 30 minutes, alternating with a 35mg/ml fortified amikacin eye drops. Systemic treatment with 100 mg doxycycline two times a day is recommended in both cases, due to its ability to block collagenase production. The use of topical corticosteroids should be avoided. The treatment protocol will need to be adjusted once the antibiogram response is obtained.

Prevention for avoiding this devastating complication includes the use of sterile material and isolating the eyelashes during surgery using adhesive surgical drape Even if treated correctly, the outcome of these complications can often be very serious with significant loss in visual acuity. In the most serious cases, the last treatment is complete anterior lamellar or perforating cornea transplant, based on the depth of the residual corneal scarring.

Sterile peripheral corneal infiltrates: presence of one or more stromal infiltrates, localized peripherally beyond the flap edge. The epithelium above is intact and presents an undamaged cornea zone between the infiltrate and limbus. It presents between the first and fifth day after surgery; visual acuity is not usually compromised. Clinically a modest hyperemia of the eye is found with quiet anterior chamber. It is generally associated with a blepharitis or a malfunction of the meibomian glands. Patients only complain about a sensation of a foreign body in the eye and increased lacrimation. It is an immune reaction caused by hypersensitivity to toxins produced by bacteria that colonize the eyelid margin (especially *Staphylococcus aureus*). Treatment involves frequent application of a topical steroid. Differential diagnosis is with an infectious form.

Dry eye: very frequent postoperative condition (5-50%) that tends to resolve in a few months. The pathogenic mechanism includes direct damage to the corneal nervous plexus, both during creation of the flap with resection of nerve fibers and by the excimer laser with direct photoablation damage. A loss of conjunctival goblet cells has also been observed, probably caused by application of the suction ring, with a decrease in mucin production and consequent dry eyes.

Postoperative dry eyes occur frequently, therefore topical artificial tears are always indicated for the first three/six months after surgery (Systane, Alcon; Ortive, Allergan). In rare cases the disturbances persist with significant patient discomfort. In the United States these cases can be treated with a topical immunosuppressant treatment (Cyclosporin A 0.05% Restasis, Allergan), this product is not available in Europe yet. Another treatment option is the off-label use of 20% autologous serum for its anti-inflammatory cytokine content. Punctal plugs represent another therapeutic option; however they cause stagnation of tears and all the pro-inflammatory cytokines. Puntal plugs use should be limited to patients who do not respond to the above treatments.

Ectasia: progressive protrusion of the corneal apex, with growing curvature radii increase and thinning of the cornea. This complication may present long after refractive surgery with a progressive worsening of the patient's visual acuity. The incidence of this complication ranges from 0.04% to 0.6%, even if it is most likely underestimated.

Risk factors for developing ectasia include: keratoconus, pellucid marginal degeneration, forme fruste keratoconus, residual stromal bed thickness less than 250μ, thin cornea, high myopia and age younger than 24 years.

Patients with refractive instability and clear family history of keratoconus are at risk. A careful evaluation of the anterior and posterior surface and corneal pachymetry is essential. Many assessment scales have been proposed which use all of these parameters to identify at-risk patients. In doubtful cases a topographic examination should be repeated over time. The use of a femtosecond laser provides a greater degree of safety, since the flap can have a very small thickness (up to 90μm), with the possibility of increasing the residual stromal bed values. In doubtful cases a surface treatment can be performed (PRK with or without crosslinking), or phakic IOL implant in cases of high ametropia.

Ectasia is treated with crosslinking, implantation of intrastromal rings or use of gas permeable contact lenses. In the worst cases a cornea transplant is the only option.

Epithelial ingrowth: a proliferation of epithelial cells in the interface between the flap and stromal bed.

Risk factors include: lengthy flap manipulation, excessive insertion of instruments in the interface, inaccurate interface cleaning and irrigation, epithelial abrasions on the flap edge and retreatments. Microkeratotome use increases the risk of this complication due to involuntary introduction of epithelial cells in the interface when performing the cut.

The clinical picture is usually asymptomatic for the patient since the cells normally grow in the peripheral areas, without involvement of the visual axis. If the epithelial growth in the interface continues towards the center it may cause a decrease in visual acuity, onset of irregular astigmatism (also seen by topography) and hypermetric shift.

Dr. Jeffrey Machat suggested a classification useful for an adequate treatment:

- Grade 1: small white peripheral aggregates, well-delineated, limited to within 2 mm of flap edge. They are nonprogressive and no treatment is required.
- Grade 2: grayish peripheral aggregates, not well-delineated, limited to within 2 mm of flap edge. They may tend to progress towards the pupil center. They require frequent monitoring, possibly photographic documentation. Treatment is indicated in the event of progression.
- Grade 3: growth extends more than 2 mm from the edge with flap involvement. Urgent treatment required.

Prevention of epithelial ingrowth includes:

- Carefully washing the interface after surgery
- Avoiding prolonged manipulations of the flap
- Applying a contact lens for significant epithelial defects
- Using a femtosecond laser to create the flap: this makes it possible to create a square flap edge; with some femtosecond models it is possible to make a flap with an inverted angle up to 150°; this makes epithelial cell infiltration more difficult.

Treatment has a high recurrence rate (approximately 10%). Direct treatment with Neodymium-laser can be used to eliminate or reduce peripheral cell aggregates. A power of 0.6-1.2 mJ is used, focused slightly posterior to the epithelial plaque to clean and a few dozen pulses are applied. The patient is checked after 2-3 weeks and the procedure is repeated if necessary. Often this treatment is sufficient for stopping the progression. If Yag laser treatment is not enough, surgery is required. It is mandatory to avoid new epithelial cells introduction into the interface. The flap needs to be lifted from the side closest to the epithelial growth using a hook (with a slit lamp) and lifted with blunt tip forceps (Buratto flap forcep). Traditional spatulas are not recommended for flap lifting due to the risk of introducing new cells in the interface. The two stromal surfaces (bed and roof) need to be carefully cleaned to remove all residual epithelial cells with a microspatula. The instrument used for cleaning (spatula, cannula, etc.) must be checked and cleaned after each passage to prevent adding epithelial cells. The flap is then repositioned and a contact lens applied. If the first surgery is not sufficient the flap needs to be lifted again and the cleaning procedure repeated with moderate scraping of the involved surfaces; some Authors suggest eliminating the epithelial cells by applying 20% to 50% ethanol or by PTK treatment of both stromal surfaces; this should be done after accurately cleaning the involved areas.

For cases of significant epithelial growth, it is advisable to act early since the stroma between the interface epithelium and surface epithelium may undergo necrosis with flap melting.

References

Alio JL, Salem T, Artola, Osman A. Intracorneal rings to correct corneal ectasia after laser in situ keratomileusis. *J. Cataract. Refract. Surg*. 2002;28:1568-1574.

Battat L, Macri A, Durson D, Pflugfelder SC. Effect of laser in situ keratomileusis on tear production, clearance, and the ocular surface. *Ophthalmology*. 2001;108:1230-1235.

Buhren J, Cichocki M, Baumeister M, Kohnen T. Diffuse lamellar keratitis after laser in situ keratomileusis. Clinical and confocal findings. *Ophthalmology*. 2002;99:176-180.

Chang MA, Jain S, Azar DT. Infections following laser in situ keratomileusis: an integration of the published literature. *Surv Ophthalmol*. 2004;49:269-280.

Choe CH, Guss C, Musch DC, Niziol LM. Incidence of diffuse lamellar keratitis after LASIK with 15 KHz, 30 KHz and 60 KHz femtosecond laser flap creation. *J. Cataract. Refract. Surg*. 2010: 36: 1912-8.

Davison JA, Johnson SC. Intraoperative complications of LASIK flaps using the IntraLase femtosecond laser in 3009 cases. *J. Refract. Surg*. 2010;26:851-857.

Hernandez-Matamoros J, Iradier MT, Moreno E. Treating folds and strie after laser in situ keratomileusis. *J. Cataract. Refract. Surg*. 2001;27:350-352.

Jain V, Mhatre K, Shome D. Flap buttonhole in thin-flap laser in situ keratomileusis: case series and review. *Cornea*. 2010;29:655-658.

Lifshitz T, Levy J, Klemperer I, Levinger S. Anterior gas bubbles after corneal flap creation with a femtosecond laser. *J Cataract Refracr Surg*. 2005;31:2227-2229.

Llovet F, de Roias V, Interlandl E, Martin C. Infectious Keratitis in 204586 LASIK procedures. *Ophthalmology*. 2010;117:232-238.

Moshirfar M, Gardiner JP, Schliesser JA, Espandar L. Laser in situ keratomileusis flap complications using mechanical microkeratome versus femtosecond laser: retrospective comparison. *J. Cataract. Refract. Surg*. 2010;36:1925-1933.

Nettune GR, Pflugfelder SC. Post-LASIK tear dysfunction and dysestesia. *Ocul Surf*. 2010;8:135-145.

Rodrìguez-Galietero A, Martinez JV, Del Buey A, Bescòs JA. Use of brimonidine before LASIK with femtosecond laser-created flaps for the correction of myopia: a controlateral eye study. *J. Refract. Surg*. 2010;26:28-32.

Schallhorn SC, Amesbury EC, Tanzer DJ. Avoidance, recognition, and management of LASIK complications. *Am. J. Ophthalmol*. 2006;141:733-739.

Sharma N, Ghate D, Agarwal T. Refractive outcomes of laser in situ keratomileusis after flap complications. *J. Cataract. Refract. Surg*. 2005;31:1334-1337.

Steinert RF, Ashrafzadeh A, Hersh PS. Results of phototherapeutic keratectomy in the management of flap strie after LASIK. *Ophthalmology*. 2004;111:740-746.

Stonecipher KG, Dishler JG, Ignacio TS, Binder PS. Transient Light Sensitivity after femtosecond laser flap creation: clinical findings and management. *J. Cataract. Refract. Surg*. 2006;32:91-94.

Stulting RD, Carr JD, Thompson KP. Complications of laser in situ keratomileusis for the correction of myopia. *Ophthalmology*. 1999;106:13-20.

Villarubia A, Palacìn E, Gòmez del Rio M, Martinez P. Description, etiology, and prevenction of an outbreak of diffuse lamellar keratitis after LASIK. *J. Refract. Surg*. 2007;21:6-10.

In: Current Understanding and New Techniques ...
Editor: Michael O'Keefe

ISBN: 978-1-62808-748-2

Chapter 3

Dry Eyes in Patients Undergoing Refractive Surgery

Ian John Dooley*

Royal Victoria Eye and Ear Hospital,
Dublin, Ireland

Abstract

This chapter discusses the effects of refractive surgery upon the ocular surface, particularly in relation to dry eye, which is the most common source of morbidity following refractive laser procedures. The procedures discussed include corneal refractive techniques such as laser-assisted in situ keratomileusis (LASIK), surface laser procedures (including laser assisted subepithelial keratectomy or LASEK and photo refractive keratectomy or PRK), corneal lenticule extraction procedures (including ReLEx and ReLEx smile) as well as intraocular lens (IOL) based procedures such as phakic IOL (pIOL) implantation, intraocular contact lens (ICL) and clear lens extraction (CLE).

Dry eye is a multifactorial disease of the tears and ocular surface that results in symptoms of discomfort, visual disturbance, and tear film instability with potential damage to the ocular surface. It is accompanied by increased osmolarity of the tear film and inflammation of the ocular surface.

Of the many tests to assess the ocular surface and dry eye, tear osmolarity is the most consistent test clinically available. It is important to remember that dry eye is a clinical diagnosis. The dry eye associated with refractive surgery is usually transient.

Post-LASIK dry eye describes a spectrum of diseases encompassing transient or persistent post-operative neurotrophic disease, tear instability, true aqueous tear deficiency, corneal and conjunctival epitheliopathy, and neuropathic pain states. This chapter compares the different rates of induced dry eye associated with each procedure. Flap based procedures such as LASIK seem to generate more dry eye effects. A detailed synopsis of the available treatments for dry eye and how to step-wise manage post-refractive surgery dry eye is contained in this chapter.

* Dr Ian John Dooley MB BAO BCh, MSc MRCOPHTH, MRCSI (Ophth) - Royal Victoria Eye & Ear Hospital, Adelaide Road, Dublin 2, E-mail: Iandooley55@hotmail.com.

Ancillary tests are useful but should be combined with careful history-taking and examination, a normal test value does not preclude the diagnosis. Meticulous preoperative identification of at-risk patients and diligent consent are crucial, if the refractive surgeon is to avoid desperately unhappy postoperative patients. Procedure which section large portions of corneal nerves, such as flap based procedures may be at higher risk of inducing dry eye.

Introduction

In this chapter, we will discuss the effects of refractive surgery upon the ocular surface, particularly in relation to dry eye, which is the most common source of morbidity following refractive laser procedures. [1-5] We will discuss corneal refractive techniques such as laser-assisted in situ keratomileusis (LASIK), surface laser procedures (including laser assisted subepithelial keratectomy or LASEK and photo refractive keratectomy or PRK), corneal lenticule extraction procedures (including ReLEx and ReLEx smile) as well as intraocular lens (IOL) based procedures such as phakic IOL (pIOL) implantation, intraocular contact lens (ICL) and clear lens extraction (CLE). Let us discuss dry eye further, before considering it in the context of refractive procedures.

Definition

In 2007 the international dry eye workshop defined, dry eye as a multifactorial disease of the tears and ocular surface that results in symptoms of discomfort, visual disturbance, and tear film instability with potential damage to the ocular surface. It is accompanied by increased osmolarity of the tear film and inflammation of the ocular surface [6].

Tear Composition

A simplified tear model states that the tear film is composed of 3 basic layers (figure 1). A deficiency of a single constituent, will have knock-on effects upon the other layers and lead to a dry eye. For example a lack of oil, due to meibomian gland dysfunction leads to exposure of the aqueous layer with resultant evaporation and dehydration of the mucin layer and resultant dry eye [7].

Clinical Features

Symptoms

The dry-eye patient may report symptoms of ocular fatigue with associated stinging or foreign body sensation, which is at its worst upon wakening or at the end of the day. Exacerbating factors include low blink rate activities, such reading, watching television and computer-use along with environmental factors such as air conditioning or windy conditions.

These may also precipitate reflex tearing with overflow epiphora. In fact, dry eye is a common source of epiphora [8].

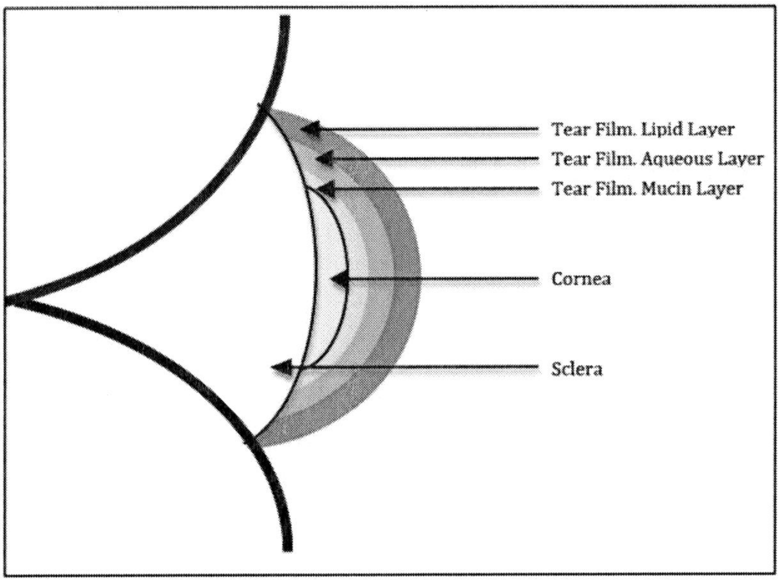

Figure 1. Schematic diagram of the anterior ocular surface depicting a stylized representation of the tear film as a three layered structure composed of mucin, aqueous and lipid layers. The innermost layer, which lies directly over the epithelial surface, is composed of mucin derived from conjunctival goblet cells, the middle aqueous layer is secreted by the lacrimal gland in the superolateral orbit and the outermost oily layer is produced by the meibomian glands, the orifices of which are visible posterior to the lashes. In reality the mucin and aqueous layers are not truly distinct, but as one travels further from the ocular surface the lower the observed mucin concentration.

Given that the tear film is the first interface between light and the eye, it is a crucial part of the visual apparatus. Therefore, an irregular tear film can cause glare and blurred vision to the patient.

Signs

The clinician may readily observe superficial punctate keratitis (SPK) on the corneal surface with stains such as fluorescein or rose Bengal, also the interpalpebral conjunctiva may also reveal staining. Conjunctival hyperaemia may be present. A tear break-up time (TBUT) of less than ten seconds is commonly associated with dry eye [6]. The clinician should also examine the eyelids for meibomian gland dysfunction, which may reveal blepharitis as a contributing factor.

The presence of conjunctival papillae may indicate allergic conjuctivitis which is commonly overlooked, it is vey prevalent, especially in the contact lens wearing population and in whom it often leads to contact lens intolerance and a request for refractive surgery. It is classically associated with the symptom of itchiness and the presence of tarsal conjunctival papillae, there may also be nodules at the limbus in extreme cases. The condition usually responds to withdrawal of the allergen (e.g. pollen, contact lenses, preserved drops, etc.), along with topical antihistamine regime. More severe cases may require a course topical steroid or topical cyclosporin regimes. It is recommended that moderate to severe allergic eye disease be controlled before further refractive surgery assessment is performed.

Classification

At its most basic dry eye can be described as aqueous deficient or evaporative [6]. Environmental factors can exacerbate an already compromised system. These factors may include: low blink rate, wide lid aperture, aging, low androgen pool, low relative humidity, high wind velocity, dusty environment and some systemic drugs (antihistamines, beta-blockers, antispasmodics, diuretics and some psychomotor drugs) [6].

Incidence

Population based studies report the prevalence of dry eye at 7.8% to 14.6% in US studies, 5.5% to 16.6% in Australian studies and 27.5% to 33.7% in Asian Studies [6]. Some of the variation may be due to different study criteria.

Effects on QOL

Dry eye can have a very detrimental effect to a patient's quality of life. This deleterious effect may be mediated via: pain and irritative symptoms; effects upon ocular as well as general health and well being; effects upon the perception of visual function; impact upon actual visual performance [9]. Although post-LASIK dry eye is usually temporary, some patients complain of severe symptoms that may negatively influence their satisfaction with the outcome [10].

Questionnaires

There are a myriad of clinical questionnaires available to diagnose and stratify patients with dry eye. The more rapidly administered include the ocular surface disease index (OSDI), which comprises 12 questions.

It is validated in the dry eye population and used as outcome measure in randomized controlled clinical trial [9]. For a more detailed questionnaire clinicians could consider the Dry Eye Questionnaire (DEQ) and Contact Lens DEQ. This questionnaire consists of 21 items, it notes contact lens wear, age, sex. It examines categorical scales of prevalence, frequency, diurnal severity and intrusiveness of symptoms in typical day of one-week recall period [9].

Tear-Film Break-up Time

Tear-film break-up time (TFBUT) was first reported by Lemp et al. in 1971 as a diagnostic feature of dry eye if the tear film broke up spontaneously in less than ten seconds. Later authors proposed reducing this cut-off to less than five seconds, which decreases the sensitivity and increases the specificity of this test (Table 1) [9].

Table 1. The sensitivity and specificity of objective clinical signs of dry eye disease [17]

Test	Cutoff	Sensitivity (n = 224)	Specificity (n = 75)
Osmolarity	>311 mOsm/L	72.8%	92.0%
TFBUT	<10 s	84.4%	43.5%
Schirmer	<18 mm	79.5%	50.7%
Corneal stain	> Grade 1	54.0%	89.3%
Conjunctival stain	> Grade 2	60.3%	90.7%

TFBUT: Tear-film break-up time. Cutoff values were located at the intersection between normal subjects and the entire subset of dry eye patients.

Conjunctival and Corneal Staining

There are several methods described to assess the ocular surface. The three most commonly used systems are the Bijsterveld system, the Oxford system and the NEI/Industry workshop system used in the CLEK study. The CLEK study methodology has the benefit of scoring staining over the visual axis. However there is no published evidence that one grading system is superior to any other (Table 1) [9].

Schirmer

The Schirmer test without anesthesia is a well-standardized test that is currently performed with the patients' eyes closed [11]. There is wide intrasubject, day-to-day, and visit-to-visit variation, but the variation and the absolute value decrease in aqueous-deficient dry eye, probably because of the decreased reflex response with lacrimal failure. It is reasonable to carry out the Schirmer test using a cutoff of ≤ 5 mm in 5 minutes (Table 1) [9].

Tear Meniscus Measurement

A non-invasive device which measures the tear film has reported to show promise in differentiating evaporative from aqueous deficient dry eye (Tearscope plus, Keeler, Windsor, Berkshire, UK) [12].

Corneal Sensation

Check corneal sensation with a cotton whisp. Patients with neurotrophic corneas are less likely to have symptomatic dry eye but are more prone to epithelial defects, which may heal poorly [13].

Osmolarity

As the tear becomes less aqueous, the relative levels of dissolved materials increases, because they cannot evaporate leading to hyperosmolarity, as the eye dries out the (crystalline) osmolarity rises. Elevated tear osmolarity is known to induce apoptosis (spontaneous cell death), serve as a pro-inflammatory stress and reduce the ability of mucin-like molecules to lubricate the ocular surface, which can result in permanent damage to the ocular surface and degradation of visual quality [14-16].

Cut off values of 308 and 311 mOsm/L have both been reported (Table 1) [2, 17]. Lemp et al., reported tear osmolarity as a new reliable metric for diagnosis and classification of dry eye [17]. Versura et al. found that the measured tear osmolarity had a 98.4% positive predictive value (PPV) for diagnosing dry eye, conferring a likelihood ratio (LR) of 10.99. These results compare very favorably with other dry eye disease diagnostic tests including: tear clearance (PPV: 95.8%; LR: 5.25); conjunctival scraping cytology (PPV: 100%; LR: ∞); Ferning test (PPV: 93.0%; LR: 3.58); corneal esthesiometry (PPV: 94.1%; LR: 4.76) and conjunctival imprint cytology (PPV: 96.0%; LR: 7.23). While conjunctival scraping cytology has a superior PPV and LR to tear osmolarity, it is considerably less convenient, therefore, tear osmolarity was proposed as the gold standard in the clinical diagnosis of dry eye [18].

There is a tear osmolarity testing device, which is commercially available (TearLab, San Diego, USA), non-invasive and suitable for the clinical setting. Tear osmolarity is a highly volatile parameter. It may rise artefactually following low blinking activities such as visual acuity testing or slit lamp examination, or it may be altered by recent eye drops. Thus the sequencing of the examination and ancillary tests in a refractive surgery assessment is important. Where possible tear osmolarity should be the first examination performed.

A study by Sullivan et al. reported poor correlation between dry eye parameters and a diagnosis of dry eye, in a retrospective study of 384 normal patients. This study casts doubt over the validity over these dry eye parameters as diagnostic tools. No correlations above $r^2 = 0.17$ were found between any signs and symptoms, except for corneal and conjunctival staining, which reported an $r^2 = 0.36$. The average r^2 for osmolarity (0.07), TBUT (0.12), Schirmer test (0.09), corneal (0.16) and conjunctival staining (0.17), meibomian grading (0.11) and OSDI (0.11) were consistently low [19]. However, tear osmolarity, while demonstrating very close agreement between eyes and in the same eyes over time in normal subjects, shows increasing variability in dry eye subjects. This is thought to be due to the instability of the tear-film in affected patients and can be used as a diagnostic hallmark of dry eye. Nonetheless, the increased variability in disease may contribute to the lack of correlation with the other signs [19].

Refractive Procedures and Dry Eye

LASIK and Surface Laser

Following LASIK dry eye affects approximately 50% of LASIK (120 micron flap) patients at 1 week, 40% at 1 month, and 20%-40% at 6 months. Although post-LASIK dry eye is usually transient, a significant cohort of patients experience severe symptoms [10]. Surface refractive laser, including LASEK and PRK, is associated with transient postoperative dry eye symptoms [3, 20]. Patients with extreme dry eye such with Sjogren's syndrome should not be considered for corneal procedures [21=.

Post-LASIK dry eye describes a spectrum of diseases encompassing transient or persistent post-operative neurotrophic disease, tear instability, true aqueous tear deficiency, corneal and conjunctival epitheliopathy, [9] and neuropathic pain states. Neural changes in the cornea and neuropathic causes of ocular surface discomfort may play a separate or synergistic role in the development of symptoms in some patients [22]. The post-LASIK neurotrophic effect and damage to goblet cells, [10] are related to the corneal flap sectioning and suction effect, respectively. These effects may not be seen in surface refractive laser patients, so theoretically LASIK would have a more profound effect on the precorneal tear film and induce more dry eye disease. This neurtophic cornea is sometimes referred to as LASIK-induced neurotrophic epitheliopathy (LINE) [23].

Corneal sensory neurons directly influence the integrity of the corneal epithelium. In the presence of neuronal destruction, epithelial cells swell, lose microvilli and produce abnormal basal lamina. This can slow or halt mitosis, which leads to epithelial breakdown. The neurotransmitters Acetylcholine and Substance P have been shown to promote corneal epithelial cell growth. An animal study found that capsaicin (which depletes substance P) led to neurotrophic keratopathy, suggesting a trophic effect of substance P. In one clinical report, a patient with neurotrophic keratopathy demonstrated complete recovery after receiving a combination of substance P and insulin- like growth factor-1 eyedrops [24]. Corneal sensation recovers one month post LASEK but can take more than 6 months in LASIK [25]. Loss of corneal innervation following a corneal flap may also affect the corneal-lacrimal gland, corneal-blinking, and blinking-meibomian gland reflex loops, resulting in decreased aqueous and lipid tear secretion and mucin expression. Because LASIK enhancement by flap lifting induces less dry eye symptoms and signs compared with the first surgery, it is suggested that other factors rather than loss of neurotrophic effect may be involved in the mechanisms of post-LASIK dry eye. These include damage of goblet cells by microkeratome suction and altered central corneal shape [10].

A study of 43 patients who had undergone bilateral femtosecond laser-assisted LASIK for myopia found corneal sensation was decreased significantly and gradually recovered over the first 3 months. No significant change was noted in TFBUT after surgery. Significant increases were noted in Schirmer values at 1 and 3 months and 6 months postoperatively in both groups. Corneal fluorescein staining increased significantly at 1 week and returned to baseline by 6 months. Conjunctival Rose Bengal staining decreased significantly by 6 months in the superior hinge group only. The OSDI significantly increased 1 week after surgery and did not completely return to baseline by 6 months postoperatively in either group [26].

It has been reported that several factors are associated with the development of post-LASIK dry eye. Higher refractive correction [1, 27-29] deeper ablation depth, [1, 28-30] narrow flap hinge [31] and female gender [28, 29] has been repeatedly reported to be associated with an increased incidence of post-LASIK dry eye. Flap thickness has both been reported to be directly related to dry eye post LASIK[32]and be unrelated [33].

The long posterior corneal nerves, which innervate the cornea, enter the eye at 3- and 9-o'clock. A superior-hinge flap transects both arms of the neuroplexus, whereas a nasal hinge transects only the temporal arm. In 2003 Donnenfield et al. found, the loss of corneal sensation and presence of dry eye syndrome were greater in eyes with a superior-hinge flap than in eyes with a nasal-hinge flap [34]. however, subsequent studies found no effect on dry eye incidence related to hinge position [1, 5, 26, 33, 35].

Albietz showed that refractive regression after LASIK was significantly related to chronic dry eye. It occurred in 27% of 45 patients with chronic dry eye and in 7% of 520 patients without. Patients with chronic dry eye had significantly worse myopic outcomes than those without, at 1 month 6 months and 1 year [28].

There is conflicting evidence regarding the effect of femtosecond laser versus microkeratome in post-LASIK dry eye. A study of 181 patients showed the incidence of LASIK-associated dry eye was statistically significantly higher in the microkeratome group (46%) than in the femtosecond group (8%) ($P < 0.0001$), as was the need for postoperative cyclosporine A treatment (24% and 7%, respectively) ($P < 0.01$) [36]. Whereas, in a study of 51 patients, there appeared to be no statistically significant difference in self-reported dry-eye symptoms between the mechanical micro-keratome group and the femtosecond laser keratome group. Also, central ablation depth, flap thickness, and age did not significantly affect the reported dryness [37].

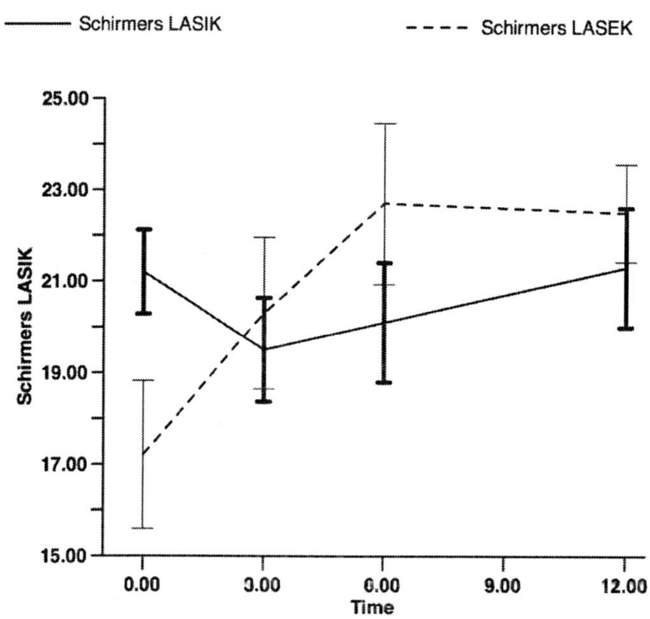

Figure 2. Double y line series, showing mean Schirmer values (mm/5min) at baseline, 3, 6 and 12 months post surgery in LASIK (bold line) versus LASEK patients (dashed line) [2].

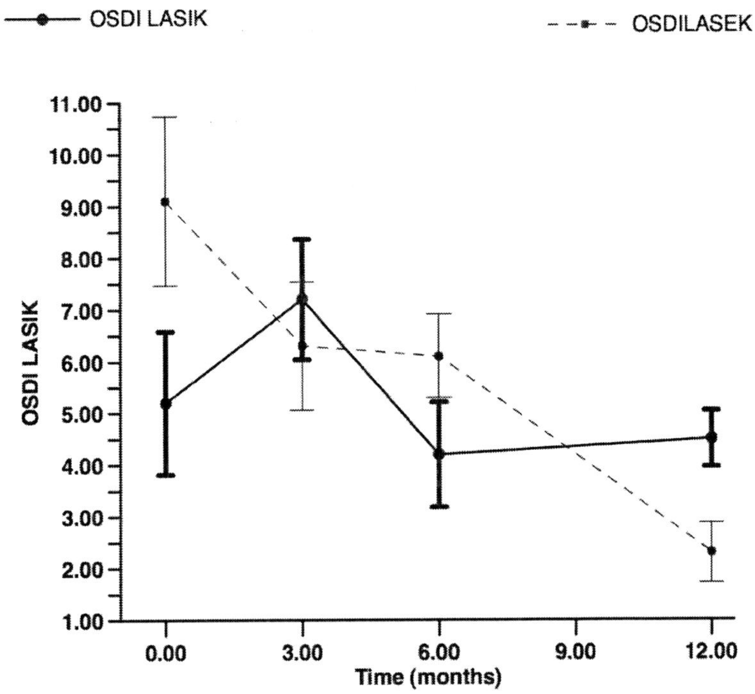

Figure 3. Double y line series, showing mean ocular surface disease index (OSDI) values (%) at baseline, 3, 6 and 12 months post surgery in LASIK (bold line) versus LASEK patients (dashed line) [2].

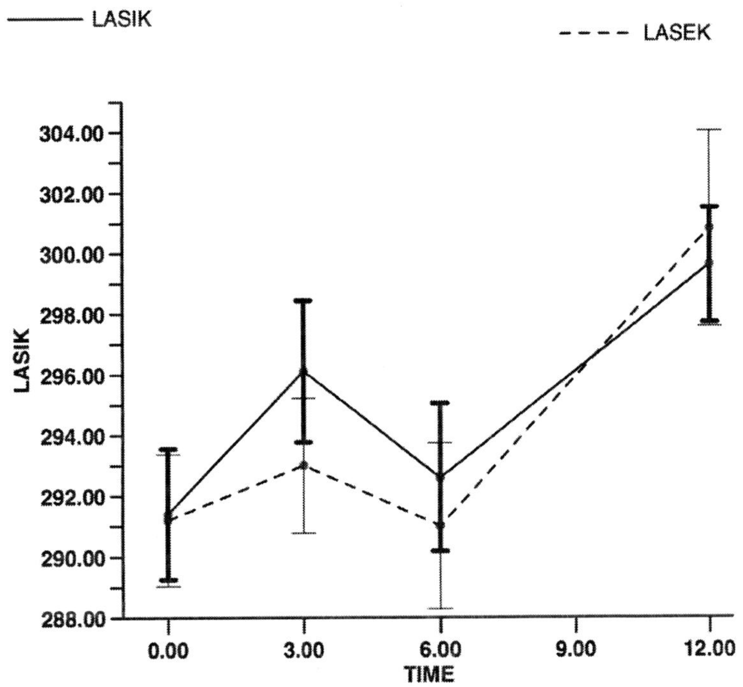

Figure 4. Double y line series, showing mean tear osmolarity values (mOsm/L) at baseline, 3, 6 and 12 months post surgery in LASIK (bold line) versus LASEK patients (dashed line) [2].

In a comparison of PRK and laser in situ LASIK with a flap thickness of 160 microns, LASIK was associated with more induced-tear dysfunction, and was of greater duration [11]. Dooley et al. compared the one-year postoperative changes in dry eye metrics between thin flap LASIK (120 microns) and LASEK eyes. This non-randomised study preoperatively had more patients with dry eye features in the LASEK group. Patients with dry eye were only offered LASEK, thus preoperatively the LASEK group had lower mean Schirmer test values (figure 2) and higher mean OSDI (figure 3), but actually had similar mean tear osmolarity (figure 4).

At three and six months postoperative the LASIK group had more dry eye features, with lower mean Schirmer test values, higher mean OSDI and higher mean tear osmolarity. By 12 months the gap was less or the trend was reversed. It would seem that LASEK is a better procedure for patients with dry eye features and the dry eye effect of both procedures are usually temporary [2].

A prospective controlled study, which examined 68 eyes in 34 patients, looked at self-reported dry eye symptoms and fluctuation of vision in LASIK versus PRK eyes. Both groups of eyes experienced significant increases in symptoms of dry eye, vision fluctuation, and foreign body sensation after LASIK and PRK at postoperative months 1, 3, and 6. However, by the 12-month postoperative visit, there was no increase in dry eye symptoms over the preoperative baseline levels in either group. At one month LASIK patients had slightly higher self reported corneal foreign body sensation compared to the PRK group ($p = 0.45$) [38].

LASEK has been reported to be a safe procedure in the context of severe preoperative dry eye related to contact-lens wear [25]. Mitomycin C used to prevent stromal haze during surface refractive laser was implicated as a possible contributing factor to chronic dry eye in a single case report [39].

Supracor (is a flap-based procedure similar to LASIK, where a stromal correction for intermediate and near vision can be incorporated with a distance correction. One would expect Supracor to have a similar incidence of dry eye to conventional LASIK, however no specific data on dry eye exists in relation to this novel procedure as yet.

Intracor is a presbyopia correcting procedure, which uses the femtosecond laser to create concentric intratromal rings. It does not involve a flap or disturbing the surface, a suction ring is employed. One would expect less dry eye than flap or surface based procedures. However, as yet there is a paucity of specific dry eye data related to this novel procedure. One prospective study of 25 eyes in 25 patients found one patient 4% had dry eyes at 3 months [40].

In recent years femtosecond lenticule extraction procedures have been developed as refractive procedures for myopia. These procedures use a femtosecond laser to create a stromal lenticule, which is extracted via conventional corneal flap (ReLEx) or via a small incision (ReLEx smile). Given the novelty of these procedures there is limited published evidence regarding post-operative dry eye rates. The small-incision procedure offers theoretical advantage over the flap based procedure, as less corneal nerves are sectioned and this should have a knock-on benefit to the ocular surface and induce less dry eye. These procedures still employ a suction-based device to fashion the lenticules, although this is described as being a lower vacuum and shorter duration than conventional microkeratome.

Shimizu presented data that show postoperative trigeminal nerve density after LASIK flap is 10% and 15% at 1 and 3 months, whereas following ReLEx smile, it was 50 % at 1 month and 60% at 3 months (unpublished data) [41]. This would suggest less likelihood of neurotrophic corneal changes and resultant dry eye in the ReLEx smile group. A paper by Sekundo et al., reported that at one week the ReLEx induced subjective dry eye symptoms in 8.3% of 108 eyes and superficial punctate keratitis (SPK) in 13.9%, compared to the ReLEx smile group, which produced no cases of subjective dry eye symptoms at one week in 38 eyes of 20 patients and SPK in only 1.1%.of cases [42]. While this initial report is promising, the small number and short duration mean limited extrapolation is possible at this juncture.

A study of simultaneous intracorneal inlay implantation and LASIK to treat presbyopia with emmetropia, hyperopia, or myopia found the dry eye symptoms increased from 21.2%, 19.2% and 27.5% preoperatively in hyperopes, emmetropes and myopes, to six-month postoperative rates of 91.7%, 100% and 74.3%, respectively. This was reported as similar to the dry eye rate reported with LASIK alone [43].

Intraocular Lens-Based Refractive Procedure Procedures

It is useful to consider phacoemulsification cataract extraction in this section as a refractive procedure. There is limited data on dry eye parameters related to PIOL, ICL implantation or CLE, while more evidence is available in relation to phacoemulsification cataract extraction.

The incidence and severity of dry eye symptoms increase after cataract surgery. In particular, phacoemulsification has been shown to reduce tear meniscus height and tear breakup time (TBUT) and increase squamous metaplasia on conjunctival impression cytology [44]. The mechanism for the exacerbation of surface disease after cataract surgery likely includes several factors: increased inflammatory mediators due to postoperative inflammation, toxicity from the use of benzalkonium chloride containing eye drops, and damage to the corneal nerves from limbal incisions [13].

Oh et al. found a significant post-operative decrease in mean goblet cell density (GCD) measured by conjunctival impression cytology, following phacoemulsification cataract extraction. This decrease was significantly and positively correlated with operative time (r^2 = 0.65). This decrease still had not recovered 3 months postoperatively. Therefore, microscopic ocular surface damage during cataract surgery seems to be one of the pathogenic factors that cause ocular discomfort and dry eye syndrome after cataract surgery [45].

These finding may be extrapolated somewhat to apply to the pIOL, ICL and CLE patient. There are quite a few similarities between the procedures: same anaesthethic options; equivalent wound placement and construction; equivalent procedure durations; similar post-operative regimes. There may also be some very important differences between the cataractous population and the refractive IOL population. The cataract patient population tend to be older than the refractive surgery population, which is significant, given dry eye incidence increases with age [46].

Also, clear lens extraction may require little or no phacoemulsification compared to standard phacoemulsification of the cataractous lens. Indeed pIOL implantation requires no phacoemulsification at all, and this difference in energy delivered to the eye, between these 3 procedures may have a role in the postoperative dryness. The emergence of femtosecond assisted refractive surgery in recent years may alter the rates of both clear lens extraction and cataract surgery induced dry eye.

Treatment

Most cases of early post-operative dry eye symptoms resolve with appropriate management, which includes optimizing ocular surface health before and after surgery. Severe symptoms or symptoms persisting after 9 months rarely respond satisfactorily to traditional treatment modalities and require aggressive management [22]. Post-refractive surgery dry eye treatments are now discussed.

Table 2. Treatment recommendations by severity level

Level 1: Education, environmental and dietary modifications Elimination of exacerbating systemic medications Tear substitutes. Drops, gels and ointments Eyelid toilet			
	Level 2: If Level 1 regime insufficient, add: Anti-inflammatory agents. Cyclosporin A Tetracyclines (meibomianitis, acne rosacea) Punctal plugs Consider secretogogues and moist chamber spectacles		
		Level 3: If Level 2 regime insufficient, consider: Serum drops Contact lenses Permanent punctual occlusion	
			Level 4: If Level 3 regime insufficient, consider: Systemic anti-inflammatory agents Surgery: Tarsorraphy; mucous membrane graft; salivary gland translocation; amniotic membrane transplantation

Modified from: International Task Force Guidelines for Dry Eye [47, 56].

Lubricants

In theory, the ideal artificial lubricant should be preservative-free, contain potassium, bicarbonate, and other electrolytes and have a polymeric system to increase its retention time.

Physical properties should include a neutral to slightly alkaline pH. Osmolarities of artificial tears have been measured to range from about 181 to 354 mOsm/L [47].

Preservatives

The preservatives added to prevent microbial growth in multidose bottles may have a significant effect upon the corneal epithelium. Benz-alkonium chloridre (BAK) has been demonstrated to be toxic to corneal epithelium. BAK can damage the corneal and conjunctival epithelium, affecting cell-to-cell junctions and cell shape and microvilli, eventually leading to cell necrosis with sloughing of 1-2 layers of epithelial cells. Less toxic preservatives, such as polyquad (polyquaternium-1), sodium chlorite (Purite®), and sodium perborate were developed to allow the use of multidose bottled lubricants and to avoid the known toxicity of BAK-containing solutions [47].

Ocular ointments and gels are also used in treatment of dry eye disease. Ointments are formulated with a specific mixture of mineral oil and petrolatum. Some contain lanolin, which can be irritating to the eye and delay corneal wound healing. In general, ointments do not support bacterial growth and, therefore, do not require preservatives [47].

Artificial Lubricant Components

It has been shown that potassium is important in maintaining corneal thickness and bicarbonate helps promote the recovery of epithelial barrier function in damaged epithelium and aid in maintaining normal epithelial utrastructure. Patients with dry eye have a higher tear film crystalloid osmolarity than normal tears. Elevated tear film osmolarity causes morphological and biochemical changes to the corneal and conjunctival epithelium and is proinflammatory [47].

Colloidal osmolality is another factor that varies in artificial tear formulations. While crystalloid osmolarity is related to the presence of ions, colloidal osmolality is dependent largely on macromolecule content. Colloidal osmolarity, also known as oncotic pressure, is involved in the control of water transport in tissues. Epithelial cells swell due to damage to their cellular membranes or due to a dysfunction in the pumping mechanism. Following the addition of a fluid with a high colloidal osmolality to the damaged cell surface, deturgescence occurs, leading to a return of normal cell physiology. Theoretically, an artificial tear formulation with a high colloidal osmolality may be of value [47].

Viscosity Agents

Macromolecular complexes added to artificial lubricants act as viscosity agents. The addition of a viscosity agent increases residence time, providing a longer interval of patient comfort in addition to protecting the ocular surface epithelium. Agents such as hydroxymethycellulose (HMC), which decrease rose bengal staining in dry eye subjects, may either "coat and protect" the surface epithelium or help restore the protective effect of mucins [47].

Punctal plugs may be absorbable or non-absorbable but have the effect of prolonging tear residence in the conjunctival sac. Beneficial outcomes in dry eye have been reported in 74 to 86% of patients treated with punctual plugs [47].

Moist Chambers

Glasses fitted with side panels to construct a moist chamber have been available for several years. They are not popular with patients, especially post-refractive surgery and supportive evidence for their use is limited [47].

Contact lenses may help to protect and hydrate the corneal surface in severe dry eye conditions. Several different contact lens materials and designs have been evaluated, including silicone rubber lenses and gas permeable scleral-bearing hard contact lenses with or without fenestration. Improved visual acuity and comfort, decreased corneal epitheliopathy, and healing of persistent corneal epithelial defects have been reported. Highly oxygen-permeable materials enable overnight wear in appropriate circumstances. There is a small risk of corneal vascularization and possible corneal infection associated with the use of contact lenses by dry eye patients [47].

Tear Stimulation

Pilocarpine and Cevilemine are 2 orally administered cholinergic agents, which have been evaluated for the treatment of KCS in Sjogrens syndrome. Both show a beneficial effect on dry eye parameters, [48] but Cevilemine seems to induce less side-effects, which includes excessive sweating [49]. Several topical agents are currently under investigation by pharmaceutical companies. They include diquafosol (P2Y2 receptor agonist), rebamipide, gefarnate, ecabet sodium (mucoussecretion stimulants), and 15(S)-HETE (MUC1 stimulant). 2% diquafosol (INS365, DE-089 [Santen, Osaka, Japan]; Inspire [Durham, NC]) has shown to reduce ocular surface staining in the treatment of dry eye in a randomized double-masked trial [47].

Serum Drops

While there is evidence that autologous serum drops are superior to ocular lubricants in the treatment of dry eyes, [50, 51] and they have been recommended in certain situations prior to LASIK, the logistical difficulties associated with their manufacture mean they remain more in the remit of healing corneal epithelial defects.

Lid Hygiene

Regular lid toilet with a mild detergent solution may reduce the bacterial load and open the meibomian orifices, if performed regularly this may improve dry eye symptoms.

Anti-Inflammatory Agents

Based on the concept that inflammation is a key component of the pathogenesis of dry eye, the efficacy of a number of anti-inflammatory agents for treatment of dry eye disease has been evaluated in clinical trials and animal models.

Cyclosporine A

Pflugfelder et al. showed an increase in goblet cell density and the production of transforming growth factor as early as 6 and 12 weeks after 0.05% cyclosporine A (CsA) emulsion therapy. There was no such increase with the use of artificial tears.[52] Microspheres, implants, and liposomes have been developed for administration of CsA subconjunctivally in order to enhance its efficiency [53].

Steroids

Corticosteroids have been shown to have beneficial effects in the management of KCS. The corticosteroid methylprednisolone was noted to preserve corneal epithelial smoothness and barrier function in an experimental murine model of dry eye. A concurrent study showed that methylprednisolone prevented an increase in MMP-9 protein in the corneal epithelium, as well as gelatinase activity in the corneal epithelium and tears in response to experimental dry eye [47].

Androgens

Preparations of topically applied androgen and estrogen steroid hormones are currently being evaluated in randomized clinical trials. A trial of topically applied 0.03% testosterone was reported to increase the percentage of patients that had meibomian gland secretions with normal viscosity and to relieve discomfort symptoms after 6 months of treatment compared to vehicle. TBUT and lipid layer thickness were observed to increase in a patient with KCS who was treated with topical androgen for 3 months. Tear production and ocular irritation symptoms were reported to increase following treatment with topical 17 beta-oestradiol solution for 4 months [47].

Tetracyclines

Tetracycline antibiotics have been demonstrated to improve dry eye parameters. These improvements may be mediated via the anti-bacterial effects, the anti-inflammatory effects and the anti-angiogenic effects of these drugs [47].

Essential fatty acids are necessary for complete health. They cannot be synthesized by vertebrates and must be obtained from dietary sources. Among the essential fatty acids are 18 carbon omega-6 and omega-3 fatty acids. In a prospective, placebo-controlled clinical trial of the essential fatty acids, linoleic acid and gamma-linolenic acid administered orally twice daily produced significant improvement in ocular irritation symptoms and ocular surface lissamine green staining. Decreased conjunctival HLA-DR staining also was observed [47].

Surgery

Salivary gland autotransplantation, may be beneficial in helping control dry eye symptoms but often has no effect upon vision.

There has been some preliminary interest in the potential use of topical nerve growth factor for the treatment of post-LASIK dry eyes. Nerve growth factor has both neurotrophic and immune-modulator effects and could be useful to treat corneal nerve damage after LASIK [54]. There may even be a role for nerve growth factor or other neurotrophins to assist with healing of corneal nerve damage in the early postoperative period [54]. However, there are still challenges in making this type of treatment accessible to the cornea. There is also a subset of post-LASIK dry eye patients with aberrant nerve regeneration and corneal neuropathy that might benefit from the tricycylic antidepressant treatment for neuropathic pain [55].

Conclusion

Dry eye remains a significant factor in refractive surgery. It is important to remember that it is a clinical diagnosis. Ancillary tests are useful but should be combined with careful history-taking and examination, a normal test value does not preclude the diagnosis. Meticulous preoperative identification of at-risk patients and diligent consent are crucial, if the refractive surgeon is to avoid desperately unhappy postoperative patients. Procedure which section large portions of corneal nerves, such as flap based procedures may be at higher risk of inducing dry eye.

References

[1] De Paiva CS, Chen Z, Koch DD, et al. The incidence and risk factors for developing dry eye after myopic LASIK. *Am. J. Ophthalmol.* Mar 2006; 141(3): 438-445.

[2] Dooley I, D'Arcy F, O'Keefe M. Comparison of dry-eye disease severity after laser in situ keratomileusis and laser-assisted subepithelial keratectomy. *J. Cataract Refract. Surg.* Jun; 38(6): 1058-1064.

[3] Herrmann WA, Shah CP, von Mohrenfels CW, Gabler B, Hufendiek K, Lohmann CP. Tear film function and corneal sensation in the early postoperative period after LASEK for the correction of myopia. *Graefes Arch. Clin. Exp. Ophthalmol.* Sep 2005; 243(9): 911-916

[4] Siganos DS, Popescu CN, Siganos CS, Pistola G. Tear secretion following spherical and astigmatic excimer laser photorefractive keratectomy. *J. Cataract Refract. Surg.* Nov 2000; 26(11): 1585-1589.

[5] Mian SI, Shtein RM, Nelson A, Musch DC. Effect of hinge position on corneal sensation and dry eye after laser in situ keratomileusis using a femtosecond laser. *J. Cataract Refract. Surg.* Jul 2007; 33(7): 1190-1194.

[6] The epidemiology of dry eye disease: report of the Epidemiology Subcommittee of the International Dry Eye WorkShop (2007). *Ocul. Surf.* Apr 2007; 5(2): 93-107.

[7] The definition and classification of dry eye disease: report of the Definition and Classification Subcommittee of the International Dry Eye WorkShop (2007). *Ocul. Surf.* Apr 2007; 5(2): 75-92.

[8] McGinnigle S, Naroo SA, Eperjesi F. Evaluation of dry eye. *Surv. Ophthalmol.* Jul-Aug; 57(4): 293-316.

[9] Methodologies to diagnose and monitor dry eye disease: report of the Diagnostic Methodology Subcommittee of the International Dry Eye WorkShop (2007). *Ocul. Surf.* Apr 2007; 5(2): 108-152.

[10] Toda I. LASIK and the ocular surface. *Cornea.* Sep 2008; 27 Suppl 1: S70-76.

[11] Serin D, Karsloglu S, Kyan A, Alagoz G. A simple approach to the repeatability of the schirmer test without anesthesia: eyes open or closed? *Cornea.* Sep 2007; 26(8): 903-906.

[12] Uchida A, Uchino M, Goto E, et al. Noninvasive interference tear meniscometry in dry eye patients with Sjogren syndrome. *Am. J. Ophthalmol.* Aug 2007; 144(2): 232-237.

[13] Movahedan A, Djalilian AR. Cataract surgery in the face of ocular surface disease. *Curr. Opin. Ophthalmol.* Jan; 23(1): 68-72.

[14] Luo L, Li DQ, Corrales RM, Pflugfelder SC. Hyperosmolar saline is a proinflammatory stress on the mouse ocular surface. *Eye Contact Lens.* Sep 2005; 31(5): 186-193.

[15] Luo L, Li DQ, Pflugfelder SC. Hyperosmolarity-induced apoptosis in human corneal epithelial cells is mediated by cytochrome c and MAPK pathways. *Cornea.* May 2007; 26(4): 452-460.

[16] Floyd AM, Zhou X, Evans C, et al. Mucin deficiency causes functional and structural changes of the ocular surface. *PLoS One.* 7(12): e50704.

[17] Lemp MA, Bron AJ, Baudouin C, et al. Tear osmolarity in the diagnosis and management of dry eye disease. *Am. J. Ophthalmol.* May; 151(5): 792-798 e791.

[18] Versura P, Profazio V, Campos EC. Performance of tear osmolarity compared to previous diagnostic tests for dry eye diseases. *Curr. Eye Res.* Jul; 35(7): 553-564.

[19] Sullivan BD, Crews LA, Messmer EM, et al. Correlations between commonly used objective signs and symptoms for the diagnosis of dry eye disease: clinical implications. *Acta Ophthalmol.* Dec 28.

[20] Horwath-Winter J, Vidic B, Schwantzer G, Schmut O. Early changes in corneal sensation, ocular surface integrity, and tear-film function after laser-assisted subepithelial keratectomy. *J. Cataract Refract. Surg.* Nov 2004; 30(11): 2316-2321.

[21] Simpson RG, Moshirfar M, Edmonds JN, Christiansen SM, Behunin N. Laser in situ keratomileusis in patients with collagen vascular disease: a review of the literature. *Clin. Ophthalmol.* 6:1827-1837.

[22] Nettune GR, Pflugfelder SC. Post-LASIK tear dysfunction and dysesthesia. *Ocul. Surf.* Jul; 8(3): 135-145.

[23] Ambrosio R, Jr., Tervo T, Wilson SE. LASIK-associated dry eye and neurotrophic epitheliopathy: pathophysiology and strategies for prevention and treatment. *J. Refract. Surg.* Apr 2008; 24(4): 396-407.

[24] Lambiase A, Rama P, Aloe L, Bonini S. Management of neurotrophic keratopathy. *Curr. Opin. Ophthalmol.* Aug 1999; 10(4): 270-276.

[25] Chen KH, Hsu WM, Lee SM, Lai JY, Li YS. Laser-assisted subepithelial keratectomy for dry eye associated with soft contact lenses. *J. Cataract Refract. Surg.* Dec 2005; 31(12): 2299-2305.

[26] Huang JC, Sun CC, Chang CK, Ma DH, Lin YF. Effect of hinge position on corneal sensation and dry eye parameters after femtosecond laser-assisted LASIK. *J. Refract. Surg.* Sep; 28(9): 625-631.

[27] Nassaralla BA, McLeod SD, Nassaralla JJ, Jr. Effect of myopic LASIK on human corneal sensitivity. *Ophthalmology.* Mar 2003; 110(3): 497-502.

[28] Albietz JM, Lenton LM, McLennan SG. Chronic dry eye and regression after laser in situ keratomileusis for myopia. *J. Cataract Refract. Surg.* Mar 2004; 30(3): 675-684.

[29] Shoja MR, Besharati MR. Dry eye after LASIK for myopia: Incidence and risk factors. *Eur. J. Ophthalmol.* Jan-Feb 2007; 17(1): 1-6.

[30] Kim WS, Kim JS. Change in corneal sensitivity following laser in situ keratomileusis. *J. Cataract Refract. Surg.* Mar 1999; 25(3): 368-373.

[31] Donnenfeld ED, Ehrenhaus M, Solomon R, Mazurek J, Rozell JC, Perry HD. Effect of hinge width on corneal sensation and dry eye after laser in situ keratomileusis. *J. Cataract Refract. Surg.* Apr 2004; 30(4): 790-797.

[32] Barequet IS, Hirsh A, Levinger S. Effect of thin femtosecond LASIK flaps on corneal sensitivity and tear function. *J. Refract. Surg.* Nov 2008; 24(9): 897-902.

[33] Mian SI, Li AY, Dutta S, Musch DC, Shtein RM. Dry eyes and corneal sensation after laser in situ keratomileusis with femtosecond laser flap creation Effect of hinge position, hinge angle, and flap thickness. *J. Cataract Refract. Surg.* Dec 2009; 35(12): 2092-2098.

[34] Donnenfeld ED, Solomon K, Perry HD, et al. The effect of hinge position on corneal sensation and dry eye after LASIK. *Ophthalmology.* May 2003; 110(5): 1023-1029; discussion 1029-1030.

[35] Ghoreishi M, Aidenloo NS, Peyman A, Peyman M, Haghdoustoskoey M. Does hinge position affect dry eye after laser in situ keratomileusis? *Ophthalmologica.* Sep-Oct 2005; 219(5): 276-280.

[36] Salomao MQ, Ambrosio R, Jr., Wilson SE. Dry eye associated with laser in situ keratomileusis: Mechanical microkeratome versus femtosecond laser. *J. Cataract Refract. Surg.* Oct 2009; 35(10): 1756-1760.

[37] Golas L, Manche EE. Dry eye after laser in situ keratomileusis with femtosecond laser and mechanical keratome. *J. Cataract Refract. Surg.* Aug; 37(8): 1476-1480.

[38] Murakami Y, Manche EE. Prospective, randomized comparison of self-reported postoperative dry eye and visual fluctuation in LASIK and photorefractive keratectomy. *Ophthalmology.* Nov; 119(11): 2220-2224.

[39] Kymionis GD, Tsiklis NS, Ginis H, Diakonis VF, Pallikaris I. Dry eye after photorefractive keratectomy with adjuvant mitomycin C. *J. Refract Surg.* May 2006; 22(5): 511-513.

[40] Menassa N, Fitting A, Auffarth GU, Holzer MP. Visual outcomes and corneal changes after intrastromal femtosecond laser correction of presbyopia. *J. Cataract Refract. Surg.* May; 38(5): 765-773.

[41] Shimizu K. The effects of refractive surgery on dry eye syndrome and corneal sensation. *Cataract and Refractive Surgery Today, Europe.* Vol Supplement to October 2012. 2012:6, 7.
[42] Sekundo W, Kunert KS, Blum M. Small incision corneal refractive surgery using the small incision lenticule extraction (SMILE) procedure for the correction of myopia and myopic astigmatism: results of a 6 month prospective study. *Br. J. Ophthalmol.* Mar; 95(3): 335-339.
[43] Tomita M, Kanamori T, Waring GOt, et al. Simultaneous corneal inlay implantation and laser in situ keratomileusis for presbyopia in patients with hyperopia, myopia, or emmetropia: six-month results. *J. Cataract Refract. Surg.* Mar; 38(3): 495-506.
[44] Li XM, Hu L, Hu J, Wang W. Investigation of dry eye disease and analysis of the pathogenic factors in patients after cataract surgery. *Cornea.* Oct 2007;26 (9 Suppl 1): S16-20.
[45] Oh T, Jung Y, Chang D, Kim J, Kim H. Changes in the tear film and ocular surface after cataract surgery. *Jpn. J. Ophthalmol.* Mar; 56(2): 113-118.
[46] Ding J, Sullivan DA. Aging and dry eye disease. *Exp. Gerontol.* Jul; 47(7): 483-490.
[47] Management and therapy of dry eye disease: report of the Management and Therapy Subcommittee of the International Dry Eye WorkShop (2007). *Ocul. Surf.* Apr 2007; 5(2): 163-178.
[48] Aragona P, Di Pietro R, Spinella R, Mobrici M. Conjunctival epithelium improvement after systemic pilocarpine in patients with Sjogren's syndrome. *Br. J. Ophthalmol.* Feb 2006; 90(2): 166-170.
[49] Ono M, Takamura E, Shinozaki K, et al. Therapeutic effect of cevimeline on dry eye in patients with Sjogren's syndrome: a randomized, double-blind clinical study. *Am. J. Ophthalmol.* Jul 2004; 138(1): 6-17.
[50] Kojima T, Higuchi A, Goto E, Matsumoto Y, Dogru M, Tsubota K. Autologous serum eye drops for the treatment of dry eye diseases. *Cornea.* Sep 2008; 27 Suppl 1:S25-30.
[51] Noda-Tsuruya T, Asano-Kato N, Toda I, Tsubota K. Autologous serum eye drops for dry eye after LASIK. *J. Refract. Surg.* Jan-Feb 2006; 22(1): 61-66.
[52] Pflugfelder SC, De Paiva CS, Villarreal AL, Stern ME. Effects of sequential artificial tear and cyclosporine emulsion therapy on conjunctival goblet cell density and transforming growth factor-beta2 production. *Cornea.* Jan 2008; 27(1): 64-69.
[53] Yavuz B, Bozdag Pehlivan S, Unlu N. An overview on dry eye treatment: approaches for cyclosporin a delivery. *Scientific World Journal.* 2012: 194848.
[54] Pepose JS, Johnson EM, Jr. Is there a role for neurotrophin treatment of the ocular surface following laser in situ keratomileusis (LASIK)? *Am. J. Ophthalmol.* Jun 2005; 139(6): 1090-1094.
[55] Ghaffariyeh A, Chamacham T. Tricyclic antidepressants: potential therapeutic alternatives for treatment of dry eye symptoms after LASIK. *J. Refract. Surg.* Oct 2008; 24(8): 770-771; author reply 771-772.
[56] Behrens A, Doyle JJ, Stern L, et al. Dysfunctional tear syndrome: a Delphi approach to treatment recommendations. *Cornea.* Sep 2006; 25(8): 900-907.

In: Current Understanding and New Techniques …
Editor: Michael O'Keefe
ISBN: 978-1-62808-748-2

Chapter 4

Corneal Ectasia

Gerard N. Kervick*
Consultant Ophthalmic Surgeon
Mater Hospital, Belfast, Northern Ireland

Abstract

Unlike many other surgical procedures that were performed and refined over many years, laser refractive surgery has progressed very rapidly in a relatively short time frame. From a start-up in the laboratory on bovine eyes a mere 30 years ago to becoming today one of the most commonly performed surgical procedures. Whilst this very rapid journey is impressive in terms of the clinical and safety profile of the procedure we know today the very speed of the advancement without carefully controlled prospective clinical trials meant there was a risk of complications developing years after the surgery which were both unexpected and detrimental to the patients vision. One such complication is corneal ectasia. It can be broadly defined as development of progressive inferior steepening of the cornea with associated irregular astigmatism and reduced UAVA and BSCVA. This complication while relatively rare can have a devastating effect on the patients vision. While there is no clear pre-operative test that can with certainty preclude its subsequent development there are a number of clinical features or 'red flags' common to many cases that subsequently develop this condition. These include both frank and form fruste keratoconus and keratoconus in the fellow eye, significant corneal asymmetry or abnormal topography, pellucid marginal degeneration, thin corneas, residual stromal bed less than 250um, attempted high myopic correction and young age. Retrospective analysis of many series of post-laser ectasia reveals a significant percentage of patients with no pre-operative 'red flags'. Therein lies the problem with this condition. It can be impossible to predict with certainty who will subsequently develop ectasia. Corneal ectasia can develop in the immediate post-operative period or many years later. While it is not possible to completely and with certainty reverse the condition the aim is to try and stabilise it and hopefully reverse some of the changes with corneal cross-linking, Intacs or a combination of both. Visual rehabilitation can be further enhanced with rigid gas permeable contact lenses or glasses. In some cases penetrating keratoplasty is required

* gkervick@aol.com

although with the advent of cross-linking this option appears to be required less than previously. Although it may be rather simplistic to say it, the best treatment is to try and avoid the condition in the first place by having a high level of suspicion when planning refractive surgery on prospective patients with any of the 'red flags' mentioned above. If in doubt then revert to some other form of refractive surgery such as surface laser, phakic lens implants or avoid refractive surgery altogether.

Introduction

Corneal ectasia following routine LASIK surgery is potentially one of the most serious complications of this procedure. It can be defined as a progressive structural corneal deformation leading to refractive and optical instability after uneventful LASIK [1]. Typically it is associated with increased irregular astigmatism, inferior steepening and reduced BCVA and BSCVA. It is probably the most feared complication of bladeless LASIK surgery akin to post-operative endophthalmitis after routine cataract surgery for the surgeon. It is rightly feared as it can have a devastating effect on the patients vision and it is not always predictable in its development and may develop in eyes with none of the usual predictable features [2]. While it most commonly occurs in LASIK for myopia it can follow routine PRK [3, 4] for myopia although this is very rare without abnormal preoperative topography [5] or hyperopic lasik [6]. The incidence of progressive corneal ectasia after LASIK has been estimated to be 0.2%. [7]. Other than obvious pre-operative keratoconus there is no one single sign that will indicate the development of the condition. For this reason a high level of vigilance is required on the part of the laser refractive surgeon to rule out patients deemed to be at risk of this complication from having surgery in the first place. Important factors in developing the condition include form fruste keratoconus, corneal asymmetry, thin corneas, reduced residual stromal bed, and young age.

We are all aware of the relatively short history of laser refractive surgery development. How it has gone from laboratory experimentation on bovine eyes in 1983 [8] to be one of the most commonly performed elective procedures in surgery today. It is estimated that some 28 million procedures have been performed world-wide to date. This is a relatively short time from start-up to its widespread use and acceptance today. One of the reasons for the rapid almost exponential growth of laser refractive surgery was due to the introduction of lasik. First performed as we know it today with ablation in the stromal bed by Pallikaris and reported in 1990 [9]. This allowed for rapid visual rehabilitation, bilateral simulataneous surgery and very little 'down time' for the patient. While there were well recognised complications associated with the surgery (discussed elsewhere in this book) particularly in the era of blade based flap creation, many if not all of these occurred in either the per-operative or the early post-operative period, flap complications, infection, inflammation, epithelial ingrowth and in cases of poorly centered flaps or decentered ablation zones, night vision problems. As a laser refractive surgeon however there was a sense that if one could perform a good flap and a well-centered ablation that within a short time period one could relax in the knowledge that the patient would recover good vision very rapidly. We grew used to the plaudits of our patients who on day one after a successful lasik procedure would read the 20/20 line on the chart unaided. It seemed there was no end to the amount of myopia that could be treated with lasik. The range of treatments often extended up to -20D and beyond

[10]. All this changed with the publication of a paper by Seiler in 1999 [11]. He reported on three patients who underwent LASIK for myopia -10.00 to -13.50D who developed central steep areas on their corneas between 1 and 8 months after surgery. He felt that this iatrogenic kerectasia was caused by too large an attempted treatment and suggested a minimum of 250um should be left in the stromal bed after LASIK. This paper was followed quickly by further papers reporting the same or a similar condition after seemingly routine LASIK surgery for myopia [12,- 17] One of the worrying aspects of this new complication was the often long latent period between the apparently normal lasik surgery and the appearance of the complication, often more than 6 years after surgery [18]. In my own practice I have had a patient who presented 7 years after routine lasik surgery with iatrogenic kerectasia. (see case report) Now as surgeons we had to worry about the potential for some of our patients to return many years after discharge with a potentially very serious complication. Having being performing laser refractive surgery since 1992 I still get a slight frisson when one of my old high myopic treatment lasik patients returns complaining of some recent change in their vision. I'm always relieved when I see at least a normal topography map regardless of any refractive error present. Glasses, after all, cannot be argued are a serious complication of laser refractive surgery given the potential for more serious issues such as ectasia.

In reviewing the early cases of iatrogentic ectasia it soon became apparent that there were often common features amongst those presenting with this condition. Pre-operative factors included, attempted high myopic corrections, residual stromal bed, form fruste keratoconus, abnormal corneal topography pre-operatively, corneal asymmetry, keratoconus in fellow eye, thin corneas and relatively young age. Rather worryingly however, in many cases there was no discernible pre-operative tell-tale signs that in retrospect would make one reconsider performing lasik in the first place. In other words, given the current diagnostic technology available to us there may well be a very small number of eyes that will slip through the net and have lasik for a low correction, with thick corneas and normal topography and still go on to develop ectasia. The best we can do as surgeons is to be very obsessive in our pre-operative assessment of all our patients. While we still don't have a treatment that can completely reverse this condition at least with the advent of corneal crosslinking (CXL) and intacs we can in many cases prevent progression and aid visual rehabilitation of the patient and limit the number of patients requiring penetrating keratoplasty which prior to the use of CXL was the only effective surgical treatment. It is likely that the incidence of the condition will reduce from its current level as we apply more stringent inclusion criteria for patients presenting for laser refractive surgery. While it could be argued that performing LASIK on the unaffected eye of a patient with unilateral keratoconus in 2000 was not unreasonable (see case report), given what we know about the condition today that would certainly not be the case now.

How to Avoid Ectasia?

One of the early criticisms of laser refractive surgery and indeed all forms of refractive surgery is that we were operating on healthy eyes, albeit these were eyes with refractive errors. It behoves us therefore as surgeons to attempt to prevent surgical complications and at the very least do no harm to the patients BCVA. While there is currently no known mechanism to predictably reverse ectasia once it has developed it is important to attempt to screen out patients who are perceived to be at risk of developing this complication. In other words the best treatment for ectasia is to try and avoid development of the condition in the first place. While for some cases of reported kerectasia there are no obvious pre-operative markers that would alert the surgeon to the potential for such a complication in many of the reported cases there are features common. These include abnormal topography, corneal thinning disorders, young age, high myopic treatment, low residual stromal bed and thin corneas.

Abnormal Corneal Topography

A major factor predisposing to LASIK-induced ectasia is unrecognized corneal thinning disorders such as keratoconus or pellucid marginal degeneration (PMD), including form fruste and early stage. In both conditions, altered collagen orientation and structure decrease the biomechanical strength of the tissue [19, 20]. There is general agreement that corneal thinning disorders are a contraindication to LASIK [21] Although various indices to detect ectatic disorders in corneal topography have been proposed [22, 23] identification of form fruste keratoconus or PMD remains difficult in some cases. A number of studies have looked at screening of abnormal corneas to eliminate form fruste keratoconus [24, 25, 26]. While it would be convenient if there was a simple topographic screening tool to rule out potential problems there is no single corneal shape that defines the cornea as normal. Therein lies the problem in relying on topographic changes exclusively. The ophthalmologist should rely on certain topographic criteria that may help in making the diagnosis of form fruste keratoconus or in identifying patients who are at risk of experiencing corneal ectasia after LASIK not exclusively but in conjunction with other factors associated with this condition.

Various attempts have been made to grade the preoperatively topography in an effort to predict those patients who might develop ectasia. Although these are certainly useful they are derived from retrospective studies, nonetheless they are helpful when used to screen out potential ectasia cases. Attempts have been made to have a pre-operative scoring system that would rule out potential cases of ectasia. Randelman et al. developed an ectasia risk scoring system [27] that correctly identified 46 of 50 cases (92%) as being at high risk for the development of ectasia. In their relatively large series they also showed that abnormal topography was the most significant factor with the highest relative risk that discriminated between ectasia cases and controls. In their studies nearly 50% of ectasia cases had defined topographic abnormalities pre-operatively, in addition to the current categories (Asymmetric Bowtie, Inferior Steep/Skewed Radial Axis, and Abnormal).

In an earlier study by the same author the availability of videokeratography has led to the identification of patients with paracentral corneas that are steeper than normal without clinical evidence of keratoconus. This has been designated as form fruste keratoconus (FFKC). It is compatible with very good spectacle corrected vision and often with low or no significant astigmatism. The long-term safety of LASIK in these patients is unknown, and a number of authors have suggested criteria and automated screening methods for identifying patients with FFKC preoperatively [28-31]. Applying the Rabinowitz/McDonnell criteria for detecting FFKC to the pre-operative topographies of patients included in this study Randelman et al. [32] found that in those patients with available preoperative topographies, 88% of affected eyes met FFKC criteria based on central K, I-S values, or both, compared with only 2% of eyes in the first control group (*P* 0.0000001, relative risk). More than 40% of ectasia cases with available topography results had abnormal preoperative patterns, including keratoconus, pellucid marginal corneal degeneration, and forme fruste keratoconus with an I-S value of more than 1.4 as defined by Rabinowitz [33] and Rabinowitz and McDonnell [34]. A further study by Tabbara [35] also attempted to develop a pre-operative risk score for patients undergoing lasik in an effort to rule out those patients who were at risk of developing ectasia. They measured keratometry, oblique cylinder, pachymetry, differences between superior and inferior corneal powers. Again there numbers were based on retrospective analysis of cases and they acknowledged in their discussion that a prospective study would be required to test the validity of their results.

Eyes with keratoconus are known to produce unpredictable refractive results and scarring after radial keratectomy, photorefractive keratectomy, and LASIK [36, 37, 38]. It is not surprising therefore that there should be absolute contraindications for having LASIK in such patients in a routine laser refractive clinical environment except in conjunction with some combined specialized corneal strengthening such as corneal cross-linking.

Thin Corneas

Relative thinness of the cornea is known to be a risk factor in developing corneal ectasia. It is unclear however what the relationship to thinness is with development of subsequent kerectasia. Does the thinness itself in isolation represent a risk or is it only a risk when taken in conjunction with topographic abnormalities or indeed attempted high corrections in such thin corneas resulting subsequently in lower residual stromal thickness (RST) after laser ? If the flap is thicker than anticipated (and unmeasured per-operatively and therefore unknown at the time of surgery) resulting in a lower RST after ablation then the problem is likely to be the thicker flap and lower RST rather than the thinner cornea per se. Without per-operative measurements however this would be unclear in any analysis of the cause. Is the absolute residual stromal bed the critical number or is it as a proportion of the overall pre-operative pachymetry? These are questions we don't have answers to at present. Given the nature of any prospective study that would be required and the large numbers required to get these answers then we are unlikely to have a definitive resolution to these anytime soon.

In talking in terms of 'thickness' or 'thinness' of the cornea, what exactly do we mean? What constitutes a thin cornea in the first place? Less than 500um? This seems to be the magic number that people use as a cut-off between 'normal' and 'thin' corneas. The average central corneal thickness (CCT) has been found to range from 537 to 550 μm. [39] Although evidence is lacking as to what is truly a safe preoperative CCT, under 500 microns has generally been accepted as a cut-off value for safe refractive surgery by a majority of surgeons. [40] Despite this, there are several publications reporting good results in these corneas, while others reports post-refractive corneal ectasia in patients with preoperative corneal thickness in the "safe" zone greater than this limit. Obviously the method employed to measure CCT may also have a bearing on the 'real' CCT. Contact ultrasonic pachymetry is probably more reliable that some of the older placeido based measuring devices.

Heretofore, refractive surgeons have accepted a minimal residual post-ablation RST of 250 μm in LASIK to reduce the risk of ectasia while recently this has crept up to 300um ; In my own practice for some years I have accepted 300um as the desired RST. Others consider a preoperative central corneal thickness of less than 500 μm to be a contraindication to both LASIK and photorefractive keratectomy (PRK). Where did these numbers come from? Are they clinically valid or just an opinion? They are certainly not derived from a peer-reviewed double-blind prospective clinical trial. Jose Barraquer in one of his many landmark papers on corneal lamellar refractive surgery recommended a RST of 300 μm for myopic keratomileusis [41].

Taken in isolation therefore there is no magic number for CCT to preclude LASIK or PRK surgery been performed all other things being equal. Obviously the CCT pre-operatively is important in deciding whether LASIK or PRK would be the preferred choice. However the ultimate decision depends on the amount of treatment required and the calculated RST. It is difficult to take the pre-op CCT in isolation when deciding who is suitable for laser surgery but rather should be taken in conjunction with the RST. In very thin corneas there is always the fear that this abnormally thin CCT represents one end of the spectrum in an abnormal corneal physiology or anatomy that may go on to develop a corneal thinning condition such as keratoconus. At this stage we have no evidence to support that but the worry remains and as such these patients should probably avoid having refractive laser correction. What this absolute number for CCT is however we don't know.

Residual Stromal Thickness

The article by Kymionis and associates [42] and the study by Binder [43] both suggest that a minimal central corneal thickness and residual stromal bed thickness are not in and of themselves sine qua non risk factors for the development of corneal ectasia [44]. They reviewed a series of their patients who had presumed low RST measurements. These cases of low RST were reconfirmed when some of these eyes underwent enhancement surgery. Recognizing that pachymetry performed immediately after the excimer ablation tends to measure the dehydrated thickness and not the normal, thicker, hydrated thickness, the real RST in these eyes most likely was higher. [45] In none of these eyes, which included 40 with a minimum two months of follow-up (average follow-up, 11.8 months) and 57 with at least one year of follow-up (mean, 28 months) did ectasia develop. Given that patients may not present with ectasia for up to 7 years post-operatively it would be useful to revisit these cases in the future and see if the incidence remains as low. Reinstein and associates also question the placement of strict limits on RST [46]. This is part due to the measurement inaccuracies of inherent in determining RST and the reproducibility of these measurements.

Recent biomechanical studies have reinforced the importance of RST after LASIK. Both stress-strain analysis [47] and cohesive tensile strength analysis [48] indicate that corneal strength is significantly greater in the anterior 40% of the corneal stroma than in the posterior 60%. Further, the corneal flap contributes minimally to the tensile strength of the cornea after LASIK [49]. Thus, LASIK reduces corneal structural integrity both by reducing overall available load bearing tissue and by shifting the load bearing responsibility to the structurally weaker posterior corneal stroma. One of the problems however in determining the importance of RST is the fact that in many cases this is not measured per-operatively. Often the flap is much thicker than anticipated, particularly in the pre-femtosecond flap era and this is only realized when re-treatment and subsequent per-operative measurements are taken [50]. Thankfully with the advent of femtosecond technology and flap creation this now seems to be less of an issue [51].

It is clear, therefore, that RST of 250 microns does not absolutely discriminate between eyes that will develop ectasia and those that will not. Rather, RST seems to be a continuous variable, with the risk of ectasia increasing with decreasing RST. This is not a linear relationship however and some eyes with significantly thinner RST will not necessarily go on to develop ectasia while the converse is also true that RSB thicker than 250 or even 300 can subsequently develop ectasia.

Age

Young patient age has been identified as a significant risk factor for ectasia in eyes without other generally accepted risk factors [27, 52]. This may be partially explained by the fact that corneal tensile strength increases with age [53] thereby imparting some protective function for older corneas. Additionally, some young patients with currently normal topographies may be destined to develop topographic abnormalities and even frank keratoconus or Pellucid Marginal Corneal Degeneration over time whether or not they undergo LASIK. There was a significantly increased odds ratio for age less than 30 in one previous study [21]. One should be cautious in attempting high myopic corrections in the younger patient for the reasons above and also the likelihood of further myopic progression in younger patients with high myopia that may require enhancement at a later stage.

Corneal Asymmetry

This is important both preoperatively and in patients presenting for enhancement. At the initial screening careful attention should be paid to any significant asymmetry between corneas particularly in cases of apparent unilateral keratoconus (as in the accompanying case report) or PMD. Keratoconus may present asymmetrically. At the very least it does indicate a likelihood of abnormality of the corneal stromal which may well go on to develop frank keratoconus whether or not laser is performed. In these cases if any laser refractive procedure is going to be performed it is probably best that it is surface treatment rather than that requiring flap creation. It will leave a significantly greater RST which should adequately support the cornea. A recent study suggests that PRK in cases of suspected keratoconus pre-operatively may not necessarily be associated with either significant progression for the condition or development of ectasia [54]. They had a mean follow-up of only 4.8 years and as my case illustrated ectasia can present significantly later than that. Still this is a very interesting paper.

Patients Presenting for Re-Treatments

It is very important to carefully screen patients presenting for enhancement surgery. The main reasons for enhancement are either primary undercorrection or later progression of the myopia. (having excluded other causes for blurred vision including dry eyes and nuclear scerosis) The latter generally applies to younger higher myopes who subsequently present with progression of myopia and undercorrection. Primary undercorrection is clear enough and the undercorrection is usually obvious from early on in the post-treatment assessments. As soon as the refraction is stable it is reasonable to perform enhancement of these patients, assuming that there is adequate residual stromal bed for treatment and the corneal topography is within normal limits of what is expected after initial treatment. With the latter group is is very important to ensure that there is refractive and topographic stability before attempting enhancement. If there is significant asymmetry between the refractions and or topography between the two eyes be very careful. In my own practice when a patient presents with a secondary or late regression (or progression of the initial treated myopia) then I suggest that the patient waits at least 6 months before having another clinical work-up. If stability is established at that point then I'm generally happy to do an enhancement. The case presented here that returned for assessment more than 7 years after initial lasik for high myopia with kerectasia illustrates the importance of careful screening of such patients prior to any decision been made about further surgery. High myopes presenting with late changes in refraction require a high level of vigilence in ensuring that the change in refraction is not related to late development of kerectasia.

Alternatives to Laser Refractive Surgery

A comprehensive refractive practice requires the ability to offer phakic lens implants as a treatment for high myopes particularly in the younger patients. Personally I do not offer laser refractive surgery as a treatment for myopia greater than a spherical equivalent of -10D, regardless of the corneal pachymetry. beyond this level I go straight to phakic lens implants if the eyes are otherwise suitable. I feel this is particularly important in the younger high myopes (less than 25 years) where there is a chance that the myopia has not completely stabilised and there is a greater likelihood that they will present later with further myopia. If a phakic lens is used as the primary treatment in such patients then it is relatively straight forward to offer laser refractive surgery at a later date on a virgin cornea if that is required.

If in Doubt Then PRK Not LASIK

The advent of mitomycin (MMC) allows us to treat higher myopes with surface laser treatment where there is a doubt about leaving sufficient tissue in the bed should LASIK be performed. MMC reduces the incidence of haze, scarring and regression (55) and is a safer option. Prior to the use of MMC there was a greater risk of poor refractive outcomes and this tended to limit treatments to lower levels of myopia because of the unpredictability of the procedure in the higher myopes. For higher myopes particularly in the younger patients where the RST is going to be borderline (i.e. less than 300um) then I immediately opt for surface treatment with MMC.

The major risk factors for keratectasia after LASIK surgery are a low residual stromal thickness (RST), retreatments, and preexisting abnormal corneal topography [50] and young age.

Treatment of Kerectasia

In an ideal world one would seek to completely reverse the ectasia after diagnosis. Unfortunately this option is currently not available to us. What we can do however is hope to prevent progression, attempt some repair and improve visual outcome either with gas permeable contact lens, spectacles, corneal cross-linking, intacs or finally penetrating keratoplasty (56) or a combination of some or all of these methods. Until relatively recently, treatment options were limited. In addition to rigid contact lenses, insertion of intra-stromal rings might help mechanically stabilize the cornea. [57, 58, 59] Insertion of single-segment Intacs has been reported to be effective in decreasing the corneal steepening and astigmatism and improving BSCVA in patients with keratoconus and to improve progressive myopia and astigmatism (regular and irregular) in eyes with post-LASIK ectasia. [60] In particular, Alio and associates [61] reported outcomes of single and double segments, but there was neither comparison nor matching of the two groups. Single-segment Intacs improved both UCVA and BSCVA by differential flattening of inferior meridian and steepening of superior meridian as reflected by change in I-S ratio [62]. However, prior to the use of corneal support with intacs and corneal crosslinking then many cases were treated by penetrating keratoplasty [63]. Thankfully this is not now the end result for many such cases.

Corneal Cross Linking

Corneal cross-linking (CXL) treatment is a relatively new, revolutionary, minimally invasive procedure aiming at the stabilization of corneal ectatic disorders. It can be particularly useful in cases of post-LASIK ectasia as well as keratoconus. Riboflavin and ultraviolet-A (UVA) crosslinking of corneal collagen increases the bio-mechanical stability of the cornea by inducing additional crosslinks between or within collagen fibers using UVA light and riboflavin as photo-mediators [64].

Its therapeutic potential for the treatment of progressive keratoconus was shown in a clinical phase I study [65]. However because it is relatively new, we don't know the long-terms effects of the treatment, whether the beneficial effects will wear off over time, will it need to be repeated? Over what time frame? Issues of long-term toxicity to endothelium, keratocytes or more worryingly, potentially to limbal stem cells need to be resolved.

When performing the CXL riboflavin solution is continually applied to the eye for 30 minutes (in most studies) and the riboflavin is then activated by illumination with UVA light for 30 minutes, during which time application of the riboflavin solution continues concomitantly. The corneal epithelium is generally removed before application of the riboflavin so that its penetration is increased. Alternative riboflavin formulations and crosslinking techniques that avoid epithelial removal are being evaluated.

How Does the CXL Work?

Experimental studies on rabbit corneas have demonstrated a significant increase in corneal collagen diameter after collagen cross-linking treatment using riboflavin and UVA, resulting in increased biomechanical stability of the cornea [66, 67]. The cross-linking effect is limited to the anterior 300 μm of the corneal stroma with decreasing anterior-posterior pattern attributable to the rapid decrease in UVA irradiance across the corneal stroma. [67] Moreover, the presence of riboflavin prevents UVA from reaching the deeper layers and protects the deep stroma, the endothelium, and the crystalline lens [67, 68]. The treatment is not recommended for corneas of 400um or less due to fears of endothelial toxicity. The treatment creates new chemical bonds (cross-links) between collagen fibrils at the level of the corneal stroma by the combined use of riboflavin and UVA irradiation. This aims to improve the biomechanical stability of the corneal tissue, halting the progression of the ectasia and in some cases reversing some of the changes. The role of riboflavin in corneal CXL is essential. It works as a photosensitizer, creating reactive oxygen species for the induction of cross-links, and simultaneously functions as a protective barrier against the harmful influence of UVA irradiation on the underlying tissues [69].

The cell damage threshold of UVA irradiation combined with riboflavin is 10 times higher than UVA irradiation alone [65] It has been proven in animal experiments and clinical studies [70, 71] that when keratocytes are exposed to UVA irradiation during treatment keratocyte apoptosis occurs. Mazotta et al. in their study [72] conclude that cell death 24 hours after treatment is found at the anterior 300 μm of the corneal stroma. This cell apoptosis follows the Lambert-Beer law, according to which smaller irradiances can lead to shallower cell death. Corneal tissue structural changes post-CXL treatments have been studied by means of corneal confocal microscopy [72, 74].

Confocal images of the cornea reveal keratocyte absence at the anterior 300 μm of the stroma 3 months after CXL treatment. A gradual keratocyte repopulation in the anterior and mid corneal stroma followed, 6 months after the procedure. Regarding the endothelium, no endothelial cell damage was evident after treatment when all preoperative inclusion criteria were met [75].

After CXL, the cornea thins and then recovers toward baseline thickness. The cause and implications of corneal thickness changes after CXL remain to be elucidated in fact the general long-term anatomic and physiologic changes in the cornea after CXL remain to be thoroughly worked out. 3 months seems to be the time of maximum corneal thinning after CXL [76]. In general, corneal thinning between baseline and 3 months was not associated with visual acuity improvement after CXL.

Complications of corneal collagen crosslinking vary by the technique used for the procedure and include delayed epithelial healing, corneal haze (may be visually significant), decreased corneal sensitivity, infectious keratitis, persistent corneal edema, and endothelial cell damage. In some cases, corneal collagen crosslinking has been used successfully in combination with other treatment methods, such as intrastromal corneal ring segments, CK, and excimer laser photoablation.

Riboflavin alone has no crosslinking effect. Its function as a photosensitizer is to serve as a source for the generation of singlet oxygen and superoxide anion free radicals, which are split from its ring structure after excitation by the UV irradiation and which then lead to physical crosslinking of the corneal collagen fibers. In the presence of riboflavin, approximately 95% of the UVA light irradiance is absorbed superficially in the anterior 300 μm of the corneal stroma. Therefore, most studies require a minimal corneal thickness of 400 μm after epithelial removal in order to prevent corneal endothelial damage. It has been suggested that patients who are deemed to have some or all of the risk factors of developing ectasia have CXL as part of their refractive treatment. This is probably extreme and certainly given the relative low incidence of the condition is exposing many such patients unnecessarily to a treatment (CXL) the long-term effects of which are unclear as yet.

Summary

Kerectasia following routine corneal refractive surgery is a potentially devastating visual condition. It is associated with progressive irregular astigmatism, inferior steepening and reduced UAVA and BSCVA. The incidence is generally reported as being about 0.2%. While there is no absolute way to prevent the condition the incidence is probably reducing as we have become more aware of pre-disposing factors such as high myopia, corneal topographic abnormalities, young age, form fruste keratoconus, thin corneas and reduced residual stromal bed thickness. In many cases it is likely multifactorial in origin. It is important to try and recognize the condition early particularly if it presents in a patient returning for enhancement surgery. Treatment has changed dramatically in recent years. In the early days then RGP contact lens followed by corneal transplant in some cases were required. In recent years the treatment of corneal cross-linking either in isolation or combined with corneal INTACS and possible RGP contact lenses have helped greatly in rehabilitating the vision and preventing progression to corneal transplantation. When planning laser refractive surgery if there is a doubt about sufficient RST following LASIK then surface treatment is probably best and in cases of high myopia (sph equiv > -10D) then phakic lens implantation is probably the safest long-term option particularly in the younger patients.

Case Report

A 35 year old female presented in 2000 for myopic LASIK Rx. Corneal maps revealed undiagnosed keratoconus in right eye (Figure 1) and a refraction of -7.0sph/-1.5 cyl @5. The appearance of the map has remained largely unchanged to the present time. The right eye was fitted with a gas permeable contact lens. She underwent LASIK on the fellow left eye. Refraction in this eye was -5.0sph/-2cyl@174. The astigmatism was regular and symmetrical (pre-op color map not available), ultrasound measured central corneal pachymetry 485um and calculated RST of 236um. The patient had a good refractive correction following LASIK. She was seen in 2003 and the accompanying scan (Figure 2) reveal normal topography following surgery. In particular there is no sign of any ectasia at this stage. The patient was lost to follow-up and re-presented in 2007 (7 years post-op) at this time she had noticed some deterioration in the vision of her left eye. There were obvious signs of ectasia developing (Figure 3). She was lost to follow-up and presented again in 2012. The ectasia (Figure 4) had progressed further. She is currently been treated with CXL.

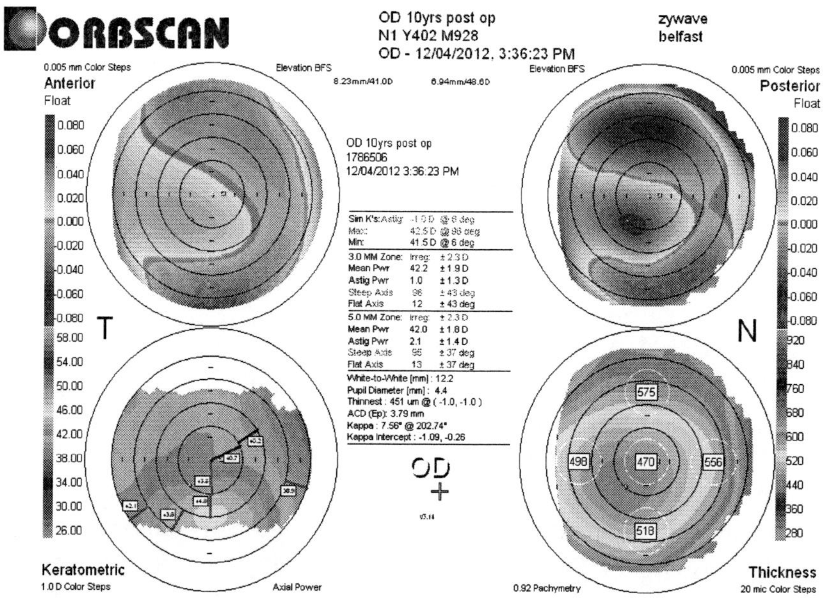

Figure 1. Orbscan of right eye with previously undiagnosed mild keratoconus.

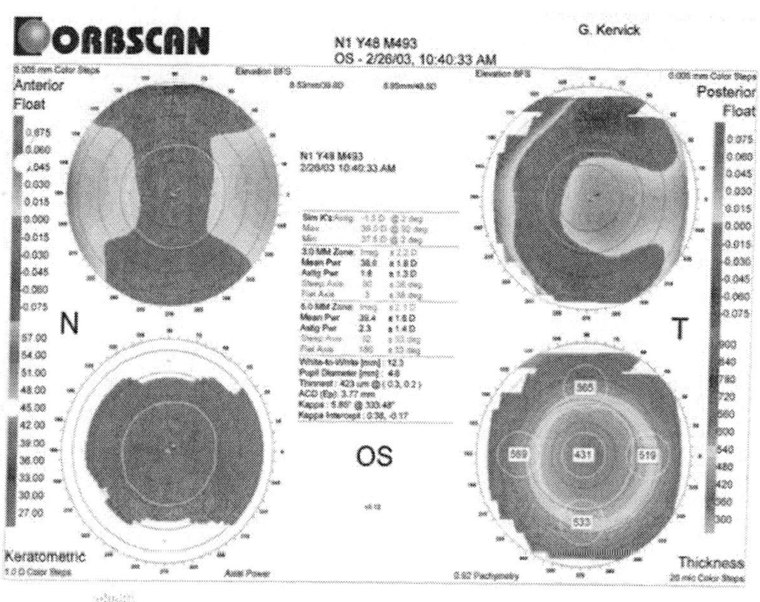

Figure 2. Map of Left eye three years post LASIK showing normal post-operative topography.

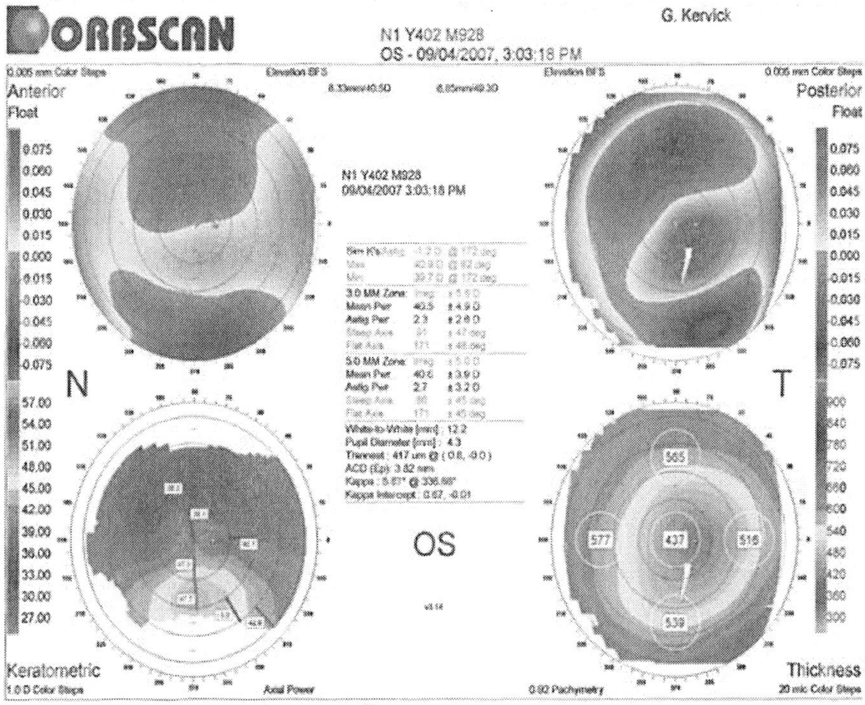

Figure 3. Left eye 7 years post-op with inferior steepening and changes typical of ectasia developing.

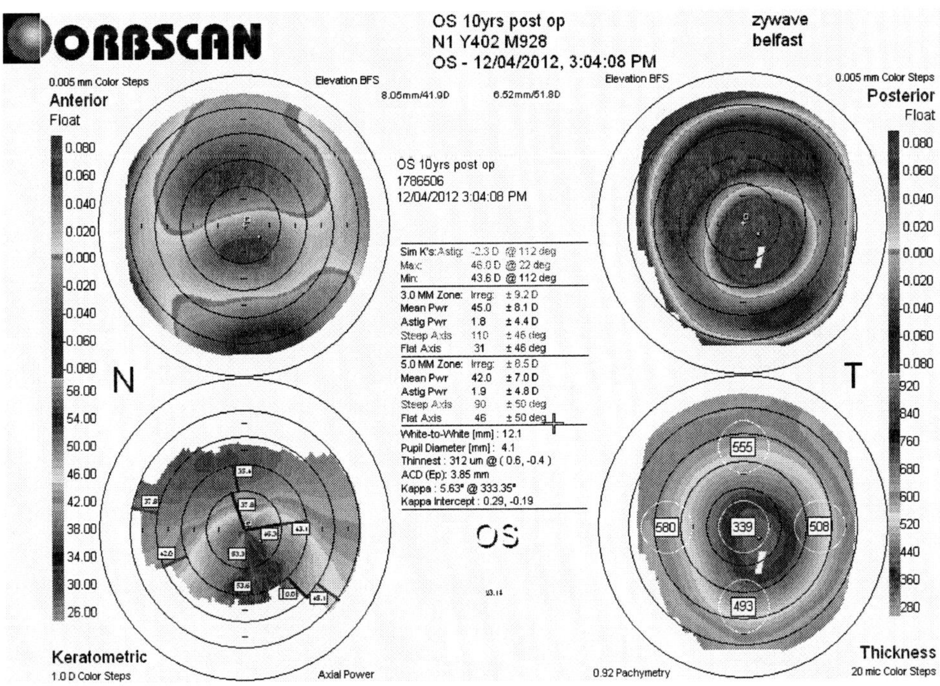

Figure 4. Left eye 12 years post-op with further progression of the etasia. The patient had been lost to follow-up between 2007 and 2012 hence the absence of any treatment offered at initial diagnosis of ectasia.

References

[1] Dupps WJ Jr. Biomechanical modelling of corneal ectasia. *J. Refract. Surg.* 2005;21:186-190.

[2] Amoils SP, Deist MB, Gous P, Amoils PM. Iatrogenic kera-tectasia after laser in situ keratomileusis for less than -4.0 to -7.0 diopters of myopia. *J. Cataract. Refract. Surg* 2000;26: 967–77.

[3] Randleman JB, Caster AI, Banning CS, Stulting RD.Corneal ectasia after photorefractive keratectomy. *J. Cataract. Refract. Surg.* 2006;32:1395–8.

[4] Malecaze F, Coullet J, Calvas P, et al. Corneal ectasia after photorefractive keratectomy for low myopia. *Ophthalmology* 2006;113:742– 6.

[5] Benito_Llopis, Alio, Ortiz, et al. Ten Year follow-up of excimer laser surface ablation for myopia in thin corneas. *AJO* 2009:147;768-773.

[6] Philipp WE, Speicher L, Göttinger W. Histological and immunohistochemical findings after laser in situ keratomileusis in human corneas. *J. Cataract. Refract. Surg.* 2003;29:808–820.

[7] Rad AS , Jabbarvand M , Saifi N . Progressive keratectasia after laser in situ keratomileusis . *J. Refract. Surg . 2004;20(suppl):S718–S722.*

[8] Trokel SL,Srinivasan R, Braren B: Excimer laser surgery of the cornea. *Am. J. Ophthalmology* 1983;96:710-715.

[9] Pallikaris IG, Papatzanaki ME, Stathi EZ, et al: Laser in situ keratomileusis. *Lasers Surg. Med.* 1990;463-468.

[10] Condon PI, O'Keeffe M, Binder P: Long-term results of laser in situ keratommilieusis for high myopia: Risk of ectasia. *J. Cataract. Refract. Surg.* 2007;33:583–590.

[11] Seiler T, Koufala K, Richter G. Iatrogenic keratectasia after laser in situ keratomileusis. *J. Refract. Surg.* 1998;14:312–317.

[12] Seiler T, Quurke AW. Iatrogenic keratectasia after LASIK in a case of forme fruste keratoconus. *J. Cataract. Refract. Surg.* 1998;24:1007–1009.

[13] Geggel HS, Talley AR. Delayed onset keratectasia following laser in situ keratomileusis. *J. Cataract. Refract. Surg.* 1999;25:582–586.

[14] Amoils SP, Deist MB, Gous P, Amoils PM. Iatrogenic keratectasia after laser in situ keratomileusis for less than −4.0 to −7.0 diopters of myopia. *J. Cataract. Refract. Surg.* 2000;26:967–97.

[15] Holland SP, Srivannaboon S, Reinstein DZ. Avoiding serious corneal complications of laser assisted in situ keratomileusis and photorefractive keratectomy. *Ophthalmology.* 2000;107:640–652.

[16] Joo CK, Kim TG. Corneal ectasia detected after laser in situ keratomileusis for correction of less than −12 diopters of myopia. *J. Cataract. Refract. Surg.* 2000;26:292–295.

[17] McLeod SD, Kisla TA, Caro NC, McMahon TT. Iatrogenic keratoconus: corneal ectasia following laser in situ keratomileusis for myopia. *Arch. Ophthalmol.* 2000;118:282–284.

[18] Chung SH, IM CY, Lee ES, et al. Clinical manifestation and pathologic finding of unilateral acute hydrops after bilateral laser in situ keratomileusis. *J. Cataract. Refract. Surg.* 2005;31:1244–1248.

[19] Rodrigues MM, Newsome DA, Krachmer JH, Eiferman RA. Pellucid marginal corneal degeneration: a clinicopathologic study of two cases. *Exp. Eye Res.* 1981; 33:277–288.

[20] Meek KM, Tuft SJ, Huang Y, et al. Changes in collagen orientation and distribution in keratoconus corneas. *Invest Ophthalmol. Vis. Sci.* 2005; 46:1948–1956.

[21] Randleman JB, Trattler WB, Stulting RD. Validation of the Ectasia Risk Score System for Preoperative Laser In Situ Keratomileusis Screening. *Am. J. Ophthalmol.* 2008;145:813-818.

[22] Schwiegerling J, Greivenkamp JE. Keratoconus detection based on videokeratoscopic height data. *Optom. Vis. Sci.* 1996; 73:721–728.

[23] Rabinowitz YS. Videokeratographic indices to aid in screening for keratoconus. *J. Refract. Surg.* 1995; 11:371–379.

[24] Rao SN, Raviv T, Majmudar PA, Epstein RJ. Role of Orbscan II in screening keratoconus suspects before refractive corneal surgery. *Ophthalmology* 2002; 109:1642–6.

[25] Rabinowitz YS, McDonnell PJ. Computer-assisted corneal topography in keratoconus. *Refract Corneal Surg* 1989;5:400–8.

[26] Klyce SD, Endl MJ. Corneal topography in modern refractive surgery. *Int. Ophthalmol. Clin* 2002;42(4):19 –30.

[27] Randleman JB, Woodward M, Lynn MJ, Stulting RD. Risk assessment for ectasia after corneal refractive surgery. *Ophthalmology*. 2008;115:37–50.

[28] Rabinowitz YS, Rasheed K. KISA% index: a quantitative videokeratography algorithm embodying minimal topographic criteria for diagnosing keratoconus [published erratum appears in J. Cataract. Refract. Surg 2000;26:480]. *J. Cataract. Refract. Surg* 1999;25:1327–35.

[29] Maeda N, Klyce SD, Smolek MK, Thompson HW. Automated keratoconus screening with corneal topography analysis. *Invest Ophthalmol. Vis. Sci.* 1994;35:2749–57.

[30] Maeda N, Klyce SD, Smolek MK. Comparison of methods for detecting keratoconus using videokeratography. *Arch. Ophthalmol.* 1995;113:870–4.

[31] Wilson SE, Klyce SD. Screening for topographic abnormalities before refractive surgery. *Ophthalmology* 1994;101:147– 52.

[32] Randleman, Russel, Ward et al. Risk factors and prognosis for corneal ectasia after lasik. *Ophthalmology* 2003;110:267-275.

[33] Rabinowitz YS. Videokeratographic indices to aid in screening for keratoconus. *J. Refract. Surg.* 1995;11:371–379.

[34] Rabinowitz YS, McDonnell PJ. Computer-assisted corneal topography in keratoconus. *Refract Corneal Surg.* 1989;5:400–408.

[35] Tabbara KF, Kotb AA. Risk factors for corneal ectasia after LASIK. *Ophthalmology.* 2006;113:1618–1622.

[36] Mamalis N, Montgomery S, Anderson C, Miller C. Radial keratotomy in a patient with keratoconus. *Refract Corneal Surg.* 1991;7:374 – 6.

[37] Ellis W. Radial keratotomy in a patient with keratoconus. *J. Cataract. Refract. Surg* 1992;18:406–9.

[38] Buzard KA, Tuengler A, Febbraro JL. Treatment of mild to moderate keratoconus with laser in situ keratomileusis. *J. Cataract. Refract. Surg* 1999;25:1600–1609.

[39] (Harper CL, Boulton ME, Bennett D, et al. Diurnal variations in human corneal thickness. *Br. J. Ophthalmol.* 1996;80:1068–1072).

[40] Kohnen T. Iatrogenic keratectasia: Current knowledge, current measurements. *J. Cataract. Refract. Surg*. 2002;28:2065–2066.

[41] Barraquer JI. In: Queratomileusis y queratofaquia. Bogota, Columbia: Litografia Arco; 1980;p. 340–342405–406).

[42] Kymionis GD, Bouzoukis D, Diakonis V, et al. Long-term results of thin corneas after refractive laser surgery. *Am. J. Ophthalmol*. 2007;144:181–185.

[43] Binder PS, Analysis of ectasia after laser in situ keratomileusis: risk factors, *J. Cataract. Refract. Surg* 2007;331530-38.

[44] Salz JJ, Binder PS, Is there a "Magic Number" to reduce the risk of ectasia after Laser In Situ Keratomileusis and Photorefractive Keratectomy? *American J. Ophthalmol*. 2007;144:284-285.

[45] Flanagan GW, Binder PS. The theoretical vs. measured laser resection for laser in situ keratomileusis. *J. Refract. Surg*. 2005;21:18–27.

[46] Reinstein D, Srivannaboon S, Archer T, Silverman R, Sutton H, Coleman D. Probability model of the inaccuracy of residual stromal thickness prediction to reduce the risk of ectasia after LASIK (Part II: quantifying population risk). *J. Refract. Surg*. 2006;22:861–870).

[47] Kohlhaas M, Spoerl E, Schilde T, Unger G, Wittig C, Pillunat LE. Biomechanical evidence of the distribution of cross-links in corneas treated with riboflavin and ultraviolet A light. *J. Cataract. Refract. Surg*. 2006;32:279–283.

[48] Randleman JB, Dawson DG, Grossniklaus HE, McCarey BE, Edelhauser HF. Analysis of quantitative cohesive tensile strength In normal human corneas: implications for refractive surgery. *J. Refract. Surg*. 2008;24:S85–S89.

[49] Seiler T, Koufala K, Richter G. Iatrogenic keratectasia after laser in situ keratomileusis. *J. Refract. Surg*. 1998;14:312–3173.

[50] Condon PI, Will keratectasia be a major complication for lasik in the long-term? *J. Cataract. Refract. Surg*. 2006;12:2124-2132

[51] Randleman JB, Hebson CB, Larson PM. Flap Thickness in eyes with ectasia after Laser in situ Keratomileusis. *J. Cataract. Refract. Surg*. 2012 May;38(5):752-7.

[52] Change in intraocular pressure measurements after LASIK the effect of the refractive correction and the lamellar flap. *Ophthalmology*. 2005;112:1009–1016.

[53] Klein SR, Epstein RJ, Randleman JB, Stulting RD. Corneal ectasia after laser in situ keratomileusis in patients without apparent preoperative risk factors. *Cornea*. 2006;25:388–403).

[54] Randleman JB, Dawson DG, Grossniklaus HE, McCarey BE, Edelhauser HF. Analysis of quantitative cohesive tensile strength in normal human corneas: implications for refractive surgery. *J. Refract. Surg*. 2008;24:S85–S89).

[55] PRK in patients with suspected keratoconus Mikael Guedj, Alain Saad, Etienne Audureau, Damien Gatinel. *J. Cataract. Refract. Surg*. 2013;39(1):66-73.

[56] Miguel A. Teus, Laura de Benito-Llopis, Jorge L. Alió Survey Ophthalm 2009;54(4)487-502 Mitomycin C in Corneal Refractive Surgery.

[57] Binder PS. Ectasia after laser in situ keratomileusis. *J. Cataract. Refract. Surg*. 2003; 29:2419–2429.

[58] Woodward MA, Randleman JB, Russell B et al. Visual rehabilitation and outcomes for ectasia after corneal refractive surgery. *J. Cataract. Refract. Surg*. 2008;34:383–388.

[59] Kymionis GD, Siganos CS, Kounis G, et al. Management of post-LASIK corneal ectasia with Intacs inserts; one-year results. *Arch. Ophthalmol.* 2003; 121:322–326.

[60] Lovisolo CF, Fleming JF. Intracorneal ring segments for iatro- genic keratectasia after laser in situ keratomileusis or photore- fractive keratectomy. *J. Refract. Surg* 2002; 18:535–541.

[61] Siganos CS, Kymionis GD, Astyrakakis N, Pallikaris IG. Management of corneal ectasia after laser in situ keratomileusis with INTACS. *J. Refract. Surg* 2002; 18:43–46.

[62] Pokroy R, Levinger S, Hirsh A. Single Intacs segment for post-laser in situ keratomileusis keratectasia . *J. Cataract. Refract. Surg.* 2004;30:1685–1695).

[63] Alio JL, Artola A, Hassanein A, et al. One or 2 Intacs segments for the correction of keratoconus . *J. Cataract. Refract. Surg.* 2005;31:943–953.

[64] M Boxer, Wachler BS. Comparison of single single segment and double segment intacs for keratoconus and post-LASIK ectasia. *Am. J. Ophthalmology.* 2006;141(5):891-895.

[65] Seitz B, Rozsival P, Feuermannova A, et al. Penetrating keratoplasty for iatrogenic keratoconus after repeat myopic laser in situ keratomileusis: histological findings and literature review. *J. Cataract. Refract. Surg* 2003; 29:2217–2224.

[66] Spoerl E, Seiler T. Techniques for stiffening the cornea. *J. Refract. Surg* 1999; 15:711–7139.

[67] Wollensak G, Spoerl E, Seiler T. Riboflavin/ultraviolet- A-induced collagen crosslinking for the treatment of keratoconus. *Am. J. Ophthalmol.* 2003; 135:620–627.

[68] Wollensak G, Iomdina E, Dittert D, Herbst H. Wound healing in the rabbit cornea after corneal collagen cross-linking with riboflavin and UVA. *Cornea.* 2007;26:600–605.

[69] Wollensak G, Wilsch M, Spoerl E, Seiler T. Collagen fiber diameter in the rabbit cornea after collagen cross-linking by riboflavin/UVA. *Cornea.* 2004;23:503–507.

[70] Wollensak G. Crosslinking treatment of progressive keratoconus: new hope. *Curr. Opin Ophthalmol.* 2006;17:356–360.

[71] Wollensak G, Spörl E, Reber F, Pillunat L, Funk R. Corneal endothelial cytotoxicity of riboflavin/UVA treatment in vitro. *Ophthalmic Res.* 2003;35(6):324–328.

[72] Caporossi A, Baiocchi S, Mazzotta C, Traversi C, Caporossi T. Parasurgical therapy for keratoconus by riboflavin-ultraviolet type A rays induced cross-linking of corneal collagen: preliminary refractive results in an Italian study. *J. Cataract. Refract. Surg.* 2006;32(5):837–845.

[73] Mazzotta C, Traversi C, Baiocchi S, et al. Conservative treatment of keratoconus by riboflavin-uva-induced cross-linking of corneal collagen: qualitative investigation . *Eur. J. Ophthalmol.* 2006;16(4):530–535).

[74] Mazzotta C, Balestrazzi A, Traversi C, et al. Treatment of progressive keratoconus by riboflavin-UVA–induced cross-linking of corneal collagen (Ultra-structural analysis by Heidelberg retinal tomograph II in vivo confocal microscopy in humans). *Cornea.* 2007;26:390–397.

[75] Mazzotta C, Balestrazzi A, Traversi C, et al. Treatment of progressive keratoconus by riboflavin-UVA–induced cross-linking of corneal collagen (Ultra-structural analysis by Heidelberg retinal tomograph II in vivo confocal microscopy in humans). *Cornea.* 2007;26:390–397.

[76] Kymionis GD, Diakonis VF, Kalyvianaki M, et al. One-year follow-up of corneal confocal microscopy after corneal cros-linking in patients with post laser in situ keratomileusis ectasia and keratoconus . *Am. J. Ophthalmol..* 2009;147(5):774–778).

[77] Vinciguerra P, Albè E, Trazza S, et al. Refractive, topographic, tomographic, and aberrometric analysis of keratoconic eyes undergoing corneal cross-linking . *Ophthalmology*. 2009;116(3):369–378).

[78] Greenstein SA, Shah VP, Fry KL, Hersh PS. Corneal thickness changes after corneal collagen crosslinking for keratoconus and corneal ectasia: one-year results. *J. Cataract. Refract. Surg.* 2011;37(4):691–700)..

In: Current Understanding and New Techniques ...
Editor: Michael O'Keefe
ISBN: 978-1-62808-748-2

Chapter 5

Refractive Surgery in Patients with Strabismus

Gillian O'Mullane[1,*] and Caitriona Kirwan[2,≠]
[1]Children's University Hospital, Dublin, Ireland
[2]Mater Private Hospital, Dublin, Ireland

Abstract

This chapter discusses the potential advantages and risks associated with refractive surgery in patients with/or a history of strabismus. A change in refractive error or an imperfect refractive outcome may result in decompensation of strabismus and diplopia. We outline the investigations which should be carried out pre-operatively to identify those who may be at risk of complications.

Introduction

For many years, refractive surgery was contraindicated in patients with strabismus. The risk of decompensation of strabismus and the development of diplopia were feared complications. The publication of successful outcomes of refractive surgery in this patient population however has prompted closer examination and the subsequent treatment of many such patients. The aim of refractive surgery is to eliminate the need for glasses while maintaining the patient's binocular status. However, refractive surgery may induce temporary blur which can challenge binocular fusion. Tests which target binocular status and determine a patients ability to tolerate binocular stress can help stratify their risk level for future postoperative problems. Patients at most risk of long term complications are those with binocular vision defects such as intermittent strabismus, microtropia, poorly compensated heterophoria and incomitancy.

* Gillian.omullane@cuh.ie
≠ caitrionakirwan@eircom.net

A comprehensive investigation of binocular function should determine: (a) the presence or absence of sensory fusion, (b) the range of motor fusion and how well it is sustained under refractive stress and (c) the size and depth of any suppression scotoma.

The clinician needs to make an informed prediction as to how refractive surgery will impact on strabismus both from a functional and cosmetic standpoint. The relationship between accommodation and convergence is vital to the understanding of esotropia and exotropia. Individual variations in the accommodative convergence to accommodation ratio (AC/A) means that a customisable approach is necessary to avoid negative outcomes.

There have been several reports of improved or recovered fusion follow refractive surgery [1-7]. Ocular alignment and binocular function remained unchanged or improved in a mixed cohort of 13 esotropes and exotropes following refractive surgery [2]. Hoyos et al. reported on LASIK treatment in nine patients with refractive accommodative esotropia [5]. All patients were postoperatively orthophoric or remained micro-esotropic. Stidham et al. noted a change in the eso-deviation in only 42% of 24 hyperopic patients (mean refractive error pre-op +7.25D; post-op +2.25D) [4]. Ten patients had a fully accommodative esotropia, of whom two became orthophoric postoperatively. Four patients had their esotropia converted to an esophoria and four patients showed no improvement at all. Nemet et al. had a successful outcome in six out of six patients, three fully accommodative and three partially accommodative [6]. Sabetti et al. found PRK and LASIK equally successful in 18 fully accommodative esotrope, all of whom had esophoria or orthophoria post treatment [7]. Attainment of orthophoria was also reported by Nucci et al., in all patients after PRK for mild to moderate hypermetropia with fully accommodative esotropia [8].

Kushner and Kowal published a review of 28 patients that had been referred to their clinic with persistent diplopia following refractive surgery [9]. In two cases the diplopia was purely monocular, in the remaining 26 it was binocular. One patient had an induced prism, one had induced torsion and two had induced aniseikonia. In 17 patients refractive control of an intermittent heterotropia was disrupted; four of these had an unintentional undercorrection, three an unintended overcorrection and in 10 patients the pre-operative assessment failed to detect refractive or prismatic management of a squint. In seven patients post-operative monovision disrupted the asymptomatic status; in three of these monovision disrupted the compensation of a heterophoria, in three with comitant heterotropia it broke down suppression and in the remaining patient, who had a superior oblique palsy, there was an increase in the angle of deviation due to enforced fixation with the paretic eye.

Patient Assessment

History

All patients should be questioned about their past ocular history with particular attention paid to previous amblyopia therapy or strabismus surgery. Patients should also be asked if they have ever experienced diplopia with or without their glasses or in any particular direction of gaze.

Refraction

The patient's current prescription should be checked for any near addition or prisms. Under or over-corrected refractive error in amblyopes and anisometropes needs careful consideration and the binocular impact of full correction should be established.

Age

Traditionally a minimum age of 18 or preferably 21 has been recommended for refractive surgery. Younger patients are less likely to have a stable refractive error and a greater degree of latent hyperopia may be present. Latent hyperopia of more than 2 dioptres is considered by many to be a contra-indication for refractive surgery as in time this latent component will become manifest, resulting in reduced acuity and a return of strabismus in accommodative esotropes. The younger patient is also more susceptible to refractive regression. Philips et al. reported that 47% of adolescent hyperopes required enhancement [10]. Children may also be more susceptible to corneal haze and regression [11].

Visual Acuity

Where amblyopia is present, further investigation is required to determine the etiology. In the absense of deprivation amblyopia or anisometropia, strabismus is likely to be the cause. It is also imperative that amblyopic patients do not have unrealistic expectations of visual outcome following refractive surgery.

Cover Test

An accurate cover test is the foundation of strabismus evaluation. It should be carried out with and without refractive correction with an accommodative near target at 33cm and a 6m Snellen target. The cover/uncover test exposes any manifest deviation. Thorough attention should be paid for small microtropic deviations which may infer a vulnerability to post-op difficulties. The magnitude of deviation, the time it takes for the deviating eye to take up fixation, and alternation of fixation should be observed.

An alternate cover test examination will reveal any latent deviation and should be sustained long enough to elicit the maximum deviation as fusional input is dissociated. The speed of recovery is particularly relevant as an indication of the patient's ability to restore fusion. In the case of hyperopia, it is important to ensure that the patient is accurately accommodating on the fixation target as the fully accommodative esotrope may have learnt to avoid accommodation without their glasses.

The presence of a vertical phoria increases the patient's probability of a decompensating strabismus. Their level of risk may be estimated by examining their vertical fusion range.

Ocular Movements

Ocular motility should be checked in the nine positions of gaze and any diplopia reported. Where there is incomitance it should be noted whether the patient prefers to fix with the paretic or non-paretic eye. An abnormal head posture might give a clue to an underlying paresis or torsion. Similarly a chin up or chin down head posture may be adopted to control and 'A' or 'V' pattern deviation.

Accommodation and Convergence

It is inadvisable to assume that normal accommodation levels exist in the pre-presbyopic patient regardless of whether they report symptoms of asthenopia. A myopic patient may routinely remove their glasses for near work masking a deficiency in accommodation. Other indicators of potential accommodation difficulties are history of trauma and certain drugs such as antidepressants and antihypertensives.

The near point of accommodation is easily measured using an RAF rule. It should be recorded monocularly and binocularly using the smallest size print the patient can read with their glasses on.

The near point of convergence is recorded as the nearest point the patient can binocularly fuse a target. Regardless of age, normal patients should have a near point of convergence of 8cm or less.

Binocular Function Assessment

Worth [12] classified three grades of binocular single vision:

- Simultaneous perception
- Fusion
- Stereopsis

Simultaneous Perception

The ability to simultaneously perceive an image from each eye is essential for fusion. In the case of diplopia, simultaneous perception occurs even though the images cannot be fused. If the factors causing diplopia can be resolved then fusion may be restored. The strabismus can be neutralised with a prism or synoptophore (figure 1) and fusional potential can be explored.

One of the simplest ways to assess simultaneous perception and sensory fusion is with Bagolini Striated lenses (figure 2). Bagolini striated lenses convert a point of light into a streak of light at the 45° meridian to one eye and the 135° meridian to the other eye. In normal bifoveal fusion the patient appreciates the two streaks as a cross or 'X' with the point of light at the centre. The patient with central suppression may appreciate an 'X' with a gap in the centre of the streak seen by the non-fixating eye (in practise this is rarely reported). The patient with a large suppression scotoma will only see one streak of light. If the patient is aware of diplopia then it is sometimes useful to combine a prism bar with Bagolini glasses to help the patient recognize when diplopia resolves and fusion occurs.

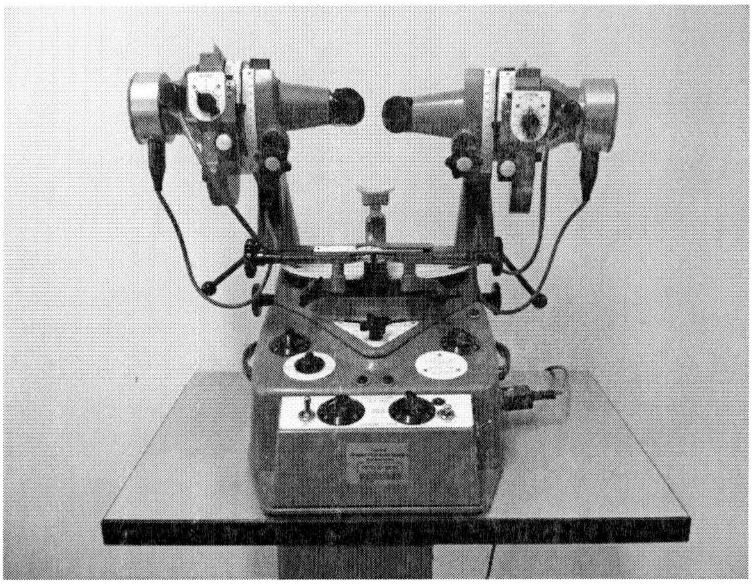

Figure 1. Synoptophore.

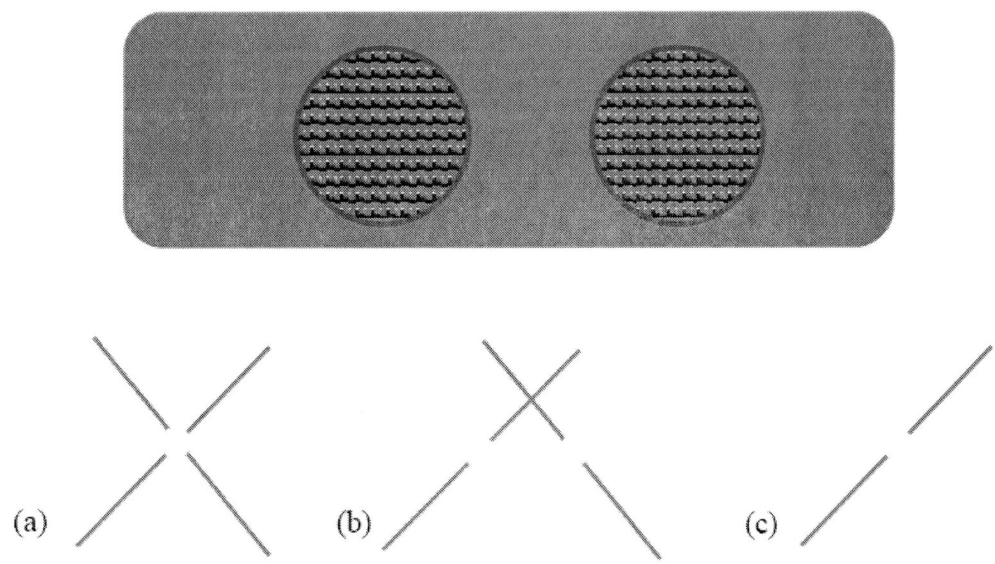

Figure 2. Bagolini lenses - circular lenses with fine striations. The lenses are placed in a trial frame at 45^0 in front of one eye and 135^0 in front of the other. A point light source is observed. The streak of light observed is at 90^0 to the striations. (a) orthotropia and normal retinal correspondance or strabismus and anomalous retinal correspondance, (b) diplopic response (c) left suppression.

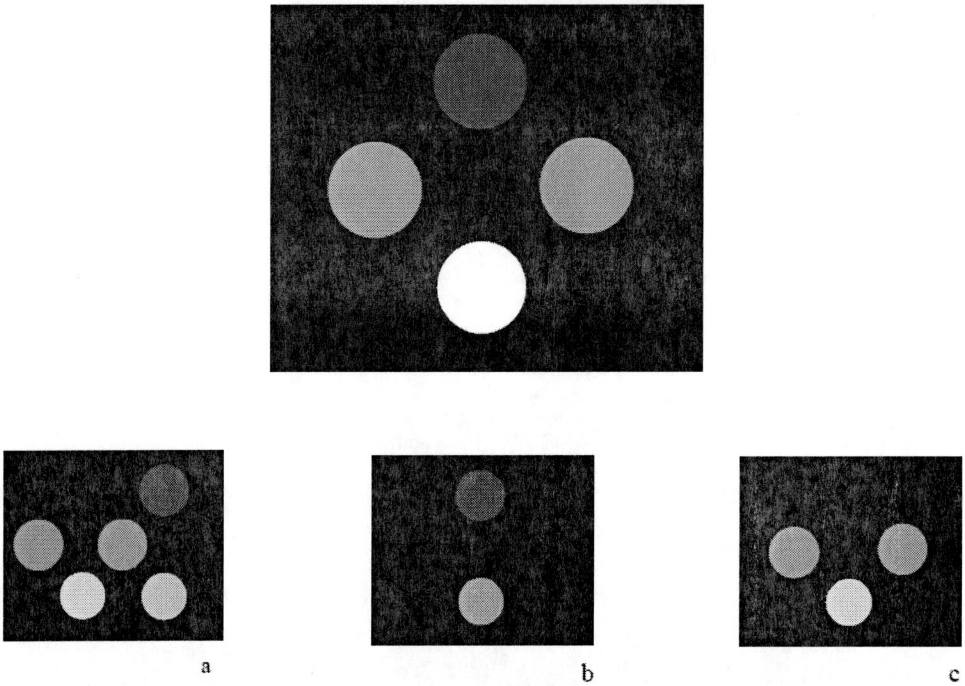

Figure 3. Worth's 4 lights. Top image shows a binocular response where 2 green and one red image are seen and the lower white light is fused as a single image (often appearing slightly red or green depending on eye dominance) a) demonstrates a diplopic response b) left suppression response (red filter in front of right eye) c) right suppression response (green filter in front of left eye).

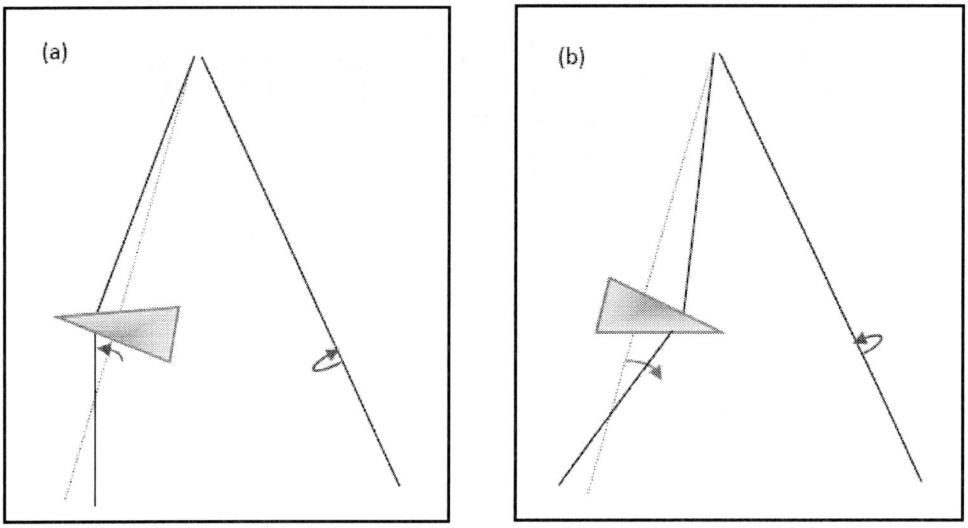

Figure 4. Motor Fusion Testing – normal response (a) Placement of a base-in prism in front of the left eye requires this eye to abduct to maintain foveal fixation. The right eye initially adducts due to Hering's law of equal innervation and then abducts to restore fusion of a single image. The prism is increased until the patient can no longer maintain a single fusional response and diplopia is reported. (b) Placement of a base-out prism in front of the left eye requires this eye to adduct to maintain foveal fixation. The right eye will initially abduct and then adduct to restore a single fusional response. The prism is increased until diplopia is reported and then decreased until recovery of fusion occurs.

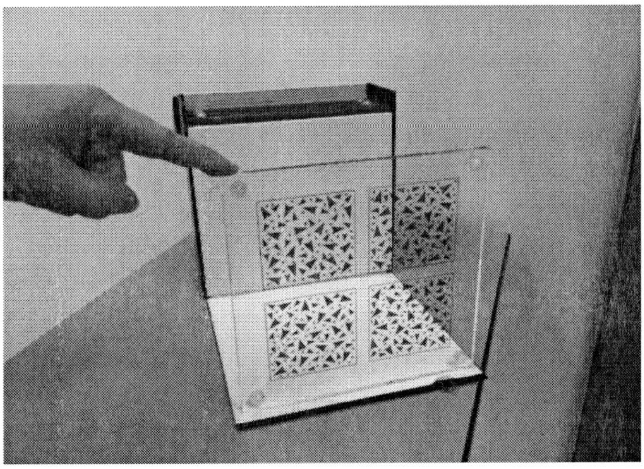

Figure 5. Frisby stereotest.

Another popular technique is the Worth's 4 lights test which comprises of one red, two green and one white light (figure 3). The patient, wears anaglyphic glasses (the red lens over one eye and the green lens over the fellow eye and is shown the four lights. With both eyes open, a patient with normal binocular vision will appreciate all four lights (the white light often seen as flickering between red and green is fused as one light). If the patient either closes or suppresses an eye they will see either two or three lights. If the patient has diplopia and cannot fuse the images of the two eyes, they will see five lights.

Motor Fusion

Motor fusion is the ability to maintain a single fused image during vergence movements. Horizontal vergence movements occur to maintain fusion when base-in and base-out prisms are introduced (figure 4). It may be recorded using a near target and/or a 6m target such as a Snellen chart. The prism strength is increased until the images can no longer be fused and diplopia occurs (break point), the prism is then reduced until binocular single vision is restored (recovery point). Positive fusional amplitude is assessed using base-out prisms and the negative amplitude with base-in prisms. The total prism, both positive and negative that can be overcome are recorded as the horizontal motor fusion amplitude. It is important to examine the base-in or negative amplitude first as otherwise it may be underestimated due to increase tonus of the convergence system [13]. Patients were reported to have a good fusion range if (a) they reached normal limits, 35Δ base-out for convergence and 14Δ base-in for divergence or (b) they satisfied Sheard's criteria by having an opposing fusional range of double their heterophoria i.e. a patient with a 10ΔBI exophoria has at least 20Δ of base-out fusion [14].

Stereopsis

Stereopsis is defined as the perception of relative depth of objects due to binocular disparity. Stereoacuity is a measure of the minimum binocular disparity required for the perception of depth. Of the commercially available tests for measuring stereoacuity those that give the least monocular clues are the most useful. These include the random-dot stereotests such as the TNO test which uses red and green anaglyph glasses to view a random dot stereogram with disparities ranging from 1980 to 15 seconds of arc. Similarly the Randot test uses Polaroid lenses to view a random dot stereogram with disparities of 500 to 20 seconds of arc. The Frisby test comprises of three transparent plastic plates of different thickness (figure 5). Four squares of randomly arranged arrowheads and dots are printed on each plate; 3 on one side and one (the target) on the other. The thickness of each plate provides disparity. The advantage of the Frisby stereotest is that it does not require the use of lenses which may have a dissociative effect on the patient. Disparities of 600 to 15 seconds of arc or less can be recorded by increasing the distance between the patient and the test plate.

Reduced steroacuity (poorer than 100 seconds of arc) may be indicative of a microtropia and abnormal retinal correspondence and requires further investigation. Particular care should be taken in these patients to ensure that they do not switch fixation post-surgery as diplopia may occur [15].

Opinion is divided as to the functional significance of stereopsis. Patients with a longstanding absence of stereopsis can perform many tasks equally well as those with stereopsis. However, sudden loss of stereopsis can adversely affect performance and lead to patient dissatisfaction [16]. Permanent loss of stereopsis has been demonstrated after correction of anisometropia and surgically induced monovision [17]. The loss of stereopsis is often disturbing, even when visual acuity outcome is excellent. Fawcett et al. found that laser in situ keratomileusis (LASIK) or photorefractive keratectomy (PRK) induced monovision had a significant effect on Random dot stereoacuity [17]. They reported stereoacuity values of 40 sec of arc for age-matched control subjects, 100 sec of arc for patients who underwent PRK or LASIK with less than 1.50 spherical D of anisometropia, and 150 sec of arc for patients who had surgically induced anisometropia of 1.50D or greater. Of 48 patients who had planned monovision, 11 complained of symptoms of abnormal binocular vision. Successful monovision was associated with a good visual outcome and reduction of stereopsis by less than 50 seconds of arc. Garcia-Gonzalez et al. reported a reduction in stereopsis with TNO test in patients with monovision [18]. However only 6 of 37 (16.2%) patients reported using glasses for near 'high demanding' tasks because they perceived a slight subjective reduction in near stereoacuity.

Suppression

Suppression refers to the cortical inhibition of perception of objects in all or part of the visual field of one eye during binocular visionvision [19]. The extent of a suppression scotoma can be measured by increasing a prism in front the deviating eye until diplopia is recognised. This should be performed in both base-in and base-out positions as well as in the vertical meridian. The suppression area should be large enough that it can encompass small changes in the angle of deviation that may occur as a result of refractive surgery. The angle of deviation may improve post-treatment [1, 2] or deteriorate [20]. The depth of suppression can be measured with a Sbisa bar (Bagolini filter bar) which is a series of red filters (numbered 1 to 17) of increasing darkness (figure 6). The lightest filter is placed in front of the fixing eye while the patient regards a near spotlight. The light gradually appears darker red as the filters are increased and this continues until diplopia is appreciated.

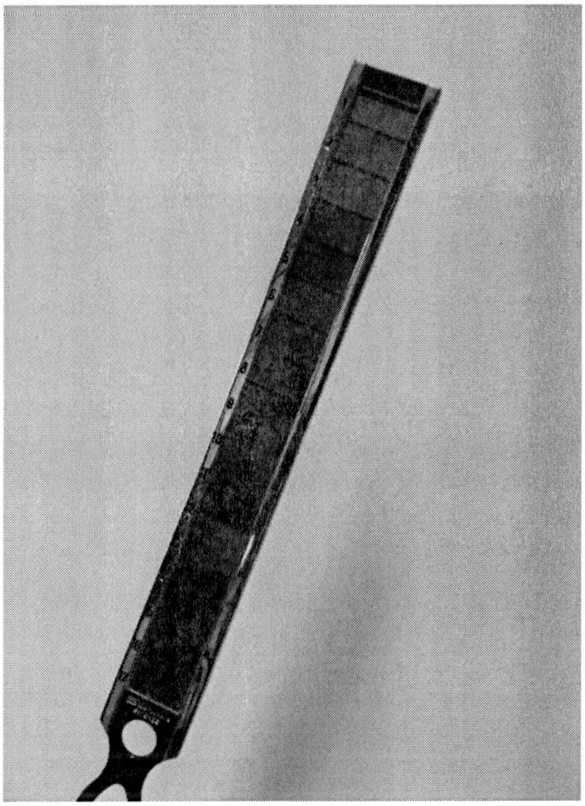

Figure 6. Sbisa bar – series of red filters of increasing density. Used to measure depth of suppression.

The filter prior to this is recorded as the density of suppression. If the spotlight is seen to change from red to white without diplopia then fixation has switched and the eye behind the filter is now suppressed. It is not clear how predictive the Sbisa bar is as a tool for assessing risk of anti-suppression [21] but logic dictates that where only a light filter (<5) is required to induce diplopia then that patient is at higher risk of anti-suppression and intractable diplopia.

4Δ Prism Test for Central Suppression

A foveal suppression scotoma is confirmed with a 4Δ prism test. The test is best performed with a small detailed target which will not subtend an image larger than the central fovea area. When the prism is placed in front of the deviating eye no re-fixation movement will be seen as the image is inside the suppression scotoma; when the prism is placed in front of the other eye a small movement will be seen. The test should be repeated base in and base out.

Refraction Stress Test

Although refractive outcomes and predictability have improved considerably in recent years, attainment of absolute emmetropia cannot be guaranteed. Excellent initial outcomes can over time be tempered by regression, myopic progression or conversion of latent to manifest hyperopia. It is important to try to predict how well a patient will cope with an imperfect or changeable refractive result. A refraction stress test is proposed where lenses of +1.00D and -1.00D are placed over the patients glasses and the prism cover test is repeated (a refractive outcome of greater than ±1.00D is likely to result in retreatment). The likelihood of any significant change in the angle of deviation and loss of binocular status is investigated. An eso tendency will be produced by an unexpected hyperopic shift and an exo tendency by an unexpected myopic shift. In patients who have a high accommodative convergence to accommodation ratio (AC/A) there can be a higher than expected change in alignment. If decompensation of strabismus, or change in binocular status are noted then this is highlighted as a risk, and in some cases, refractive surgery may be contraindicated. The stress test does not predict the outcome where there is an unexpected astigmatic or anisometropic result. The test may be adapted where there is an increased risk of residual or incorrect refractive outcome, particularly with high refractive errors.

Ocular Dominance

Ocular Dominance can be determined by using the 'Hole' test. The patient is requested to look at a target through a circular ring positioned so that both eyes are used simultaneously. Covering each eye in turn results in loss of alignment when the dominant eye is covered.

Ocular dominance can also be determined by the "finger pointing" test, whereby the patient, using binocular vision, points to an object using the index finger of his or her dominant hand. The eye in alignment with the object and the finger is considered to be the dominant eye.

Hyperopia

Typically hyperopic patients are more at risk of strabismus than myopes and may fall into one of the following categories:

- Fully accommodative esotropia: defined as orthophoria or esophoria at near and distance with hyperopic correction, esotropia without hyperopic correction
  - A common sub-group of fully accommodative esotropes are those who are 'controlled to a microtropia' with their hyperopic correction.
- Convergence excess esotropia: where an excessive amount of convergence is exerted in relation to accommodation. The patient will have an esotropia on accommodation and be straight for distance.
- Partially accommodative esotropia: the angle of the esotropia is reduced with hyperopic correction but there is no binocular function and suppression is present.
- Non accommodative esotropia: refractive status is not the primary aetiology of the strabismus.

- Residual esotropia or consecutive exotropia: a patient who has had previous strabismus surgery.

Fully accommodative esotropes are a group particularly suited to refractive surgery with the potential to correct both the refractive error and the strabismus simultaneously. However as with all hyperopes, treatment of the appropriate refractive error is of paramount importance to ensure the best outcome in the long term. Full correction of the manifest hyperopia, the maximum plus that permits threshold visual acuity, should be performed. If there is a discrepancy between the manifest hyperopia and cycloplegic refraction then the difference is termed latent hyperopia. With increasing age, latent hyperopia becomes manifest and will likely result in a reoccurrence of the esotropia and reduced acuity. A trial of the full cycloplegic refraction is advisable where there is a significant latent hyperopic component. If the latent component remains over 2D then refractive surgery may be inadvisable.

The patients risk of developing a decompensating phoria post treatment can be estimated by measuring their motor fusion amplitude and carrying out a refraction stress test. It is important to differentiate between a true fully accommodative esotropia with bifoveal binocular fixation and one which is controlled to a microtropia with extrafoveal fixation. This is especially true when the angle of deviation is very small, or in the case of a microtropia 'with identity', where no manifest deviation is seen. Patients with a central suppression scotoma and abnormal retinal correspondence are especially vulnerable to fixation switch diplopia [9] and/or decompensation of strabismus. A small manifest deviation coexisting with binocular fusion is confirmatory of a microtropia with anomalous retinal correspondence. If a manifest deviation is not seen, a sub-optimal stereopsis response (poorer than 100 seconds of arc) and a negative response to the 4Δ prism test will confirm central suppression.

It is imperative that the ocular dominance in these patients is maintained to avoid fixation switch which can result in diplopia as they may not be able to suppress the image from the dominant eye [15]. Once fixation switch occurs, it is not always reversible even if the image is degraded in the non-dominant eye. Where possible both eyes should be treated on the same day or within as short an interval as possible. Temporary diplopia and on-going symptoms have been reported in patients where there has been a delay between the refractive correction of both eyes [22-26]. Pre-operatively a strong base-in, or negative fusion reserve, would suggest the patient has a sufficient degree of flexibility in their binocular system to sustain fusion.

Convergence excess esotropia is identified by an excessive accommodative convergence response (AC) to an accommodative demand (A), a high AC/A ratio. The patient may be esophoric or orthophoric for distance and have a constant or intermittent esotropia for near. An additional hyperopic correction for near or prisms may be incorporated into the patient's lenses to help them to control the esotropia at near. This information may not be forthcoming and requires careful evaluation of their current lenses in relation to their pupil position. A trial of single vision or non-prismatic lenses may be worthwhile. Relevant patients should be warned that refractive surgery will not eliminate the need for reading glasses/prisms or that strabismus surgery may be necessary.

Partially Accommodative Esotropia or esotropia with an accommodative element is typified by a persistent manifest deviation for near and distance when the accommodative component is corrected. In longstanding cases there is rarely any potential for binocular function but this can be verified with prismatic correction of the deviation in combination with Bagolini lenses or with a Synoptophore. In most cases there will be a suppression scotoma in the deviating eye. The size of this suppression scotoma should be sufficient to allow for a reasonable variation in the angle of strabismus. The refraction stress test will indicate any change in the magnitude of the deviation and the patient should be made aware if there is likely to be any negative impact on the cosmesis of their strabismus.

Non-Accommodative Strabismus

This category may include infantile esotropia, paretic nerve palsies, neurogenic and mechanical restrictions. In most cases it is unlikely the deviation will be altered by refractive surgery. However an individual approach must be taken.

The patient may have a fixation preference and it is usually best to manage the patient so that they continue to fix with that eye to avoid fixation switch diplopia [15]. If the patient has suppression then the size and depth of the scotoma should be recorded to establish the likelihood of diplopia occurring if there is any change for better or worse in the angle of deviation post-refractive surgery. In many cases the angle of deviation post refractive surgery has been reported as better than the pre-operative deviation with glasses [1]. The patient should be made aware of the risks and benefits to their cosmetic appearance and sensory status.

If the patient has diplopia per-operatively then it is unlikely to resolve with refractive surgery and the opportunity to resolve it with prisms is lost with the removal of glasses. However for small angle ($<10\Delta$) strabismus with diplopia, monovision may be a feasible alternative for presbyopic diplopic patients who are dissatisfied with other conservative treatment options [27, 28]. It is thought that the induced foveal blur in the deviating eye may help the patient to suppress the diplopic image. Bujak et al. recently reported that 50 to 85% of subjects experienced an objective improvement in their diplopia with induced monovision [28]. Furthermore, 4 of the 11 subjects who had been dissatisfied with previous prism correction found relief from their diplopia through monovision.

Consecutive Exotropia and Residual Esotropia

More often than not the adult strabismic hyperope presents with a complicated history of strabismus surgery. There is an increased probability of incomitance. The patient's refraction may have been manipulated by under or over correction to modify their deviation. As surgery aims to correct the maximum hyperopic error the alignment of the eyes should be measured with full correction in place. In the case of consecutive exotropia with under corrected hyperopia an increase in the angle of deviation is likely. The patient may wish to forego refractive surgery if there is likely to be a negative impact on their cosmetic appearance or they may wish to follow up with strabismus correction. A post-op diplopia test is advisable to expose any contra-indications for subsequent strabismus surgery.

Myopia

Refractive surgery aims to correct the least minus required for threshold acuity. Patient satisfaction results for myopia correction have been reported as 95.3% [29]. The majority of myopic patients will fall into a category of low risk of diplopia post-refractive surgery, that is, those who have myopia with low levels of anisometropia (<4D), no history of strabismus or diplopia, and only a minimal phoria with a good fusional amplitude [20]. However any refractive surgery may cause a loss of fusion. Before there was general acceptance that bilateral surgery could be performed on the same day, fusional disruption was more common [30]. The potential for sensory problems argues for simultaneous refractive surgery.

In a small percentage of cases, an overcorrection or unplanned hyperopia may result from refractive surgery [31]. In this instance an accommodative esotropia may result [24]. A preoperative refraction stress test may indicate how vulnerable the patient is to this outcome.

Some myopes may habitually underuse their accommodative facilities if they remove their glasses for near work or wear under-corrected lenses. Furthermore, high myopes may experience a base-in effect from their concave lenses which will reduce their need to converge at a near target. It is possible these patients might experience convergence or accommodation insufficiency. However, to the best of our knowledge this has not been reported in the literature. It has not been volunteered in follow up of studies [32] or meta-analysis of patient satisfaction [29].

Unless monovision is planned the myopic patient should clearly understand the future implications of presbyopia and the potential future need for reading glasses. It is worth assessing the accommodation amplitude even in young pre-presbyopic patients as other factors may cause poor accommodation.

Case Report 1

A 33 year old myopic female presented with a history of bilateral fourth nerve palsies and spinal injury following a serious road traffic accident 10 years previously. She has a moderate right exotropia of 35ΔBO and a right hypertropia. She had learnt to cope with constant diplopia and did not find it troublesome. Her pre-op refraction was -3.00/-0.50 x 115 OD; -3.75 OS; Post LASIK refraction was -0.50/+0.25 x 131 OD; +0.75/+0.25 x126 OS with good distance acuity. Unfortunately, the patient was complaining of considerable difficulty with near vision and was reading N10 at 48cm. This improved with the use of a +2.00D near addition. The patient had not mentioned that she had been removing her glasses for reading since the accident and had most likely suffered a loss of accommodation due to the head injury.

Exotropia

In cases of intermittent or constant exotropia overcorrecting minus lenses may be used to stimulate accommodative convergence. If there is a difference between the patients current prescription and their cycloplegic refraction, then there is a risk the patient will suffer a loss of fusion and a decompensating exotropia after refractive surgery.

Anisometropia

The foveal blur created by anisometropia is the probable cause of most cases of microtropia or monofixation. Microtropia is described as a small manifest strabismus of 10Δ or less with abnormal retinal correspondence. There is a foveal suppression scotoma and the extrafoveal fixation point acquires the identity of the fovea for the purposes of retinal correspondence. Microesotropia is more common than microexotropia [33, 34]. The sub-classification of 'microtropia with identity' describes where no manifest deviation may be seen on cover test and the eccentric fixation point in the deviating eye supersedes the drive to fixate with the fovea. Those with microtropia usually have weaker motor fusion and are at higher risk of decompensating strabismus. There is no evidence as to whether the likelihood of decompensation is better in those with a stable eccentric fixation point as in microtropia with identity. Stereoacuity is worse (poorer than 100 seconds of arc) in patients with microtropia than those with bifoveal fixation.

Vuori et al. reported a statistically significant improvement in the best corrected acuity of a group of myopic anisometropes 8 to 13 months after refractive surgery [35]. They postulated that the slow improvement in best corrected acuity may be related to cortical plasticity. Nemet et al. reported a complete resolution of exotropia after LASIK for myopic anisometropia [6]. A preoperative contact lens is predictive of a positive outcome in patients with anisometropia.

Holland et al. described a patient with high anisometropia and amblyopia who developed persistent diplopia after LASIK [25]. Failure to fuse the images due to aniseikonia was thought to be responsible. Diplopia secondary to aniseikonia is characterised by 2 images, differing in size and not displaced in space. It has been estimated that aniseikonia of as little as 3% may disrupt fusion [36]. According to Knapps rule, axial anisometropia may result in aniseikonia if corrected in the corneal but not in the spectacle plane [37]. Kushner & Kowal estimated that correction of >4D of anisometropia in the corneal plane may result in aniseikonia and intractible diplopia [9]. It would therefore be judicious to perform a contact lens trial in habitual spectacle wearers with significant anisometropia considering keratorefractive surgery.

It is not uncommon for high levels of anisometropia to present uncorrected especially if there is co-existent amblyopia. A balancing lens may be worn for cosmetic reasons. Refractive correction may improve the visual acuity of the anisometropic eye but induce aniseikonia.

Case Report 2

A 41 year old male presented for refractive surgery assessment. His spectacle correction was plano OD and +0.25/-1.25 x 80 OS. With this his vision was 2/60 OD and 20/15 OS respectively. He had a minimal right exotropia and no binocular fusion or diplopia. His full refraction was -6.50/-2.50 x 109 OD; +0.25/-1.25 x 80 OS which resulted in a corrected VA of 20/60 OD and 20/15 OS. With this refraction is place he had a small exotropia of 12ΔBI and constant diplopia which could not be resolved. Refractive surgery of the right eye was contra-indicated.

Monovision

Monovision has been reported as successful in 88% [38] and 92.5% [39] of patients with presbyopia. However, in patients with a previous history of strabismus or those with significant heterophoria, care should be taken in recommending monovision. Where monovision is chosen, the risk of strabismus may be lowered by creating no greater than 1.5D of anisometropia. Typically the dominant eye is corrected for distance and the non-dominant eye for near. Factors which suggest a poor outcome include a strong sighting preference, aniseikonia and reduced stereopsis. Deterioration in stereoacuity and a subjective loss of depth perception as a result of monovision have been reported [17].

Stereopsis has been found to decline with increasing levels of anisometropia (as simulated with trial lenses) with some patients showing marked reduction with only 1D of anisometropia [40]. Results from a post-refractive surgery have shown marked variability in individual tolerance levels for anisometropia [41]. Loss of stereopsis appears to be strongly correlated with patient dissatisfaction with monovision. Zane et al. reported 12 cases where strabismus occurred after 2 years of monovision, suggesting that while a trial of monovision with contact lens prior to surgery may suggest that the patient can tolerate monovision, it is not a guarantee [42].

Steroblind patients with alternating strabismus and suppression can in some cases make ideal candidates for monovision to overcome presbyopia (may be the case with infantile esotropia). Their absence of stereovision precludes them from difficulties that a loss of stereoacuity may cause. They may however complain of a positional change when switching fixation, the magnitude of which will depend on their angle of strabismus. Only patients who can seamlessly alternate fixation should be considered suitable and a trial with contact lenses or glasses may be advisable. However, patients with a constant non-alternating strabismus may not be accustomed to suppressing the image from their dominant eye when they fixate with their non-dominant eye. Monovision should be avoided in these patients as fixation switch diplopia may occur [9, 15].

Monovision may be intentionally used to disrupt simultaneous perception in patients with small angle diplopia as discussed previously. The induced foveal blur from the surgically induced anisometropia presumably degrades the foveal image and helps the patient develop monocular suppression [27, 28].

Case Report 3

A 48 year old female prsesnted with a constant alternating esotropia. Her refractive error was -5.00D OD and -2.75D OS. When fixing with her left eye, she had a moderate right esotropia of 35ΔBO and when fixing with her right eye, she had a small left esotropia of 14ΔBO. Her uncorrected left eye had a very useable range of near vision N5 with a near point of 20cm. The possibility of correcting the right eye only to give monovision was considered. When simulated with lenses, the patient felt she was able to alternate fixation quite naturally without diplopia and had good near and distance acuity. Following right LASIK, the patient had good unaided acuity at near and distance and a cosmetically improved esodeviation.

Conclusion

Evidence has shown that refractive surgery may be performed successfully on patients with strabismus. Those with fully accommodative esotropia have the potential not only to attain emmetropia but also ocular alignment. Refractive error may in many instances influence the angle of deviation, so in cases where both refractive surgery and strabismus surgery are planned it is very important to perform refractive surgery as the initial procedure. Obtaining a detailed ocular history is an essential component of refractive surgery assessment. In those patients with strabismus or a history or strabismus surgery, a thorough orthoptic evaluation is required to determine the risk of decompensation post refractive surgery. In this way, the best advise may be offered to these often complex patients.

References

[1] Kirwan C, O'Keefe M, O'Mullane, GM, Sheehan C. Refractive surgery in patients with accommodative and non-accommodative strabismus: 1-year prospective follow-up. *Br. J. Ophthalmology*. 2010;94:898-902.

[2] Godts D, Trau R, Tassignon M J. Effect of refractive surgery on binocular vision and ocular alignment in patients with manifest or intermittent strabismus. *Br. J. Ophthalmol.*, 2006;90:1410-1413.

[3] Wasserman B, McCoy C. Improved binocularity after laser in situ keratomileusis. *Arch. Ophthalmol.* 2007;125(9):1293-4.

[4] Stidham DB, Borissova O, Borissova V, Prager TC. Effect of Hyperopic laser in situ keratomileusis on ocular alignment and stereopsis in patients with accommodative esotropia. *Ophthalmology*. 2002;109:1148-1153.

[5] Hoyos JE, Cigales M, Hoyos-Chacon J, Ferrer J, & Maldonado-Bas A. Hyperopic laser in situ keratomileusis for refractive accommodative esotropia. *J. Cataract Refract. Surg*. 2002;28(9):1522-9.

[6] Nemet P, Levenger S, Nemet A. Refractive surgery for refractive errors which cause strabismus. A report of 8 cases. *Binocul. Vis. Strabismus Q.* 2002;17(3):187-190.

[7] Sabetti L, Spadea L, D'Alessandri L, Balestrazzi E. Photorefractive keratectomy and laser in situ keratomileusis in refractive accommodative esotropia. *J. Cataract Refract. Surg.;*2005:31(10):1899-903.

[8] Nucci P, Serafino M, Hutchinson AK. (2003). Photorefractive keratectomy for the treatment of purely refractive accommodative esotropia. *J. Cataract Refract. Surg.* 2003;29(5):889-894.

[9] Kushner BJ, Kowal L. Diplopia after refractive surgery: occurence and prevention. *Arch. Ophthalmol.* 2003;121(3):315-21.

[10] Phillips C, Prager TC, McClellan G, Mintz-Hittner HA. Laser in situ keratomileusis for high hyperopia in awake, autofixating pediatric and adolescent patients with fully or partially accommodative esotropia. *J. Cataract Refract. Surg*. 2004;30(10):2124-2129.

[11] O'Keeffe M, Kirwan C. Pediatric Refractive Surgery. *J. Pediatr. Ophthalmol. Strabismus*. 2006;43(6):333-336.

[12] Worth C. The orthoptic treatment of convergent squint in young children. *Transactions of the ophthalmological society of the United Kingdom*. 1901;21:245-258.

[13] Rosenfield M, Cuiffreda KJ, Ong E, Super S. Vergence adaptation and the order of clinical vergence range testing. *Optom. Vis. Sci.*1995;72(4):219-223.

[14] Sheard C. Zones of ocular comfort. *Am. J. Optom. 1930;7*:9-25.

[15] Kushner BJ. Fixation switch diplopia. *Arch. Ophthalmol. 1995;113(7)*:896-899.

[16] O'Connor, A. R., Birch, E. E., Anderson, S., & Draper, H. The functional significance of stereopsis. *Invest. Ophthalmo. Vis. Sci.* 2010;51(4):2019- 2023.

[17] Fawcett SL, Herman WK, Alfieri CD, Castleberry KA, Parks MM, Birch EE. Stereoacuity and foveal fusion in adults with longstanding surgical monovision. *Journal of American Association for Pediatric Ophthalmology and Strabismus*. 2001;5(6):342-347.

[18] Garcia-Gonzalez M, Teus MA, Hernandez-Verdejo JL. Visual outcomes of LASIK-induced monovision in myopic patients with presbyopia. *Am. J. Ophthalmol.* 2010;150(3):381-386.

[19] Jampolsky A. Characteristics of suppression in strabismus. *AMA Arch. Ophthalmol.* 1955;54(5):683-696.

[20] Kowal L, Battu R, Kushner, B. Refractive surgery and strabismus. *Clin. Exp. Ophthalmol.* 2005;33(1):90-96.

[21] Newsham D, O'Connor A. Intractable diplopia resulting from treatment of amblyopia and use of the spisa bar in the UK to assess the risk. *Invest. Ophthalmol. Vis. Sci.* 2010;51(10): 5288.

[22] Marmer RH. Ocular deviation induced by radial keratomy. *Ann. Ophthalmol.* 1987;19(12):451-452.

[23] Schuler E, Silverberg M, Beade P, Moadel K. Decompensated strabismus after laser in situ keratomileusis. *J. Cataract Refract. Surg.* 1999;25(11):1552-1553.

[24] Kim SK, Lee JB, Han SH, Kim EK. Ocular deviation after unilateral laser in situ keratmileusis. *Yonsei Med. J.* 2000;41(3):401-406.

[25] Holland D, Amm M, de Decker W. Persisting diplopia after bilateral laser in situ keratomileusis. *J. Cataract Refract Surg*. 2000;26(10):1555-7.

[26] Furr BA, Archer SM, Del Monte MA. Strabismus misadventures in refractive surgery. *Am. Orthopt. J.* 2001;*51*:11-15.

[27] London R. Monovision correction for diplopia. *J. Am. Optom. Assoc.* 1987;58(7):568-570.

[28] Bujak MC, Leung AK, Kisilevsky M, Margolin E. Correction for small-angle Diplopia. *Am. J. Ophthalmol.* 2012;154(3):586-592.

[29] Solomon KD, Fernandez de Castro LE, Sandoval HP, Biber JM, Groat B, Neff KD, Ying MS, French JW, Donnenfeld ED, Lindstrom RL, Joint LASIK Task Force. LASIK World literature Review: Quality of life and patient satisfaction. *Ophthalmology*. 2009;116(4):691-701.

[30] Mandava N, Donnenfeld ED, Owens PL. Ocular deviation following excimer laser photorefractive keratectomy. *J. Cataract Refract. Surg*. 1996;22(4):504-505.

[31] Alio JL, Muftuoglu O, Ortiz D, Perez-Santonja JJ, Artola A, Ayala MJ, Garcia MJ, de Luna GC. Ten-year follow-up of laser in situ keratomileusis for myopia of up to −10 diopters. *Am. J. Ophthalmol.* 2008;145(1):46-54.

[32] O'Doherty M, O'Keefe M, Kelleher C. Five year follow up of laser in situ keratomileusis for all levels of myopia. *Br. J. Ophthalmol*. 2006;90(1):20-3.

[33] Lang, J. Lessons learned from microtropia. In J. M. S.Moore (Ed.), *Orthoptics, Past, Present and Future. Transaction of the third international orthoptic congress.* 1976 (pp. 183-190). Miami: Symposia Specialists.

[34] Arnoldi, K. Monofixation with eso-,exo-, or hypertropia: is there a difference? *Am. Orthopt. J.* 2001;51:55-66.

[35] Vuori E, Tervo TM, Holopainen MV, Holopainen JM. (2007). Improvement of visual acuity following refractive surgery for myopia and myopic anisometropia. *J. Refract. Surg*. 2007;23(5):447-455.

[36] Katsumi O, Tanino T, Hirose T. Effect of anisekonia on binocular function. *Invest. Ophthalmol. Vis. Sci.* 1986;27:601-604.

[37] Benjamin WJ. Patients with anisometropia and anisekonia. In Borish's Clinical Refraction. Philadelphia, PA: WB Saunders;1998:1134-1159.

[38] Jain S, Arora I, Azar DT. Success of monovision in presbyopes: Review of the literature and potential applications to refractive surgery. *Surv. Ophthalmol.* 1996;40(6):491-499.

[39] Miranda D, Kreuger RR. Monovision laser in situ keratomileusis for pre-presbyopic and presbyopic patients. *J. Refract. Surg.* 2004;20(4):325-8.

[40] Brooks SE, Fischer N, Johnson D. Anisometropia and binocularity. *Ophthalmology* 1996;103(7):1139-1143.

[41] Kirwan C, O'Keefe, M. Stereopsis in refractive surgery. *Am. J. Ophthalmol.* 2006;142(2):218-22.

[42] Zane F, Pollard M C, Greenberg MB, Elliot J, Hsu V. Strabismus precipitated by monovision. *Am. J. Ophthalmol.* 2011;152(3):479-482.

In: Current Understanding and New Techniques …
Editor: Michael O'Keefe
ISBN: 978-1-62808-748-2

Chapter 6

Pediatric Refractive Surgery

William F. Astle[1,2], Santa Heede[*,4], Peter T. Huang[3,†] and Emi Sanders[1,#]
[1]Alberta Children's Hospital, Vision Clinic, Calgary, Alberta, Canada
[2]Division of Ophthalmology, Pediatric Surgery, Department of Surgery, University of Calgary, Calgary, Alberta, Canada
[3]Ophthalmology, Department of Surgery, University of Calgary, Calgary, Alberta, Canada
[4]Charite – Universitatsmedizin Berlin, Klinik fur Augenheilkunde, Kinderaugenheilkunde und Strabologie, Berlin, Germany

Abstract

The goal of this chapter is explore and detail the current use of refractive surgery in the treatment and management of abnormal refractive errors in the paediatric population.

There are many recent advances in the area of refractive surgery. Dramatic improvements have been made in laser equipment, intraocular lens design, and diagnostic tools, influencing the safety and efficacy of refractive surgery in the pediatric population. Recent research into this complex field associated with other ocular pathology, neurological issues and other special needs and considerations will be discussed.

The challenges presented by the requirement for general anaesthesia are addressed. With this sub-population, general anaesthesia is necessary, however as this population typically have some cormorbidity, this has been seen as an obstacle. Considerations and solutions to these issues are presented and discussed.

Treatment modalities including advanced surface ablations; Photorefractive keratectomy (PRK), laser in situ keratomileusis (LASIK), and laser-assisted subepithelial keratectomy (LASEK), along with anterior and posterior chamber phakic lenses, sulcus fixated intra-ocular lenses', clear lens extraction with refractive lens exchange are detailed. Specifics regarding each modality and considerations for undertaking each are

* santa.heede@gmx.de
† huangp@telus.net
# Emi.Sanders@albertahealthserices.ca

presented and discussed. Such treatments have all been shown to be safe procedures in children, with no more complications than would be expected with adults.

The care and vision of children with complex refractive situations combined with other issues has always presented a challenge to paediatric ophthalmologists. However, this sub-population of children who have previously failed traditional treatment, may benefit significantly from these emerging treatments –used individually, or in combination. Congenital high ametropia (myopic and hyperopic), extreme refractive conditions, over -15.0 D, anisometropic amblyopia – hyperopic, myopic and astigmatic, infantile nystagmus, refractive errors associated with strabismus, and visual autism secondary to multiple associated neurobehavioral disorders, are just some of the conditions in which refractive surgery should be assessed as an option when traditional treatment fails.

Refractive surgery is emerging as a safe and effective treatment option for the pediatric population.

Introduction

The field of cataract and refractive surgery is advancing at startling rates. The rapid ongoing advancements in new intraocular lens design, dramatic improvements in laser equipment, improved diagnostic equipment, and a plethora of new and ever expanding research into the field has improved our ability to effectively treat patients with the most complex combinations of refractive disorders. This is true even when faced with associated complex pathological disorders that may accompany the abnormal refractive state.

Never has this been so true in the field of pediatric ophthalmology, where in the past, many complex refractive disorders in children were not effectively treated as the equipment, surgical armamentarium, and overall clinical understanding and knowledge was not available. Recent advances in amblyopia therapy, as shown in the many PEDIG studies, for example, have demonstrated that children with complex forms of amblyopia previously thought to not be treatable, can be effectively improved with various combinations of glasses, contact lenses, patching, and atropine drops. There is now conclusive evidence of successful resolution of amblyopia, and improvement in fusional ability even in older children in their teens, who have never been previously treated [1-5].

However, there is a subset of children who may still fail these more traditional forms of treatment. This is especially true of children with concurrent medical diagnoses such as autism, cerebral palsy, developmental delay, and with other ocular disorders (including cornea, retina, and optic nerve disorders), which may contribute to these treatment failures. In the past there was no effective treatment for these children if traditional methods failed. Although many treatment failures are due to noncompliance or secondary to cognitive or communication limitations, it is important to recognize that refractive error complications, including severe myopia, anisometropia, or astigmatism, can contribute to aniseikonia, leading to image disparity, rejection of optical corrections, and the subsequent development or maintenance of amblyopia in an otherwise normal child [6-9]. Thus, with a concurrent medical diagnosis and an empty reserve of alternative refractive error care, many children (neurologically impaired or simply noncompliant) will fail to develop normal vision. In the past few years, refractive laser surgery techniques have been shown to be a good last-resort treatment in children who have failed with traditional treatment approaches [10-19].

Photorefractive keratectomy (PRK), laser in situ keratomileusis (LASIK), and laser-assisted subepithelial keratectomy (LASEK) have been used effectively to treat bilateral high myopia [10, 12, 13, 16], anisometropia [10, 13, 19], and high astigmatic refractive errors [12]. As a result, the clinical indications for laser refractive surgery in children continue to broaden, and the results overall are excellent.

The same findings are true when employing phakic intraocular lenses (pIOL's) to correct anisometropia, and congenital high myopic and hyperopic refractive errors in children. Lenses such as Verisyse ™ (Abbott Medical Optics Inc, Santa Ana CA USA), Artisan, Artiflex (Ophtec, Groningen Netherlands), and Implanted Contact Lenses (ICL's) have been used for the same purposes as outlined for laser refractive treatments in children. These surgical implants have been effectively used to restore vision for more than 20 years in Europe and Asia, and these lenses and surgical techniques have now made their way to North America [20-22].

In addition, implantation of posterior chamber intraocular lenses (IOLs) in children is becoming more common and accepted [23-33]. Despite the demonstrated efficacy and safety of paediatric IOL implantation, one of the most difficult challenges faced with paediatric cataract surgery is the choice of implant power to use, as children's eyes continue to grow over time, the 'myopic shift' must be considered[28, 34-45]. Although good data are present in the literature analysing growth patterns of normal phakic eyes in children [42], surgical predictions of appropriate IOL power become increasingly complicated in children under age 6 years, especially those children under 1 year of age [27, 43]. Rapid growth of the eye in children, especially in the first year of life, increased tissue reactivity, decreased scleral rigidity, and documented alterations in growth patterns of aphakic and pseudophakic eyes make paediatric cataract surgery particularly challenging [25, 27, 34, 43, 46-49].

With improvements in surgical technique, ongoing improvements in IOL design and surgical instrumentation, our ability to implant in small eyes and very young children has been realized, and will hopefully continue to advance. However, the ability to calculate the appropriate IOL power for any given pediatric eye is still not accurate and consistent enough in all circumstances, unlike that seen in adult IOL power calculations [44]. The values for axial length (AL), anterior chamber depth (ACD), and keratometry (K) readings, the different tissue dynamics in young eyes, plus variability in growth factors and disease presentation in the pediatric eye are much different than in adults. Yet, the standard, well tested regression and theoretical formulas used in adults are still the only tools available to pediatric cataract surgeons at present. As many others have noted [26, 34-37, 38, 45-53], a consistently accurate pediatric IOL formula is needed that addresses all of the issues and potential inaccuracies involved in pediatric cataract surgery with IOL's.

Consequently, refractive surprises in pediatric cataract surgery are still common, and for all the reasons discussed are not always avoidable, considering our present understanding of pediatric eye growth parameters and the predictive formulas available. However, new secondary sulcus fixated IOL's such as the Sulcoflex IOL © (Raynor Intraocular Lenses Limited, East Sussex UK) can aid is successful resolution of a refractive surprise in children after successful primary intraocular lens implantation. Other new adjustable power IOL's are being trialed in the adult cataract and refractive world that may have potential uses in children, and femtosecond lasers may be tremendously useful new tools in pediatric refractive conditions as well [54-56].

With this background, the goal of this chapter is to look at each of these new techniques in more detail, and discuss how all of these newer refractive surgical techniques can be used to reverse more complex refractive disorders in children, effectively restoring vision in children, thought to be treatment failures in the past.

Co-Morbidity and Special Needs Issues

Traditional treatment methods to correct and rehabilitate the refractive status of children with complex forms of refractive problems include glasses and contact lenses. However, these more traditional forms of treatment fail in a subset of children, especially those with concurrent medical diagnoses such as autism, cerebral palsy, progressive childhood encephalopathies, severe developmental delay, hearing impairments, and other ocular disorders, including cornea, retina, and optic nerve disorders, that may contribute to their inability to wear glasses or contact lenses. As outlined in detail by Tychsen [56] and others [10, 12, 22, 57] many children with various syndromic issues find it difficult, if not impossible, to wear glasses and contact lenses. Severe long term uncorrected visual refractive impairments in children have been shown to induce behaviors similar to autism may promote inappropriate fearfulness, decreased interest in the outside world and cause a major negative impact on social interactions. Tychsen [56] has named this group of behaviors as "visual autism". These large refractive errors and associated visual loss rarely present alone, but exist in common with strabismus, amblyopia, retinopathies and optic neuropathies, as well as a myriad of other organ and limb disorders. A child affected by extremely poor vision in the face of multiple other congenital challenges can be reduced to an extremely low level of overall functional ability.

While the majority of children with significant refractive errors respond well to standard forms of treatment, the subset previously discussed, generally do not. These children are best served by the newer forms of refractive surgery now available. The effect of refractive surgery in this complex group cannot be quantified in the standard ways used for adults. In many cases, true levels of post-operative visual acuity cannot be objectively quantified in this complicated group of children, although changes in refractive error pre and post surgery generally can be. Many papers [1-103] now demonstrate significant functional improvement post refractive surgery for these children. The positive changes are usually of a behavioral and social nature, being able to negotiate better in their environments, improved awareness and attentiveness, plus improved ability to feed themselves, play games, watch TV and computer screens, with improved social interaction skills overall. Tychsen [56] has demonstrated that scores for eye tracking, finding and avoiding, depth perception and reading improved 73% in children with bilateral ametropia and 58% in children with anisometropia post laser refractive surgery. Many others [1-103] have demonstrated improved visual acuity, fusional ability and positive improvement to standard treatment was noted. Pediatric refractive surgery fills a crucial void for children that in the past did not respond to traditional treatments and were dismissed by health care workers as functionally blind.

General Anesthesia Issues

Anesthesia in this group of children and the environment can present challenges. Most of these children have some cormorbidity, such as cerebral palsy, ex-prematurity, autism, and developmental delay. Not all lasers center are designed for general anesthesia so equipment may have to be brought in from outside. Nevertheless, the general anesthesia techniques required for these children, are standard techniques delivered in a standard way (Figure 1).

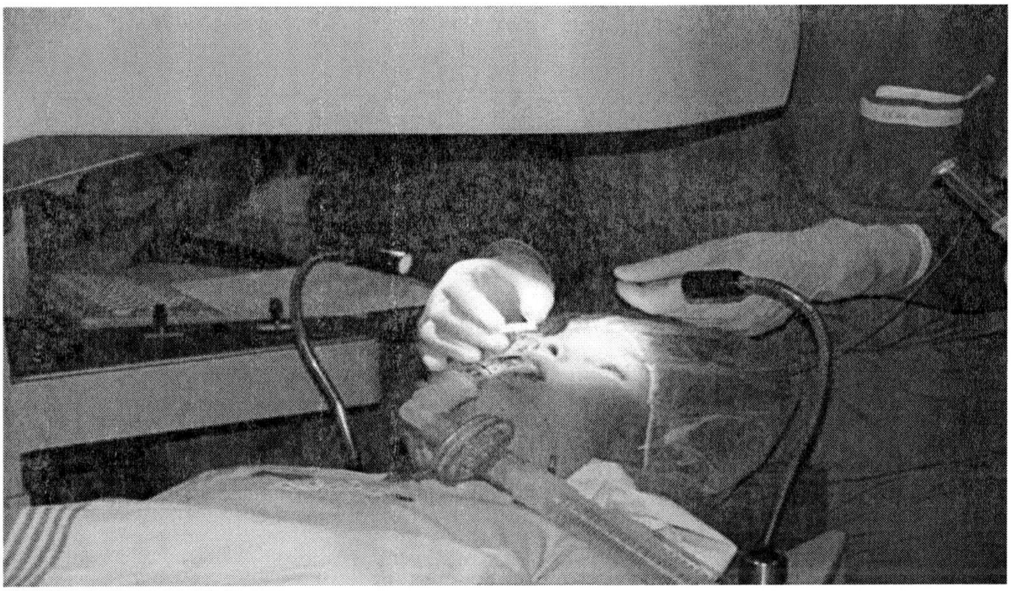

Figure 1. LASEK surgery in a child under general anaesthesia (usually a laryngeal mask or nasopharyngeal airway).

Flammable agents should be avoided in the laser room, but oxygen can be allowed in the inhaled mixture of gases. For the anesthetic technique, whether the procedure is corneal or intraocular most of these children will not be manageable with conscious sedation. General anesthesia and definitive airway management will generally provide safer and more reliable conditions. As venous access is not always easy, Astle et al. [13, 14] perform inhalation inductions with sevoflurane before establishing an intravenous catheter and securing the airway with a laryngeal mask airway or nasopharyngeal airway. None of their patients required intubation. A combination of sevoflurane and/or propofol usually provides good operative conditions and a rapid, smooth recovery. Ketamine should probably be avoided [58, 59], because of concerns about eye movements, emergence delirium, vomiting, and airway secretions. However, the key to success is having a well-trained team, comprehensive anesthesia and monitoring equipment rather than the drugs themselves.

Treatment Modalities

Advanced Surface Ablations (ASA) - PRK, LASEK, LASIK

Early studies on laser refractive surgery in children, in the 1990's, supported the general notion that Photorefractive keratectomy (PRK) and laser in situ keratomileusis (LASIK) in children were safe procedures, with no more complications than would be expected in adults. In all the studies cited [14, 58,59, 61-64]laser treatments, regardless of technique consistently and effectively reduced the SE refractive error over the long term (usually 1 year post treatment) and the children's vision was maintained or improved. Also, most studies involved older children, out of the most effective age range for treating amblyopia. Despite the older age group, however, the overall improvement in visual acuity in these children was positive.

As a result of the success with these early studies, there is now a plethora of literature demonstrating the safety and success of laser refractive surgery in children, regardless of technique. This is especially true in the treatment of children who have failed with traditional treatment approaches. [5–14] PRK, LASIK, and laser-assisted subepithelial keratectomy (LASEK), which came into vogue in the year 2000, have been used effectively to treat bilateral high myopia, [5, 7, 8, 11] anisometropia, [5, 8, 14] and high astigmatic error. [7] All recent studies show that refractive laser surgery for these complex groups of children is effective and safe. Target refractions are achieved with minimal myopic regression, and complications, including negligible subepithelial corneal haze. The findings for PRK9, [14] and LASEK [5, 8, 11] are similar. Functionally, refractive laser surgery improves uncorrected visual acuity and best corrected visual acuity (BCVA), [5, 7–9, 11, 14] restores stereopsis and binocular fusion in some patients, [7, 11] and has a positive effect on patients' visual and social functions in their environment. In some children, these improvements eliminate a constellation of signs that previously prompted a diagnosis of autism. [5, 8, 9].

There have been many studies comparing surface ablations that imply LASEK treatments may potentially decrease the amount of postoperative haze encountered in children as compared to PRK [13-14, 65-67]. The exact mechanism for the decrease in corneal haze noted in LASEK is open to debate in the literature. Replacement of the epithelial flap after the ablation may decrease the loss of stromal keratocytes and the release of corneal stromal cytokines responsible for stromal fibrosis [d, 13, 13.9, 13.10]. Another theory is that the epithelial flap prevents inflammatory cells present in the tear film from causing direct damage within the corneal stroma. This may decrease the loss of stromal keratocytes and decrease fibroplastic hyperplasia in the cornea [13, 13.9, 13.12, 13. 15]. Espana et al. [13.15] performed an immunofluorescence study to determine the location of the anatomic cleavage plane created in a LASEK epithelial flap. The cleavage plane of the ethanol-induced flap is located in the epithelial basement membrane between the lamina lucida and the lamina densa. The authors also note that the repositioned epithelial flap facilitates corneal epithelial healing, decreases chemotaxis, reduces inflammation, and produces less postoperative pain and haze formation. The action of ethanol in splitting the epithelial basement membrane does not affect the basement membrane anchored to Bowman's layer deeper in the cornea (Figure 2). Corneal haze, especially in treating children with refractive errors above -15.00D, has really been the only complication noted in most studies employing surface ablation treatments in children. As an example, Astle et al. [66] now always add 0.02% mitomycin, painted on the stromal surface for 30 sec, post laser ablation, prior to replacing the epithelial flap, for any child being lasered for +/- 5.00 D or more. This has virtually eliminated the haze problem in almost all cases. (WA Astle, personal communication, February 1, 2013).

The literature notes potential advantages of LASIK over PRK in adults.3,6 In adults, LASIK allows more rapid restoration of vision, minimal pain and discomfort postoperatively, and an intact Bowman's membrane with potentially less haze. In addition, in adults having LASIK, there appears to be a more predictable outcome with higher levels of myopia. Laser in situ keratomileusis, however, has a surgical learning curve, requires more complex instrumentation, and has more potentially serious long-term complications associated with flap complications, corneal ectasia, halos, and glare [66]. Macular hemorrhage has been reported in eyes with high myopia and permanent optic neuropathy post-LASIK, presumably due to the intraocular pressure increase induced by the instruments during the procedure [17-18].

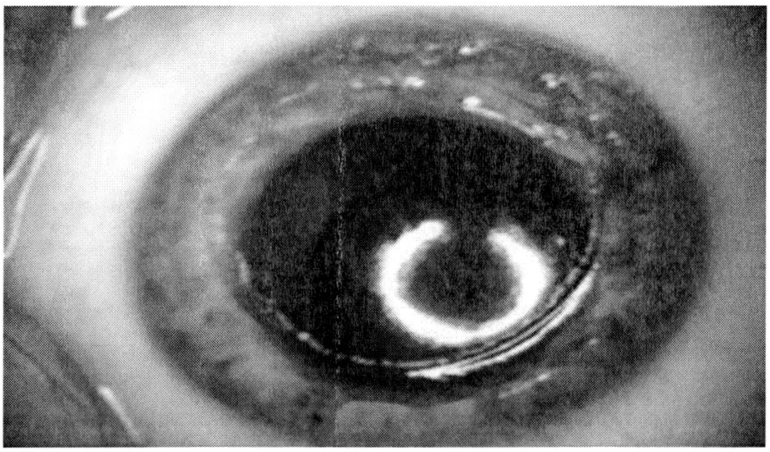

Figure 2. Pediatric eye undergoing LASEK surgery.

Nevertheless, despite these potential issues with LASIK, there are now many studies in the literature [65] documenting excellent success in treating children with LASIK [39, 54, 65, 73-74].

Astle et al. [65] published their long term results for 56 eyes of 39 patients undergoing PRK or LASEK under general anesthesia. These patients were followed for a minimum of 3.5 years with excellent results and no significant haze or other long term complications. They have now analyzed their entire cohort of patients now followed for over 14 years with the same excellent results [Astle WA, (2012, September). Can the refractive surgeon help? PRK, LASEK and LASIK in children. D. Epstein and KK Nischal (Chair), ESCRS/WCPOS. Symposium conducted at the XXX Congress of the European Society of Cataract and Refractive Surgeons, Milan]. The series has now expanded to 446 eyes of 274 patients that had either PRK or LASEK under general anesthesia. The mean age at surgery was 6.5 years (range 1.0 to 17.4 years).

The mean pre laser range was from -27.00 D to +13.50 D, showing the tremendous new potential treatment range when laser is employed. At the final postoperative examination (mean 8.9 years), the mean spherical equivalent was -1.65 D in all patients. Refraction and corneal clarity were stable over the long term in all eyes, and there have been no cases of corneal ectasia, or corneal decompensation. In children that could be measured, visual acuity improved from 0 to 16 lines, with no patient developing worse vision secondary to the laser treatment. 20.96 % of patients had no documented stereo visual acuity pre-operatively. Fine stereo vision improved post laser from 18.75 % to 40.44 % for the entire cohort of 274 patients. No patient lost binocular fusion post operatively. On a quality-of-life questionnaire, no family recorded negative opinions of the procedure or negative social or functional outcomes postoperatively.

These studies [1-102] demonstrate how safe and effective laser procedures can now be over the long term with these complex children. While there is still some controversy over which laser surgical technique is better in children, at this point in laser technology and laser surgical technique, PRK, LASEK and LASIK have all been employed successfully in correcting even extreme refractive errors in children[13, 65-67]. This gives the pediatric laser surgeon options for treatment when faced with more complex refractive disorders in children. As all modern laser techniques seem to be equally effective in children, the choice of technique will depend on the laser surgeons' comfort with the techniques, keeping in mind a child's concomitant health problems, any coexisting behavioral issues, and the type of refractive disorder being treated.

Posterior Chamber Phakic Lenses- Implanted Contact Lenses (ICL's)

Lesueur amd Arne [21] successfully implanted Staar Surgical phakic ICL's (Visian ICL, Monroria CA, USA) in 11 eyes of children (age 3 – 16 years) with myopic anisometropic amblyopia ranging from -8.00 D to -18.00D pre-surgery. Best corrected visual acuity improved to 20/63 post implant for the amblyopic eyes and there was fusional improvement documented in 6 of 11 children. Mean SE refraction improved from -12.71 D pre implantation to +0.71 D post implantation, effectively eliminating the ansiometropia enough to allow for resolution of the amblyopia in almost all cases.

Proponents of ICL implantation note that the technique is reversible, and there is potentially less risk of corneal endothelial loss with the ICL in the posterior chamber, than with phakic anterior chamber IOL's. If necessary, corneal refractive surgery can be secondarily applied if any refractive augmentation is required. The potential risks of ICL's are glaucoma, cataracts and uveitis, but in the small series documented by Lesueur and Arne [21], neither complication occurred. Newer ICL designs can correct from -23.00D to +20.00D and could prove very useful in older children experiencing less myopic shift. ICL design over time may increase the successful use of these lenses for high refractive errors in children.

Sulcus Fixated IOL's (Sulcoflex ©)

In the past standard posterior chamber IOL's designed for in-the-bag placement were occasionally placed in the sulcus in conjunction with the in-the-bag IOL. The problem with this type of situation was that the sulcus fixated IOL was the wrong design and platform for placement in the sulcus, having been designed for in-the-bag placement. Consequently, secondary complications occurred with these second IOL's, such as inter-lenticular opacification, optic deformation, uveal damage, pigment dispersion, secondary inflammation, glaucoma, and even hemorrhage.

However, now when a pseudophakic patient presents with a secondary refractive surprise, the Sulcoflex IOL © (Rayner Intraocular Lenses Limited, East Sussex UK) meets the design characteristics and optical needs to improve a patient's vision without the potential secondary complications outlined. The sulcoflex IOL is made of hydrophilic acrylic material, that avoids any potential uveal trauma. The haptic length is 14 mm which allows for centration stability and the undulated haptics are designed to give the IOL rotational stability. The IOL has a 10^0 posterior angulation that allows for uveal clearance, and a 6.5 mm optic that will avoid pupillary capture. The IOL has a round edge design that avoids any uveal chaffing and also avoids any potential dysphotopsia or edge glare. The sulcoflex IOL is designed with a concave posterior surface so there is not optic touch with the in-the-bag IOL and no potential for distortion. With present designs, the sulcoflex IOL can correct up to 10 D of power change (myopic and hyperopic), and is available in toric formats as well as multifocal designs [54] (Figures 3 and 4).

Khan and Muhtaseb [54] have published documented success with Sulcoflex secondary IOL's in adults, and note that by 2011 over 1000 Sulcoflex IOLs have been implanted successfully in adults without significant complications. WA Astle(personal communication, February 1, 2013) have implanted 20 sulcoflex IOL's in children under 18 years of age, with successful restoration of vision, improvement in amblyopia, relief of anesikonia, with no complications post implant.

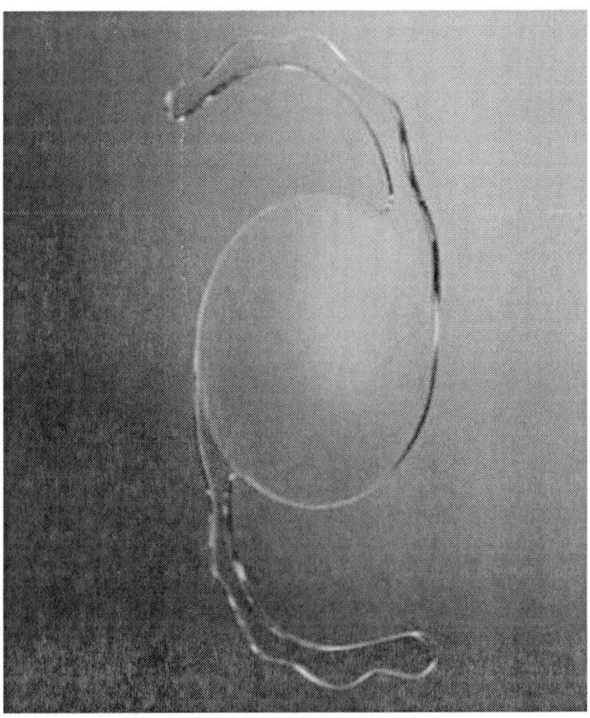

Figure 3. Rayner Monofocal Sulcoflex Intraocular lens.

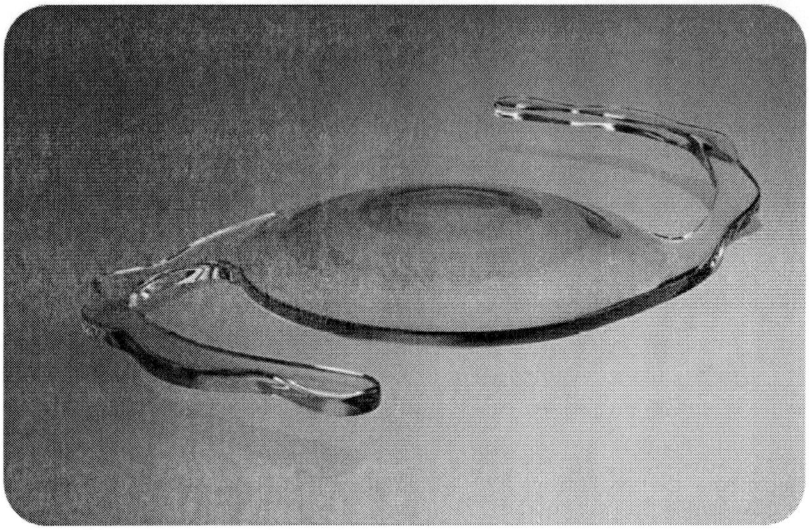

Figure 4. Rayner multifocal sulcoflex intraocular lens.

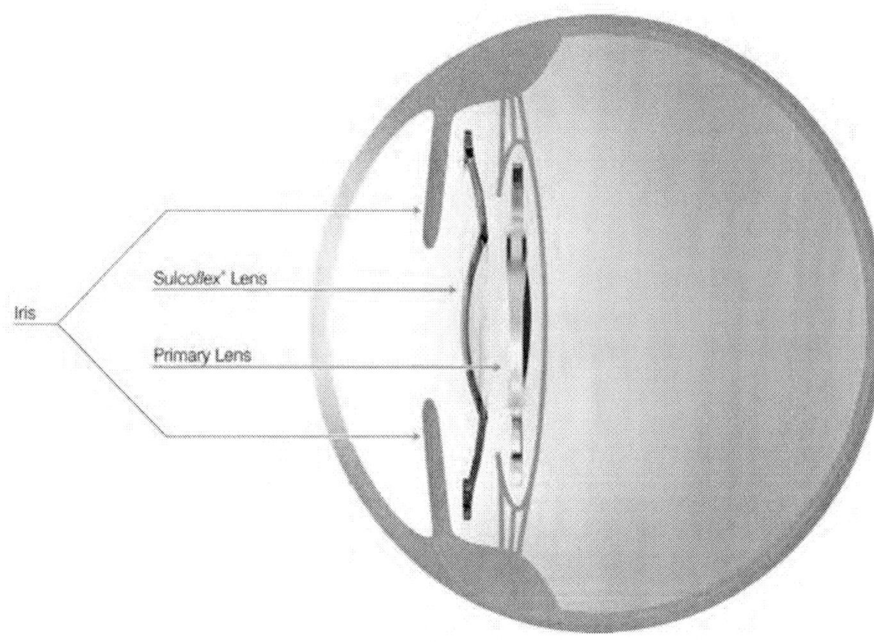

Figure 5. Sulcoflex supplemental lens is implanted anterior to the primary lens, with haptics to hold it in place in the sulcus.

The Sulcoflex secondary implanted sulcus fixated IOL (Figure 5) is ideal in pseudophakic children that experience a significant, unanticipated myopic shift that affects both fusion and vision, as well as older children with secondary mid-range refractive changes associated with aneisikonia with the potential need for multifocal ability. This lens represents a significant improvement in the ability to successfully deal these types of problems, where no previous therapy was available. In addition, implantation of a sulcoflex IOL is reversible, and exchange of IOL powers is also possible. Secondary augmentation with laser refractive surgery, if required, is also an option, if further augmentation is required. The sulcoflex IOL represents a safe effective option to augment refractive error issues in children, and is a significant positive step forward in helping children with more complex anisometropic issues.

Clear Lens Extraction (CLE) / Refractive Lens Exchange (RLE)

CLE / RLE has been employed effectively in children, especially is extreme refractive situations, over -15.00 D. Another good indication is a child with a high refractive error, combined with a shallow anterior chamber (less than 3.2 mm), making it unsafe to consider a phakic IOL (Artisan etc.) While removing the lens may affect a child's ability to accommodate, older children could be considered for a mutifocal IOL, or secondarily be implanted at a later date if needed, with a multifocal IOL like a multifocal sulcoflex. As outlined by Paysse et al. [55], the major potential complication in pediatric CLE with high myopia is the long-term risk of retinal tears and detachment. This has been estimated to be 0.26% to 2.2% post surgery with CLE in adults. At this time, there is no long term data on retinal detachment risk with CLE in children. Nevertheless, CLE/RLE is a successful option in these more complex highly myopic situations where ASA and pIOL's are thought to be less viable options to achieve appropriate refractive change [10, 16, 22, 55-57].

pIOL's: Artisan / Verysise / Artiflex ("Iris – Claw" Lenses)

As outlined in many more recent papers [55-56, 75-84], pIOL's such as the Artisan / Verisyse have been safely and reliably implanted in adults, since 1991. In particular, the experience with these IOL's is extensive now throughout Europe, especially the Netherlands. As noted by Cleary et al. [20] in 2012, Artisan and Verisyse IOL's were initially developed in the late 1970's, and have undergone some refinements over the years, being modified to a bi-convex design in 1997. The original lenses were 3 piece rigid PMMA IOL's with an optic diameter of 5 mm and overall diameter of 8 mm. The lens powers range from +2.00 D to + 30.00 D for hyperopic correction and from -1.00 to -23.50 D for the myopic IOL's. In addition, all Artisan lenses are now available in toric design and can correct up to 7.50 D of cylinder.

There is now a foldable version available that can be implanted through a 3.0 mm incision, known as the Artiflex pIOL, available from -14.50 D to +20.00D. Artiflex pIOL's are now also available in toric design, correcting up to 5.00D of cylinder, further improving the use and indications of pIOL's for more complex forms of refractive error. These IOL's are designed to hold a knuckle of iris on each side of the pupil, to keep the lens centered and in proper position, (Figure 6) and the surgical technique to implant these lenses is an easily mastered bi-manual technique.

Lesueur and Arne [21, 75], and Ben Ezra et al. [76] effectively treated anisometropic amblyopic children with Artisan lenses in 1999 - 2000, without any serious complications. Saxena and co-workers documented the successful implantation of an Artisan lens for a child with anisometropic amblyopia, correcting -15.00 D of myopia, and reversing the patient's amblyopia while improving stereo vision [77]. Endothelial cell counts decreased 11.9 % in this child 19 months post-operatively, without any obvious corneal decompensation.

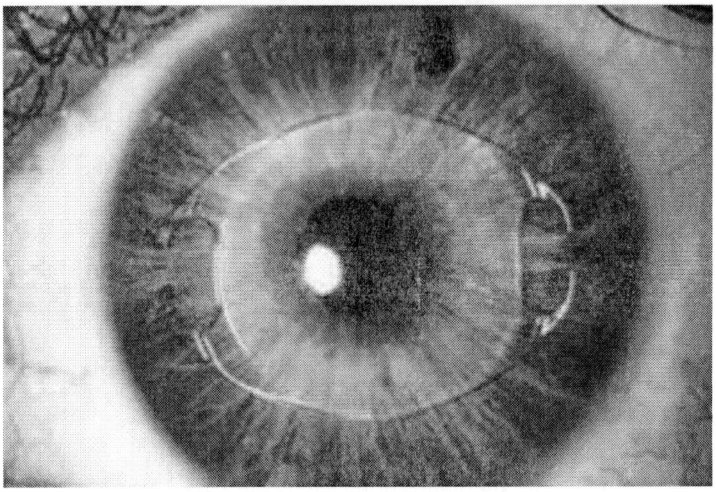

Figure 6. Artisan Intraocular lens.

Lifshitz and Levy [78] had the same success implanting a -14.00 D Artisan pIOL in a child that was pseudophakic after successful cataract surgery at 8 weeks of age, but subsequently experienced a large unexpected myopic shift. The secondary implantion of the Artisan lens to correct this large anisometropic refractive error was uneventful and improved the patient's amblyopia. Assil and co-workers implanted a -16.00 D Verisyse pIOL in a 3 year old child with myopic anisometropic amblyopia [79]. The child's vision improved from 20/1200 to 20/30 with standard patching treatment post implant. There were no significant complications noted with the implantation. Tychsen et al. in 2008 implanted 18 eyes of 12 children with Artisan/Verisyse pIOL's for high myopia ranging from -10.00 to -22.75 D [22]. 86% of eyes were within +/- 1.00 D of emmetropia post implantation, and Tychsen found that these children improved substantially in their visual function [22]. Many of the children that had substantial neurobehavioral problems pre-operatively, also improved post implantation because of better visual function. No eyes in their series experienced corneal edema or other significant complications. Only one pIOL had to be re-positioned secondary to partial dislocation from the iris knuckle. Alio et al. in 2011 experienced the same findings as Tychsen, implanting 10 children with anisometropic amblyopia that were not responding to traditional amblyopia treatments [80].

All 10 children improved post implant, without significant complications from the surgery or long-term from the implants themselves. Pirouzian et al. in 2009, had almost identical results as described implanting 6 patients with Verisyse pIOL's for myopic anisometropic amblyopia [81-82]. All children improved both visually and with improved stereopsis.

In 2012, Cleary and co-workers published their results with implantation of Artisan pIOL's following lensectomy for ectopia lentis [20]. Artisan lenses were implanted in 8 eyes of 5 children. Logmar BCVA improved from 0.21 pre-operatively to 0.04 post-operatively. There was a mean endothelial cell loss over time of 14.2% in the implanted eyes, with no significant post-operative complications.

In 2006, Odenthal and co-workers evaluated possible endothelial cell loss with implantation of Artisan pIOL's post cataract surgery [83]. Their analysis showed that the

Artisan lens does not cause excessive, dangerous endothelial cell loss and seems to be a safe, effective procedure.

Based on the extensive literature in adults, and now 15 – 20 years of experience in children, pIOL's are a safe effective option for correcting high refractive errors in children, including myopes, hyperopes and those with complex astigmatic combinations as well. Success has been documented with children having ametropia in phakic, aphakic and pseudophakic conditions. pIOL's are definitely an option to consider when faced with a child with high ametropia not responding to more traditional treatments.

Treatment Strategies for Consideration

There are many complex refractive situations that can be improved by choosing the appropriate refractive surgical modality, singly or in combination. While the surgical indications continue to expand as our knowledge and the technical tools expand and improve, a few patterns for successful treatment of these children have emerged in the literature.

Anisometropic Amblyopia – Hyperopic, Myopic and Astigmatic

Anisometropic amblyopia can now be treated effectively, and is especially suited to those children who have not responded to more traditional treatments [16, 19, 65-66, 74-75, 79-80, 81-82, 84]. Fortunately, this group of children tends to have fewer other associated medical problems, but the loss of fusion can be a significant functional problem even for children without other associated neurobehavioral or structural disorders.

The long-term success with pIOL's in anisometropia was outlined in detail in the previous pIOL section, demonstrating excellent improvement in eliminating anisometropia and anesikonia, thus allowing traditional amblyopia treatments to effectively reverse any residual amblyopia post surgery. pIOL's are a viable alternative from -23.50D to +30.00D with astigmatic correction available, and in rigid or foldable designs.

There are also multiple papers documenting success with ASA laser procedures in treating anisometropic amblyopia of all forms. Nucci and Drack in 2000 found that LASIK and PRK can be performed safely and effectively in children with myopic anisometropic amblyopia [11]. The average pre laser refractive difference was -7.96 D in 14 eyes of 14 patients. The average refraction post laser was -0.46 D at 2 months, and -0.67 D at 20 months. All patients experienced a small myopic shift, but all patients post laser were within ranges that allowed for amblyopia treatments to be effective. Vision and stereopsis improvement was noted in their study. Autrata and Rehurek in 2003 [84] used PRK effectively for 21 eyes with high myopic anisometropia, with a mean SE of -8.93 D pre-operatively, improving to -1.66 D post laser, which is within a refractive range where resistant amblyopes may now respond to traditional amblyopia therapies. BCVA improved in 14 of 21 eyes treated, as well as improved stereopsis. Tychsen, Packwoodand Berdy in 2005 treated 35 myopic anisometropes resistant to amblyopia therapy, with LASEK and PRK [16]. The myopia ranged from -3.25 D to -24.25 D pre laser. 89% of patients were within 1.00 D of targeted refraction and visual acuity improved in 97% of eyes lasered.

Tychsen and Hokel in 2006 found the same results with LASEK and high myopia in children with associated neurobehavioral disorders [10]. Paysse and co-workers in 2006 concluded that PRK for severe anisometropic amblyopia in children results in stable reduction of refractive error and definite improvement in both stereopsis and vision. 11 children were treated for both myopia and hyperopic anisometropic amblyopia ranging from -13.70 D to + 4.75 D [19]. Both stereopsis and UCVA improved post laser. Astle et al. in 2007 reported on 53 children with various forms of anisometropic amblyopia resistant to standard treatment [47]. All 53 eyes underwent LASEK.

The mean preoperative anisometropic difference was 6.98 D in the entire group, 9.48 D in the anisomyopic group, 3.13 D in the anisoastigmatic group, and 5.50 D in the anisohyperopic group. One year after LASEK, the mean anisometropic difference decreased to 1.81 D, 2.43 D, 0.74 D, and 2.33 D, respectively. Postoperatively, 63.6% of children had an improvement in best corrected visual acuity (BCVA) and the remainder had no noted change. Of 33 children, 39.4% had positive stereopsis preoperatively and 87.9% had positive stereopsis one year after LASEK. In 2010, Astle et al. evaluated a larger cohort of hyperopic anisometropes, lasering 18 eyes of 18 children ranging from +1.75 D to +7.75 D pre laser [47, 66]. 83% of eyes were within 1.00D of targeted refraction, stereopsis improved by 22%, and 64.7% of eyes experienced improved vision one year post laser, adding appropriate amblyopia treatment to the post – op regimen.

Anisometropia secondary to other pathology such as lid and orbital hemangiomas, long standing chalazions, ocular and orbital dermoids, and congenital ptosis, can be successfully treated in the same way [12, 85].These forms of anisometropia whether myopic or hyperopic, are usually associated with oblique astigmatism, which is intensely amblyopiogenic. As shown by France [86] even as little as 1.00D of oblique astigmatism has a 90% chance of inducing significant amblyopia in a child. In these situations, treating the underlying lid or orbital disease, with subsequent laser or pIOL for the residual refractive error, in resistant eyes, can be very safe and effective in restoring a child's vision and stereopsis.

Based on the extensive literature available on the successful refractive treatment of anisometropic amblyopia in all forms, all surgical treatments will work in almost all situations. The final decision on which refractive modality to employ can be left to the experience of the surgeon involved, and gives the refractive surgeon options to consider for all of these complex pediatric conditions.

Refractive Surgery in Children with Coexisting Ocular Pathology

As has been demonstrated in the literature, refractive errors in children rarely present in isolation. In many cases, these children present with multiple ocular disorders that can limit the ultimate visual and fusional results obtainable. However, it has been noted that even faced with significant optic nerve disorders, such as optic atrophy, optic nerve hypoplasia, infantile nystagmus syndromes, and all forms of ocular albinism as more common examples, elimination of the refractive component of the child's problem can have dramatic positive effects on a child's long term visual and functional improvement [13, 14, 16, 22, 47, 55-58, 65-66]. This can be true even in children with severe optic nerve lesions and marked secondary nystagmus. In terms of nystagmus, the improved visual acuity post refractive surgery, can then significantly dampen the child's nystagmus, further improving the overall visual and fusional result [12, 56]. This improvement post refractive surgery has been noted in many other difficult cases that some would consider previously to be inoperable situations.

Most of these children have high refractive errors associated with large astigmatic errors. Regardless of surgical technique employed, these children usually do extremely well post surgery, as their vision, fusion, and nystagmus dramatically improves. This subgroup of children rarely wear glasses and contacts well, and refractive surgery is usually very successful in rehabilitating even the most complex child.

Refractive Surgery Associated with Strabismus

The effect of refractive surgery on ocular alignment is controversial. Nemet et al. [87] performed LASIK in eight adult patients with stable refractive error and strabismus. Ocular alignment improved in all of their cases after LASIK. Conversely, retrospective studies have shown significant decompensation of the preexisting exodeviation with loss of binocular function after refractive surgery for moderate to high myopia [88-89]. However, Nucci et al. [90] performed PRK in 27 young adults with purely refractive accommodative esotropia and concluded that PRK is an effective treatment for esotropia associated with mild to moderate hyperopia. There have also been a few reports in both children and adults [91-94], that hyperopic LASIK significantly reduced esotropia in patients with accommodative esotropia.

Astle et al. noted that the pre-laser strabismus noted in their cases tended to improve after LASEK, allowing for less strabismus surgery to be required [91]. It is important to remember this fact, and be sure to measure carefully post laser refractive surgery, prior to making a final decision on the amount of strabismus surgery to undertake.

Hutchison published a review in 2012 documenting the successful treatment of residual accommodative esotropia with laser refractive surgery [95]. Refractive surgery is especially effective in restoring vision and fusion without the need for optical correction in older children (16-18 years of age) who do not experience enough myopic shift with growth to completely eliminate the need for hyperopic correction. Overall the surgical results in this group are excellent. ASA procedures work extremely well in these situations, and pIOL's are also an excellent option.

Elimination of the refractive component for these patients provides considerable visual and functional improvement, even those with co-existing ocular and medical disorders. If required, with improved UCVA overall post refractive surgery, subsequent strabismus surgery is more likely to be successful in restoring stereopsis, even with patients having complex co-existing medical issues. Based on these positive results in the literature, refractive surgeons and pediatric ophthalmologists should consider the combination of laser refractive surgery with strabismus surgery, as a surgical alternative in patients with these more complex pediatric medical problems [67].

Congenital High Ametropia (Myopic and Hyperopic)

There are now many papers [10-16,] demonstrating the successful use of almost all of the refractive surgery modalities discussed previously. Tychsen [56], and Paysse et al. [55], have documented an excellent strategy to consider when faced with children with high ametropia, especially bilateral situations. Their premise is to consider refractive laser for refractive errors in the mid ranges from -10.00 D to +6.00D. If a child is over -10.00D, the surgeon should consider a pIOL if the anterior chamber depth is appropriate (> 3.2 mm), or a Clear Lens Extraction / Refractive Lens Exchange if the anterior chamber depth is too shallow. In children over +6.00D, one could again attempt a pIOL if the anterior chamber depth is appropriate. This would be seem to be an excellent strategy for all pediatric refractive surgeons to employ as a starting point for making an appropriate surgical plan for a pediatric patient undergoing a refractive procedure.

However, these surgical indications can blurred by improvements in technology. Astle et al., [10, 12-14, 16, 19, 22, 47, 55-57, 58, 65-67, 97] have demonstrated that PRK and LASEK can be effective even as high as -27.00D to +14.00D. As an example of these successful extremes, one child documented by Astle et al., [12, 14, 65], a congenital high myopic child initially labeled at 6 months of age as severely developmentally delayed, underwent PRK laser at 11 months of age for -25.00 D of effect. This patient at time of publication is now 14 years old, with no corneal ectasia, clear corneas bilaterally, and wearing glasses of -6.00D OU. The patient's BCVA is 20/60, limited by retinal issues from his bilateral high myopia, but he is now functional normally in public school. Surprisingly, at age 14, his pachymetry readings are 433 microns, and well out of the range for possible corneal ectasia. These kinds of startling findings in children demonstrate not only how effective refractive surgery can be for children, but as demonstrated in a recent PEDIG study [96]pediatric corneas may be thicker than adult corneas, thus allowing for success in extreme refractive error situations, where adults would potentially have complications, or not be treatable. Further study will help to clarify some of these interesting observations in these complex children.

As outlined by Tychsen [22], refractive surgery of any kind in a high myopic situation magnifies the new image post surgery, reversing any image minification that may cause anesikonia for these patients. For children with bilateral congenital myopia, the combined effect of this additional magnification and improved UCVA can have dramatic positive effects on their ability to function.

In addition, pediatric patients may have different treatment goals than those for a typical adult group. The main goal with children is to keep the eyes balanced throughout the refractive process. As long as significant anisometropia does not remain after surgery, a slight overcorrection or undercorrection is not a concern. As an example, because of the known tendency in children for a myopic shift to occur after laser treatment, the surgeon could aim for an initial post-LASEK hyperopic correction, depending on the age of the child and balancing with the fellow eye [12-14, 47, 58, 65-67, 97].

In children, a true myopic shift secondary to refractive surgery may be indistinguishable from myopic changes that occur with normal axial length changes as children grow [47, 65, 98-99]. Goss [100] [c.23] found that, on average, normal phakic pediatric eyes have a myopic shift of 0.50 D per year. Gordon and Donzis [98] and Moore [99] report that children's eyes continue to undergo significant growth with a myopic shift until 16 to 18 years of age. This regression may be due to an axial myopic shift related to normal growth patterns in pediatric eyes or possibly destruction of Bowman's membrane during laser treatments, which initiates a more vigorous healing response.

Therefore one can anticipate a myopic shift will occur in children post refractive surgery and its occurrence should not be considered a complication or contraindication to refractive surgery [10, 19, 55]. Paysee et al., [19] and Tychsen and Hoekel [10] report refractive regression rates of approximately 1.00 D per year after laser surgery in children. The mean regression rate noted by Astle et al., [65] was 1.46 D per year.

Specific Ocular Diagnosis	Concomitant Medical conditions and associated ocular pathology
Anisometropic Amblyopia – Hyperopic, astigmatic, myopic (or combinations thereof) – Post-cataract surgery anisometropia with/without myopic shift Bilateral high refractive errors Older Children who have not outgrown refractive errors associated with: – Accommodative esotropia – other strabismic disorders – residual hyperopia – accommodative esotropia with residual hyperopia and/or astigmatism – Exotropes where correction of residual refractive error restores fusion	– Ocular, lid and orbital hemangiomas – Goldenhar's syndrome – Ocular dermoids – Autism – Cerebral Palsy-Severe developmental delays – Progressive childhood encephalopthies – Congenital motor nystagmus/infantile nystagmus syndrome – Oclulo-cutaneous Albinism – Down's Syndrome – Various strabismic disorders (commonly esotropia)

Figure 7. Refractive surgery in children- Surgical indications.

In extremes, combinations of treatments could also be considered to achieve even higher refractive results if necessary. The choice of technique in a given situation can still be left to the experience of the surgeon, but as our technology improves, more surgical options and indications are available. As noted in Figure 7, all of the potential pediatric ophthalmic and associated medical conditions that can be successfully treated with refractive surgery with our present technology are documented. The list of potential surgical indications is sure to enlarge as our expertise and technology continues to expand over time.

Conclusion – Pediatric Refractive Surgery - Thoughts for the Future

The speed of technological change in Ophthalmology is astounding, with multiple new potential treatments for children, developing on a monthly basis. New excimer laser platforms will be quicker, and take less tissue to achieve the desired refractive outcome. New diagnostic tools will help map not only the cornea, but the entire eye, making treatments even more accurate. Better understanding of the growth parameters of the pediatric eye, in phakic, aphakic and pseudophakic conditions will also aid both in prediction of appropriate refractive power long-term, but also in more accurate treatment algorithms for children.

In the near future, femtosecond laser technology could yet again positively change the success parameters in dealing with children with extremes refractive error problems. These lasers will undoubtedly become essential tools in treating complex pediatric refractive errors. As a complement to these new tools, improved medical treatments may help further augment long term refractive success in more complicated situations. For example, the use of mitomycin has virtually eliminated corneal haze as a complication with advanced surface ablations, and corneal cross linking has been shown in adults [101] to stabilize and improve corneas prone to ectasia post laser. Treatments such as this could help in pediatric groups more potentially prone to ectasia and keratoconus, such as children with Down's syndrome.

For many children, laser refractive surgery may not be the optimal treatment for their refractive error. New advances in pIOL's, like the Artiflex design with toric capability is an excellent example in IOL design improvements, allowing these lenses to be implanted through very small incisions (2.5 – 3.0 mm). The newer light adjustable IOL's [102] sulcoflex IOL's, and Cachet [103] soft foldable implants may further add to the refractive surgeons' armamentarium in dealing with both large and small refractive errors in children. Further testing over time will further define their potential uses in children. In addition, all of the technologies discussed in this chapter can be used alone or in combination to achieved a desired refractive outcome, even in the most extreme cases.

The days of wondering whether these refractive treatments are safe and appropriate for children are long gone, evidenced by the huge amount of literature supporting the safe and effective use of these new technologies in correcting pediatric refractive errors over the past 20 years. As a profession, we should now move on to analyzing which of these new refractive treatments are most effective in a given circumstance for our patients, thus improving our surgical indications for the treatments. Pediatric Ophthalmologists and refractive surgeons who embrace these new technologies, and employ them in appropriate ways, will be astounded at how well even the most difficult pediatric patient will respond.

We are practicing in a very exciting time, where the Pediatric Ophthalmologist with an open mind can achieve dramatic results for even the most complex child, never before thought possible. Not only do these new technologies and treatments correct a child's refractive error, vision, and stereopsis effectively over the long term, but these new treatments can positively change the trajectory of a child's life, improving their overall quality of life dramatically and permanently. Pediatric refractive surgery works and is here to stay.

References

[1] Holmes JM, Lazar EL, Melia BM, Astle WF, Dagi LR, Donahue, SP, Frazier MG, Hertle RW, Repka MX, Quinn GE, Weise KK, Pediatric Eye Disease Investigator Group. Effect of age on response to amblyopia treatment in children. *Arch. Ophthalmol.* 2011; 129(11): 1451-7.

[2] Scheiman MM, Hertle RW, Beck, RW, et al., Pediatric Eye Disease Investigative Group. Randomized trial of treatment of amblyopia in children aged 7 to 17 years. *Arch. Ophthalmol.* 2005; 123(4): 437-47.

[3] Scheiman MM, Hertle RW, Kraker RT, et al., Pediatric Eye Disease Investigative Group. Patching vs atropine to treat amblyopia in children aged 7 to 12 years: a randomized trial. *Arch. Ophthalmol.* 2008; 126(12): 1634-42.

[4] Quinn GE, Beck RW, Holmes JM, Repka MX. Recent advances in the treatment of amblyopia. *Pediatrics* 2004; 113(6): 1800-2.

[5] Wallace D, Chandler DL, Beck RW, Arnold RW, Bacal DA, Birch EE, Felius J, Frazier M, Holmes JM, Hoover D, Klimek DA, Lorenzana I, Quinn GE, Repka MX, Suh DW, Tamkins S, Pediatric Eye Disease Investigator Group. Treatment of bilateral refractive amblyopia in children 3 to <10 years old. *Am. J. Ophthalmol.* 2007; 144(4): 487-96.

[6] Campos EC, Enoch JM. Amount of aniseikonia compatible with fine binocular vision: some old and new concepts. *J. Pediatr Opthalmol. Strabismus* 1980; 17:44-47.

[7] Kutschke PJ, Scott WE, Keech RV. Anisometropic amblyopia. *Ophthalmology,* 1991; 98:258-263.

[8] Weakley DR Jr. The association between nonstrabismic anisometropia, amblyopia and subnormal binocularity. *Ophthalmology* 2001; 108:163-71.

[9] Parks MM. The monofixation syndrome. *Trans Am. Ophthalmol. Soc.*, 1969;67:609-57. Available at: http://www.ncbi.nlm.nih.gov/pmc/articles/PMC1310353/pdf/taos00032-0625.pdfhttp://www.ncbi.nlm.nih.gov/pmc/articles/PMC1310353/. Accessed January 6, 2013.

[10] Tychsen L, Hoekel J. Refractive surgery for high bilateral myopia subepithelial keratectomy (LASEK). *J. AAPOS* 2006; 10:364-70.

[11] Nucci P, Drack AV. Refractive surgery for unilateral high myopia in children. *J. AAPOS,* 2001; 5:348-51.

[12] Astle WF, Papp A, Huang PT, Ingram A. Refractive laser surgery in children with coexisting medial and ocular pathology. *J. Cataract Refract. Surg.* 2006; 32:103-8.

[13] Astle WF, Huang PT, Ingram AD, Farran RP. Laser-assisted subepithelial keratectomy in children. *J. Cataract Refract. Surg.* 2004; 30:2529-35.

[14] Astle WF, Huang PT, Ells AL, Cox RG, Deschenes MC, Vibert HM. Photorefractive keratectomy in children. *J. Cataract Refract. Surg.* 2002; 28;932-41.

[15] Autrata R, Rehurek J. Laser-assisted subepithelial keratectomy and photorefractive keratectomy versus conventional treatment of myopic anisometropic amblyopia in children. *J. Cataract Refract. Surg.* 2004; 30:74-84.

[16] Tychsen L, Packwood E, Berdy G. Correction of large amblyopiognic refractive errors in children using the excimer laser. *J. AAPOS* 2005; 9:224-33.

[17] Loewenstein A, Lipshitz I, Varssano D, Lazar M. Macular hemorrhage after excimer laser photorefractive keratectomy. *J. Cataract Refract. Surg.* 1997; 23:808-10.

[18] Lee AG, Kohnen T, Ebner R, Bennett JL, Miller NR, Carlow TJ, Koch DD. Optic neruropathy associated with laser in situ keratomileusis. *J. Cataract Refract. Surg.* 200; 26:1581-4.

[19] Paysse EA, Coats DK, Hussein MAW, Hamil MB, Koch DD. Long-term outcomes of photorefractive keratectomy for anisometropic amblyopia in children. *Ophthalmology* 2006; 113:169-76.

[20] Cleary C, Lanigan B, O'Keefe M. Artisan iris-claw lenses for the correction of aphakia in children following lensectomy for ectopia lentis. *Br. J. Ophthalmol.* 2012; 96: 419-21.

[21] Lesueur LC, Arne JL. Phakic intraocular lens to correct high myopic amblyopia in children. *J. Refract. Surg.* 2002; 18: 519-23.

[22] Tychsen L, Hoekel J, Ghasia F, Yoon-Huang G. Phakic intraocular lens correction of high ametropia in children with neurobehavioral disorders. *J. AAPOS* 2008; 12: 282-89.

[23] Wilson M. Intraocular lens implantation: has it become the standard of care for children? *Ophthalmology* 1996; 103:1719-20.

[24] Wilson M, Bluestein E, Wang X. Current trends in the use of intraocular lenses in children. *J. Cataract Refract. Surg*. 1994; 20:579-83.

[25] Wilson ME, Peterseim MW, Englert JA, Lall-Trail JK, Elliott LA. Pseudophakia and polypseudophakia in the first year of life. *J. AAPOS* 2001; 5:238-45.

[26] Plager DA, Kipfer H, Sprunger DT, Sondhi N, Neely DE. Refractive change in pediatric pseudophakia: 6-year follow-up. *J. Cataract Refract. Surg*. 2002; 28: 618-23.

[27] Lambert SR, Buckley EG, Plager DA, Medow NB, Wilson ME. Unilateral intraocular lens implantation during eh first six months of life. *J. AAPOS* 1999; 3:344-9.

[28] Dahan E, Drusedau M. Choice of lens and dioptric power in pediatric pseudophakia. *J. Cataract Refract. Surg*. 1997; 23(suppl. 1):618-23.

[29] Gimbel H, Basti S, Ferensowicz M Debroff B. Results of bilateral cataract extraction with posterior chamber intraocular lens implantation in children. *Ophthalmology* 1997; 104:1737-43.

[30] Plager DA, Lipsky SN, Snyder SK, Sprunger DT, Ellis FD, Sondhi N. Capsular management and refractive error in pediatric intraocular lenses. *Ophthalmology* 1997; 104:600-7.

[31] Rosenbaum A, Masket S. Intraocular lens implantation in children. *Am. J. Ophthalmol.* 1995; 120:105-7.

[32] Crouch ER, Pressman SH, Crouch ER. Posterior chamber intraocular lenses: long-term results in pediatric cataract patients. *J. Pediatr. Ophthalmol. Strabismus* 1995; 32:210-8.

[33] Cheng K. Treatment of pediatric cataracts. *Ophthalmol. Clin. North Am*. 1996; 9: 239-47.

[34] McClatchey S, Parks M. Myopic shift after cataract removal in childhood. *J. Pediatr. Ophthalmol. Strabismus* 1997; 34:239-47.

[35] McClatchey S, Parks M. Theoretic refractive changes after lens implantation in childhood. *Ophthalmology* 1997; 104: 1744-51.

[36] McClatchey SK, Dahan E, Maselli E, Gimbel HV, Wilson ME, Lambert SR, Buckley EG, Freedman SF, Plager DA, Parks MM. A comparison of the rate of refractive growth in pediatric aphakic and pseudophakic eyes. *Ophthalmology* 2000; 107:118-22.

[37] Superstein R, Archer S, Del Monte M. Minimal myopic shift in pseudophakic versus aphakic pediatric cataract patients. *J. AAPOS* 2002; 6:271-6.

[38] Crouch E, Crouch E, Pressman S. Prospective analysis of pediatric pseudophakia: myopic shift and postoperative outcomes. *J. AAPOS* 2002; 6:277-82.

[39] Weakley DR, Birch E, McClatchey SK, Felius J, Parks MM, Stager D Jr. The association between myopic shift and visual acuity outcome in pediatric aphakia. *J. AAPOS* 2003 Apr; 7(4): 86-90.

[40] Inatomi M, Kora Y, Kinohira Y, Yaguchi S. Long-term follow-up of eye growth in pediatric patients after unilateral cataract surgery with intraocular lens implantation. *J. AAPOS* 2004; 8:50-5.

[41] Enyedi L, Peterseim M, Freedman S, Buckley E. Refractive changes after pediatric intraocular lens implantation. *Am. J. Ophthalmol*. 1998; 126:772-81.

[42] Gordon R, Donzis P. Refractive development of the human eye. *Arch. Ophthalmol.* 1985; 103:785-9.

[43] Neely D, Plager D, Borger S, Golub R. Accuracy of intraocular lens calculations in infants and children undergoing cataract surgery. *J. AAPOS* 2005; 9:160-5.

[44] Eibschitz-Tsimhoni M, Archer SM, Del Monte MA. Intraocular lens power calculation in children. *Surv. Ophthalmol.* 2007 52(5), 474-82.

[45] Wilson ME, Bartholomew LR, Trivedi R. Pediatric cataract surgery and intraocular lens implantation. Practice styles and preferences of the 2001 ASCRS and AAPOS memberships. *J. Cataract Refract. Surg.* 2003; 29(9):1811-20.

[46] Dahan E. Intraocular lens implantation in children. *Curr. Opin. Ophthal.* 2000; 51-55.

[47] Astle WF, Ingram AD, Isaza GM, Echeverri P. Paediatric pseudophakia: analysis of intraocular lens power and myopic shift. *Clinical and Experimental Ophthalmology* 2007; 6(3):244-51.

[48] Mezer E, Rootman DS, Abdolell M, Levin AV. Early post-operative refractive outcomes of pediatric intraocular lens implantation. *J. Cataract Refract. Surg.* 2004; 30(3): 603-10.

[49] Eibschitz-Tsimhoni M, Tsimhoni O, Archer SM, Del Monte MA. Discrepancies between intraocular lens implant power prediction formulas in pediatric patients. *Ophthalmology* 2007; 114(2):383-6.

[50] Eibschitz-Tsimhoni M, Tsimhoni O, Archer SM, Del Monte MA. Effect of axial length and K measurement error on intraocular lens implant power prediction formulas in pediatric eyes. *J. AAPOS* 2008; 12(2):173-6.

[51] Moore DB, Zion B, Neely D. Accuracy of biometry in pediatric cataract extraction with primary intraocular lens implantation. *J. Cataract Refract. Surg.* 2008; 34(11):1940-7.

[52] Lin AA, Buckley EG. Update on pediatric cataract surgery and intraocular lens implantation. *Curr. Opin. Ophthalmol.* 2010; 21(1):55-59.

[53] McClatchey SK, Parks MM. Theoretic refractive changes after lens implantation in childhood. *Ophthalmology* 1997; 104(11):1744-51.

[54] Khan MI, Muhtaseb M. Performance of the Sulcoflex piggyback intraocular lens in pseudophakic patients. *J. Refract. Surg.* 2011; 27(9): 693-6.

[55] Paysse EA, Tychsen MD, Stahl E. Pediatric refractive surgery: Corneal and intraocular techniques and beyond. *J. AAPOS* 2012; 16: 291-7.

[56] Tychsen L. Refractive surgery for children: excimer laser, phakic intraocular lens, and clear lens extraction. *Curr. Opin. Ophthalmol.* 2008; 19: 342-8.

[57] Tychsen L. Refractive surgery for special needs children. *Arch. Ophthalmol.* 2009; 127(6): 810-13.

[58] Astle WF, Hackenbergova L, Huang PT, Ruddell S. Improvement in vision and stereopsis after laser-assisted subepithelial keratectomy (LASEK) for children with albinism. *Clinical & Surgical Ophthalmology* 2011; 29(1): 10-15.

[59] Agarwal A, Agarwal A, Agarwal T, et al. Results of pediatric laser in situ keratomileusis. *J. Cataract Refract. Surg.* 2000; 26: 684-89.

[60] Alio JL, Artola A, Claramonte P, et al. Photorefractive keratectomy for pediatric myopic anisometropia. *J. Cataract Refract. Surg.* 1998; 24: 327-330.

[61] Singh D. Photorefractive keratectomy in pediatric patients. *J. Cataract Refract. Surg.* 1995; 21: 630-2.

[62] Nano HD Jr, Muzzin S, Fernandez Irigaray L. Excimer laser photorefractive keratectomy in pediatric patients. *J. Cataract Refract. Surg.* 1997; 23: 736-9.

[63] Rashad KM. Laser in situ keratomileusis for myopic anisometropia in children. *J. Refract. Surg.* 1999; 15: 429-35.

[64] Haw WW, Alcorn DM, Manchee EE. Excimer Laser refractive surgery in the pediatric population. *J. Pediatr. Ophthalmol. Strabismus* 1999; 36: 173-7.
[65] Astle WF, Fawcett SL, Huang PT, Alewenah O, Ingram A. Long-term outcomes of photorefractive keratectomy and laser-assisted subepithelial keratectomy in children. *J. Cataract Refract. Surg.* 2008; 34:411-6.
[66] Astle WF, Huang PT, Ereifej I, Paszuk A. Laser-assisted subepithelial keratectomy for bilateral hyperopia and hyperopic anisometropic amblyopia in children: one-year outcomes. *J. Cataract Refract. Surg.* 2010; 36: 260-7.
[67] Astle WF, Huang PT, Ereifej I, Paszuk AM. Laser-assisted subepithelial keratectomy (LASEK) combined with strabismus surgery: improved combination for restoring vision and fusion. *Clin. Surg. Ophthalmol.* 2009; 27:8-11.
[68] Shahinian L Jr. Laser-assisted subepithelial keratectomy for low to high myopia and astigmatism. *J. Cataract Refract. Surg.* 2002; 28: 1334-42.
[69] Autrata R, Rehurek J, Holousova M. [Photorefractive keratectomy in high myopic anisometropia in children]. [Czechoslovakian] *Cesk. Slov. Oftalmol.* 1999; 55: 216-21.
[70] Lee JB, Seong GH, Lee JH, et al. Comparison of laser epithelial keratomileusis and photorefractive keratectomy for low to moderate myopia. *J. Cataract Refract. Surg.* 2001; 27:565-70.
[71] Azar DT, Ang RT, Lee J-B, et al. Laser subepithelial keratomileusis: electron microscopy and visual outcomes fo flap photorefractive keratectomy. *Curr. Opin. Ophthalmol.* 2001; 12: 323-8.
[72] Espana EM, Grueterich M, Mateo A, et al. Cleavage of corneal basement membrane components by ethanol in laser-assisted subepithelial keratectomy. *J. Cataract Refract. Surg.* 2003; 29: 1192-7.
[73] Dvali ML, tsintsadze NA, Mirtskhulava SE. Features of hyperopic LASIK in children. *J. Refract. Surg.* 2005;21: S614-S616.
[74] Utine CA, Cakir H, Egemenoglu A, Perente I. LASIK in children with hyperopic anisometropic amblyopia. *J. Refract. Surg.* 2008; 24: 464-72.
[75] Lesueur LC, Arne JL. Phakic posterior chamber lens implantation in children with high myopia. *J. Cataract Refract. Surg.* 1999; 25:1571-75.
[76] BenEzra D, Cohen E, Karshai I. Phakic posterior chamber intraocular lens for the correction of anisometropia and treatment of amblyopia. *Am. J. Ophthalmol.* 2000; 130: 292-6.
[77] Saxena R, van Minderhout HM, Luyten GPM. Anterior chamber iris-fixated phakic intraocular lens for anisometropic amblyopia. *J. Cataract Refract. Surg.* 2003; 29: 835-8.
[78] Lifshitz T, Levy J. Secondary artisan phakic intraocular lens for correction of progressive high myopia in a pseudophakic child. *J. AAPOS* 2005; 9:497-8.
[79] Assil KK, Sturm JM, Chang SH. Verisyse intraocular lens implantation in a child with anisometropic amblyopia: four-year follow up. *J. Cataract Refract. Surg.* 2007; 33: 1985-6.
[80] Alio JL, Toffaha BT, Laria C, Pinero DP. Phakic intraocular lens implantation for treatment of anisometropia and amblyopia in children: 5-year follow up. *J. Refract. Surg.* 2011; 27:494-501.
[81] Pirouzian A, Ip KC, O'Halloran HS. Phakic anterior chamber intraocular lens (Verisyse TM) implantation in children for treatment of severe ansiometropia myopia and

amblyopia: six-month pilot clinical trial and review of literature. *Clin. Ophthalmol.* 2009; 3: 367-71.

[82] Pirouzian A. Pediatric phakic intraocular lens surgery: review of clinical studies. *Curr. Opin. Ophthalmol.* 2010; 21: 249-54.

[83] Odenthal M Th P, Sminia ML, Prick LJJM, Gortzak-Moorstein N, Volker-Dieben HJ. Long-term follow-up of the corneal endothelium after artisan lens implantation for unilateral traumatic and unilateral congenital cataract in children: two case series. *Cornea* 2006; 25:1173-7.

[84] Autrata R, Rehurek J. Clinical results of excimer laser photorefractive keratectomy for high myopic anisometropia in children: Four-year follow up. *J. Cataract Refract. Surg.* 2003; 29: 694-702.

[85] Frank RC, Cowan BJ, Harrop AR, Astle WF, McPhalen DF. Visual development in infants: visual complications of periocular haemangiomas. *J. Plast. Reconstr. Aesthet. Surg. 2010;63:1-8.*

[86] France LW. Evidence-based guidelines for amblyopgenicrisk factors. *Am. Orthopt. J.* 2006; 56:7-14.

[87] Nemet P, Levinger S, Nemet A. Refractive surgery for refractive errors which cause strabismus. A report of 8 cases. *Binocul. Vis. Strabismus Q* 2002; 17:187-90.

[88] Snir M, Kremer I, Weinberger D, et al. Decompensation of exodeviations after corneal refractive surgery for moderate to high myopia. *Ophthalmic Surg. Lasers Imaging* 2003; 34:363-70.

[89] Yap E-Y, Kowal L. Diplopia as a compication of laser in situ keratomileusis surgery. *Graefes Arch. Clin. Exp. Ophthalmol.* 2001; 29:268-71.

[90] Nucci P, Serafino M, Hutchinson AK. Photorefractive keratectomy for the treatment of purely refractive accommodative esotropia. *J. Cataract Refract. Surg*. 2003; 29: 889-94.

[91] Astle WF, Huang PT, Ereifej I, Paszuk AM. Laser-assisted subepithelial keratectomy (LASEK) combined with strabismus surgery: improved combination for restoring vision and fusion. *Clin. Surg. Ophthalmol*. 2009;27:8-11.

[92] Hoyos JE, Cigales M, Hoyos-Chacon J, et al. Hyperopic laser in situ keratomileusis for refractive accomodative esotropia. *J. Cataract Refrac. Surg*. 2002; 28:1522-9.

[93] Phillips CB, Prager TC, McClellan G, et al. Laser in situ keratomileusis for treated anisometropic amblyopia in awake, autofixating pediatric and adolescent patients. *J. Cataract Refract. Surg.* 2004; 30: 2522-8.

[94] Stidham DB, Borissova O, Borissov V. Effect of hyperopic laser in situ keratomileusis on ocular alignment and stereopsis in patients with accommodative esotropia. *Ophthalmology* 2002; 109: 1148-53.

[95] Hutchinson AK. Refractive surgery for accommodative esotropia: past, present, and future. *Eur. J. Ophthalmol.* 2012; 22:871-77.

[96] Pediatric Eye Disease Investigator Group, Bradfield YS, Melia BM, Repka MX, Kaminski BM, Davitt BV, Johnson DA, Kraker RT, Manny RE, Matta NS, Weise KK, Schloff S. Central corneal thickness in children. *Arch. Ophthalmol.* 2011; 129:1132-8.

[97] Astle WF, Rahmat J, Ingram AD, Huang PT. Laser=assisted subepithelial keratectomy for anisometropic amblyopia in children: Outcomes at 1 year. *J. Cataract Refract. Surg.* 2007; 33: 2028-34.

[98] Moore AT. Refraction in childhood. *Trans Ophthalmol. Soc. UK* 1985; 104:648-52.

[99] Gordon RA, Donzis PB. Refractive development of the human eye. *Arch. Ophthalmol.* 1985; 103: 785-9.

[100] Goss DA. Variables related to the rate of childhood myopia progression. *Optom. Vis. Sci.* 1990; 67:631-6.

[101] Kymionis GD, Kiakonis VF, Kalyvianaki M, Portaliou D, Siganos C, Kozobolis VP, Pallikaris Al. One-year follow-up of corneal confocal miscroscopy after corneal cross-linking in patients with post laser in situ keratosmileusis ectasia and keratoconus. *Am. J. Ophthalmol.* 2009; 147:774-8.

[102] Hengerer FH. [Current state of the "light-adjustable lens"]. [German]. *Klinische Monatsblatter fur Augenheilkunde* 2012; 229; 784-93.

[103] Mastropasqua L, Toto L, Vecchiarino L, Doronzo E, Mastropasqua R, Di Nicola M. AcrySof cachet phakic intraocular lens in myopic patients: visual performance, wavefront error, and lens position. *J. Refract. Surg.* 2012; 28:267-74.

In: Current Understanding and New Techniques ...
Editor: Michael O'Keefe
ISBN: 978-1-62808-748-2

Chapter 7

Intraocular Lens Power Calculations Post Refractive Surgery

Grainne Brosnan[*]
Mater Private Hospital, Dublin, Ireland

Abstract

This chapter provides a review of intraocular lens power calculation for the post refractive surgery patient. Biometry methods are described including, ultrasound, immersion and optical biometry. The effect of these methods on the final IOL power value is defined. Corneal power is difficult to measure accurately in the post refractive surgery eye, as the Gullstrand-ratio has been altered. Methods to overcome this obstacle are specified. A brief history of formula development and progression is included, with particular emphasis on the effect of formula choice. Methods of IOL power calculation both historical and non historical are outlined. Eight methods of calculation widely known from earlier days to the most current available are considered. It is anticipated that the content will assist practitioners involved in IOL power calculation for the post refractive patient and draw attention to the errors related to the process. Errors such as biometry methods, employed data, formula application, technology application and user dependency are all addressed. The chapter endeavours to simplify a complex task by allowing the practitioner to use methods available whatever the clinic setting and technology accessible. It is not always necessary to invest in expensive equipment in order to complete IOL calculation for the post refractive patient.

Introduction

Refractive surgery has increased in popularity worldwide over the last 20 years. Increasingly, these patients are now presenting for cataract surgery. Most refractive surgery involves modification of the corneal curvature which in turn presents difficulty in determining

[*] gbrosnan@materprivate.ie.

its actual keratometric power. This is a major issue that challenges biometry measurement and correct intraocular lens (IOL) power calculation prior to cataract surgery. Post refractive surgery patients have a great desire to be spectacle free and expect to be so after cataract surgery.

This places increased demands on the cataract surgeon to avoid a refractive surprise and the possible threat of litigation. This chapter provides guidelines to optimize predictability of refractive outcome in these patients.

Biometry Methods

Biometry involves measurement of axial length, keratometry (power of the cornea) and anterior chamber depth (ACD). This data together with an IOL formula are used to calculate the correct lens power for the desired post operative refraction (target refraction). Advances in technology have helped achieve results which are more accurate than before. The developments of various biometry techniques have helped solve outstanding issues. This is definitely the case in relation to axial length measurement.

Ultrasound biometry (A-scan ultrasonography) was for many years the only method available to obtain axial length. Contact between the probe and the cornea is essential, but inadvertent indentation of the eyeball may result in underestimation of axial length. The degree of error is user dependant. An underestimated axial length leads to overestimation of the IOL power required.

This biometry method evolved to an immersion technique, which still relies on contact with the eyeball using a scleral shell. Fluid, normally balance salt solution is placed in the shell (Prager) allowing the probe to be suspended and therefore corneal contact is not necessary. Although the cornea remains untouched results are still susceptible to changes in sound velocity. Longer eyes are especially vulnerable and there is the issue of contact between the shell and the eyeball.

However this method is still widely used today and has advantages in certain situations such as in the presence of a dense cataract. Optical biometry devices are unable to measure axial length in the presence of mature cataracts and so the immersion technique is essential to obtain a reading. Another benefit is that measurements can be obtained while the patient is in a reclined position. Optical biometry devices require the patient to sit still with the head aligned and this may be difficult for some patients.

Today biometry is mostly performed using a non-contact technique. The IOL Master (Carl Zeiss Meditec) uses laser interferometry to measure both axial length and keratometry. The Lenstar LS 900 (Haag-Streit) optical biometer uses optical low-coherence reflectometry to obtain seven measurements of the eye including axial length. Standard IOL formulas (SRK-T, Holladay 1, Hoffer Q and Haigis) are incorporated into the software of both machines with differing formulas presented for eyes post refractive surgery. Now that this technology has provided true precision with regard to axial length measurement, the challenge to obtain reliable keratometry readings and to apply the appropriate formula remains.

Keratometry

Keratometry values can be generated from many instruments and these include simulated keratometry, autokeratometry and manual keratometry. Corneal power is measured differently depending on the instrument, but the central most significant part of the cornea is not yet measurable using any of the techniques. Topography for example, measures more peripherally than centrally and so the anterior radius of curvature value may be steeper than the centre especially in the oblate cornea post laser for myopia. Although an invaluable tool to determine the steep axis of regular astigmatism, manual or autokeratometry provide a more accurate central corneal power when calculating IOL power prior to cataract surgery [1]. In contrast the IOL Master (Carl Zeiss Meditec), an autokeratometer applies a computer algorithm to the 2.5mm corneal zone measured. This radial figure is the first error encountered when measuring keratometry using traditional methods on a cornea post refractive surgery.

Corneal power is derived from the anterior radius value. A constant ratio (Gullstrand-ratio) between the anterior and posterior radius is assumed by many devices in order to calculate a corneal power figure. However refractive lasers intentionally change this ratio by modifying the cornea. This is demonstrated by a flattening of the cornea during a myopic treatment and a steeper cornea produced from a hyperopic treatment.

These errors are further exaggerated when an IOL formula is applied. This is because the derived corneal power is employed by some formulas for the effective lens position (ELP) post-operatively. These are intrinsic errors of the traditional methods, devices and calculations used to obtain biometry and calculate an accurate intraocular lens power. Haigis [2] describes these three independent error sources related to keratometry values when calculating an IOL for previously treated myopic eyes as:

- the radius measurement error
- keratometery index error
- IOL formula error

The error attributed to flawed corneal radius measurement is small and equivalent to less than a few tenths of a diopter. This is mainly due to the fact that nearly all refractive surgeons are treating corneas with larger ablation zones than in the early days. Both the keratometry index error and the formula error will be addressed in this chapter and are applicable to all methods whether historical or non historical.

Formulas and Intraocular Lens calculation

Fundamental knowledge and understanding of IOL formulas is necessary to appreciate the errors that occur during IOL calculation in an eye post refractive surgery. A brief history of formulas and their progressions is appropriate. There are two classifications of IOL power calculation formulas, Regression and Theoretical. Regression formulas are derived from linear regression analysis of large number of clinical data and were widely popular in the 1980's. Two such formulas are Sanders, Retzlaff and Kraff (SRK) and Binkhorst 11; these formulas are regarded as first generation formulas. Improvements continued at a rapid pace and so second, third and fourth generation formulas were developed. Estimated lens position (ELP) was incorporated although the method of deriving this value differed between the formulas. In 1998 Holladay [3] published the first theoretical vergence formula using a two variable predictor of ELP, axial length and corneal power. SRKT, Holladay 1, and Hoffer Q are the most popular formulas of this nature. It became apparent with implementation of this new generation of formulas that some were more accurate than others in certain circumstances. This was mostly noticed in eyes outside normal parameters. Hoffer [4] reported when comparing his Hoffer Q formula with the Holladay 1, the results were comparable in the normal range of eyes with axial lengths ranging from 22.0 to 24.5 mm. Longer eyes above 24.5mm showed less reliable results and shorter eyes less than 22.0mm were more accurate. In 2008 Aristodemou et al. [5] published the efficacy of the Hoffer Q formula for short eyes as statistically significant. Table 1 below is a guideline given for application when calculating IOL power with the IOL Master machine (Carl Zeiss Meditec).[6] The company describe formula selection as a medical decision and emphasises that it cannot recommend formulas but can reference surgeon results.

Table 1.

	Axial length	*Formula*
Short eyes	Less than 22.0mm	Hoffer Q or Haigis
Normal eyes	22.0mm to 25.0mm	Holladay, Haigis, SRKT and HofferQ
Long eyes	Greater than 25.0mm	Holladay, Haigis or SRKT
Eyes post Laser refractive surgery (PRK, LASIK or LASEK)		Haigis L, corneal K's correction after refractive corneal surgery

Reference: Carl Zeiss Meditec AG, 2010, p.74. User manual IOLMaster with Advanced Technology. Jena, Germany.

Fourth generation formulas predict ELP using four or more variables. Olsen et al. included axial length (AL), keratometry (K), pre operative anterior chamber depth (ACD) and lens thickness in 1995. [7] Later Holladay employed seven factors, the four used above with the addition of horizontal corneal diameter, pre operative refraction and age. The more information supplied regarding the anterior segment, the more reliable the ELP. The Holladay 2 formula is available with the Holladay IOL Consultant Software program. The Haigis formula differs from the above mentioned as it does not use corneal power (K) to predict ELP and therefore has an advantage when applied to eyes post refractive surgery.

Methods to Calculate IOL power post Laser Surgery

There are many articles in the literature which offer solutions to problems associated with IOL power calculation post refractive surgery. All processes can be divided according to the data required. Methods requiring prior refractive surgery data are known as the Historical group and methods accepting only current data are referred to as the Non historical group. Table 2 outlines methods addressed in this chapter.

Clinical History Method (Historical)

This method was first described by Holladay [8] and later by Hoffer [9] in order to estimate a figure of true corneal power. The method assumes that if the corneal change due to the flattening affect of the laser could be calculated and added to the pre laser power of the cornea, an effective corneal power could be established.

Table 2.

Historical Methods	Non Historical Methods
Clinical history method	Hard contact lens method
Aramberri double K	BESST2 and Pentacam
Koch and Wang nomogram	Barasio and IOLMaster
Feiz nomogram	Haigis L and IOLMaster
Masket method	Shammas post Lasik formula
ASCRS calculator	ASCRS calculator

The formula shown below requires the availability of data from the facility that performed the refractive surgery and therefore this method is classed as historical in nature.

$$K_{pre} + R_{pre} - R_{post} = K\text{ (estimated)}$$

The pre-operative keratometry reading (K_{pre}), the pre-operative refractive error spherical equivalent (SE) (R_{pre}) and the stable post-operative refraction (R_{post}) are all necessary to complete the calculation. It is important to mention here that the post-operative refraction should be one that has been recorded once the refraction has stabilised following the refractive procedure.

This is before any impact from cataract development, as to avoid the interference of cataract induced myopia. It is also essential to review all the refractive notes (patient file) in order to rule out any enhancement laser treatments. For example:

A patient with a pre refractive surgery average keratometry value of 44.00 diopters (D), a pre operative refractive error of -4.00D, and a stable post operative refraction of -0.25D with no evidence of laser enhancement, the equation would be as follows.

$$44.00D + (-4.00D) - (-0.25D) = 40.25D$$

Theoretically, avoiding the wrong corneal power reading generated by keratometers and topographers should yield more accurate IOL calculations. Unfortunately, correcting the K value for the post refractive eye with the clinical history method minimizes, but does not eliminate hyperopic results post operatively completely [10]. This is because the K value is entered into an IOL program, traditionally a third generation formula. However these types of formula use axial length and keratometry to estimate the ELP and assumes that a flat cornea equals a shallow ACD and so positions the lens closer to the cornea than is necessary. It is obvious that the ACD of an eye post refractive surgery is the same as it was pre operatively, it is only the cornea that has been altered. In 2003 Aramberri provided a solution to this problem with the Double K Correction method.

The Double-K Correction Method (Historical)

As indicated in the name this method employs two K values with one of the third generation IOL formulas. The first keratometry value determined is the pre refractive surgery value and this is applied to the ELP calculation (K_1). Secondly, a post refractive keratometry is determined which is used separately for the vergence formula IOL power calculation (K_2). The K_1 value is retrieved from either topography or keratometry results recorded prior to laser treatment. To obtain K_2 the Clinical History Method is applied. Again this method is dependant on patient data available. In 2003 Aramberri reported that using this method produced predictability of IOL calculations similar to results of cataract surgery in eyes with no previous refractive surgery, 90% within ±1.0 diopter [11]. This was concluded from a study of nine patients where the SRK/T formula was applied with the double K correction method. It is evident that a working knowledge of third generation formulas is necessary in order to apply the double K method. Information from the refractive facility where the surgery was performed is also required, in order to apply the two K values to the formula.

Nomograms devised by Koch and Wang [12] adopting Aramberri's double K method were published the same year, for those less familiar with formulas. The nomogram assumes a pre refractive surgery K of 43 diopters and the Alcon SA60AT intraocular lens for implantation. Values are applied to Hoffer Q, SRKT, and Holladay 1 formula for IOL adjustment in relation to the amount of refractive treatment induced. For example nomogram values are proportion to the amount of laser treatment received and are added in myopic cases or subtracted in hyperopic cases. An earlier nomogram produced by Feiz et al. is based on the change in refraction produced by a myopic laser assisted sub epithelial keratomilesis (LASIK) or photorefractive keratectomy (PRK) treatment independent of pre-operative corneal power [13].The spherical equivalent (SE) value of the change in refraction is calculated and biometry is performed with the IOL master (Carl Zeiss Meditec). To calculate IOL power the SRK/T formula is selected. This result is then adjusted by the addition of the nomogram value. (Table 3) This nomogram is for post myopic LASIK and PRK treatments only.

Table 3.

Induced change by LASIK/PRK (diopters in SE)	Addition to IOL power in diopters
1.00	0.36
1.50	0.66
2.00	0.96
2.50	1.26
3.00	1.55

Masket Method (Historical)

The Masket regression formula was published in 2006 as a method requiring knowledge of the amount of laser treatment induced in dioptres but independent of the double K correction method. [14] Masket developed a correction factor based on the premise that there is correlation between the amount of laser induced during refractive surgery and the amount of refractive surprise post cataract surgery. This method is similar to the Feiz nomogram but has an advantage, as it may be applied to eyes post myopic and hyperopic laser treatments.

Simulated keratometry readings are measured on the post refractive eye. Masket himself used an IOL Master (Carl Zeiss Meditec). The Hoffer Q formula is advised for eyes less than 23.0mm and the Holladay 1 formula for axial lengths greater than 23.0mm. Once the IOL calculation power is obtained the following is applied:

(Laser treatment in diopters) x (-0.326) + 0.101. = Post LASIK IOL adjustment

Hill reported a Modified Masket formula which is slightly different. It is based on data produced as a result of validating the original method.[15] There is still the need for the spherical equivalent figure of treated laser.

(Laser treatment in diopters) x (-0.4385) + 0.0295 = Post LASIK IOL adjustment

The American Society of Cataract and Refractive Surgeons (ASCRS) Calculator (Both History and no History)

In the last decade many IOL calculators have become available on line. The American Society of Cataract and Refractive Surgeons (ASCRS) site calculates IOL power for eyes that have had previous laser-assisted in situ keratomileusis (LASIK), photorefractive keratectomy (PRK) or radial keratotomy (RI). It generates results for both myopic and hyperopic refractive treatments. Many methods of calculation are included, and utilised depending on what information is entered. A result can be produced irrespective of the situation, such as:

- with no previous data,
- using the keratometry values prior to LASIK and PRK and surgically induced change
- change in manifest refraction post refractive surgery

The calculator employs Aramberri's double-K method with the Holladay1 formula, as described earlier to estimate the effective lens position using the pre-refractive corneal power. If this cannot be applied from the information entered, a default of K 43.86D is used [16]. An evaluation of the ASCRS calculator by Wang and associates in 2010 reported that the method based on pre LASIK/PRK and the change in refraction was inferior to the method using partial pre operative data or no data at all [17]. The calculator advises that it serves as a tool for IOL power calculation and it is the responsibility of the surgeon to independently determine the power of intraocular lens for implantation. It warns that there is no guarantee that every result will be accurate and has a disclaimer which must be accepted to access the calculator page.

More recently, the ASCRS IOL calculator in conjunction with optical coherence tomography (OCT) measurement was described as a better method than the hard contact lens method in the absence of prior refractive data for post myopic LASIK eyes [18].An advantage of Web-based calculators is that methods are easily updated, in fact the ASCRS calculator now uses seven methods which increases to twelve depending on the imputed data. Another web-based calculator the OcularMD Post Lasik IOL Calculator uses up to eleven methods, including all previously mentioned approaches.[19]

The no history methods or those that do not require pre-operative data of keratometry or refractive change are evolving all the time and can produce varied results depending on the method of calculation used. However both calculators provide an average of the results which is of great advantage when faced with the situation of no previous data available or equipment such as Pentacam (Oculus Opikgerate GmbH) and optical biometers.

The Hard Contact Lens Method (No History)

When past refractive data is unavailable the hard contact lens method can be applied. Holladay first described this method in order to determine a K value. In theory, when a hard contact lens with the same power as the cornea is applied to the eye there is no change in refraction. Therefore a change in refraction can determine the change in corneal power. However a best corrected vision of at minimum 20/80 is a prerequisite to attempt this method [20]. This may not always be the case when a patient initially arrives for cataract assessment. If a manifest refraction can be preformed and recorded with confidence, consequently a plano rigid contact lens of known base curve is placed on the eye and a second manifest refraction preformed. If a myopic refraction is achieved, the amount of change is equal to the additional steepness of the contact lens, and the opposite applies for a hyperopic change. For example:

- the first refraction recorded results in -2.00D
- plano contact lens of base curve 40.00D applied
- second refraction recorded results in : -3.00D
- calculated corneal power : 40.00D – 1.00D = 39.00D

Boarasio, Edmondo, Smith and Stevens (BESSt2) Calculator (No History)

The Boarasio, Edmondo, Smith and Stevens (BESSt and BESSt2) formula was specifically developed for use independent of pre-refractive data and so employs corneal radii measurements from a Pentacam (Oculus Opikgerate GmbH). The calculation requires both anterior and posterior radii measurements in addition to corneal pachymetry. It is recommended for eyes post LASIK, PRK in both instances of myopic or hyperopic treatments. BESSt2 is an advanced formula which incorporates additional improvements including Aramberri's Double-K adjustment for predictable effective lens position (ELP) estimation. The calculated corneal power, together with the SRK/T or Hoffer Q formulas produces an IOL power. An axial length measurement is also necessary.

It has been reported that outcomes of smaller standard deviations are achievable when the BESSt formula is applied, compared to methods using pre-refractive data [21]. Specifically the Clinical History Method whether the double-K adjustment is utilised or not and the Holladay 2 formula with the topographic K values. More recently, the Borasio Myopic Regression and Borasio Hyperopic Regression formula (BMR and BHR) is another approach presented which requires only IOL Master measurements in conjunction with the SRK/T formula. This method differs from the above as there is no need for Pentacam measurements. The BMR and BHR formulas are part of the EyePro 2012 which is available on the iPhone / iPad technology. [22] The BESSt2 IOL Calculator is software used with the Pentacam system.

The Haigis L formula (No History)

The Haigis formula differs from other third generation formulas. Corneal power is not used to estimate effective lens position, therefore the only error which must be corrected is the keratometer index error [23]. This formula has incorporated a correction curve specifically for the IOL Master (Carl Zeiss Meditec) machine which eliminates this error. Version four and subsequent models of the machine provide the Haigis L formula along with traditional IOL formulas. The practitioner selects the formula based on individual patient requirements, therefore knowledge of whether the previous refractive treatment was myopic or hyperopic in nature is esstential. This formula is not to be used for eyes post Radial Keratotomy treatments.

Shammas Post Lasik Formula (No History)

This formula is also referred to as a no history method, as it does not rely on pre-operative data or knowledge of the extent of myopic laser induced. It was first described in 2003 and employs a corrected K value which is clinically derived, (cd) using a regression equation as follows:

$$K_{cd} = 1.14K_{post} - 6.8$$

This equation was developed as a result of a retrospective analysis of 200 eyes using pre and post-operative data [24]. The results produced a method to calculate corrected corneal power without the necessity to track down previous patient data. This K value is used in the Shammas post LASIK formula. The error associated with third generation formulas (SRK/T, Holladay 1 and Hoffer Q) is not applicable with this formula as it does not rely on corneal curvature to estimate the effective lens position. This is also true for the Haigis formula. In 2007 the Shammas Post LASIK formula was reported as a viable alternative when compared to the following formulas, SRK/T, Holladay 1, Hoffer Q, Haigis and Holladay 2 [25]. Calculations used the Aramberri double K correction method for ELP estimation where appropriate (SRK/T, Holladay 1, Hoffer Q and Hollady 2). All K values were derived using the no history method as described in the formula above.

Table 4. Summary of: Intraocular lens power calculations after myopic laser refractive surgery: a comparison of methods in 173 eyes by McCarthy et al. presented by HJ Shammas at the ESCRS Satellite Education Program 2011

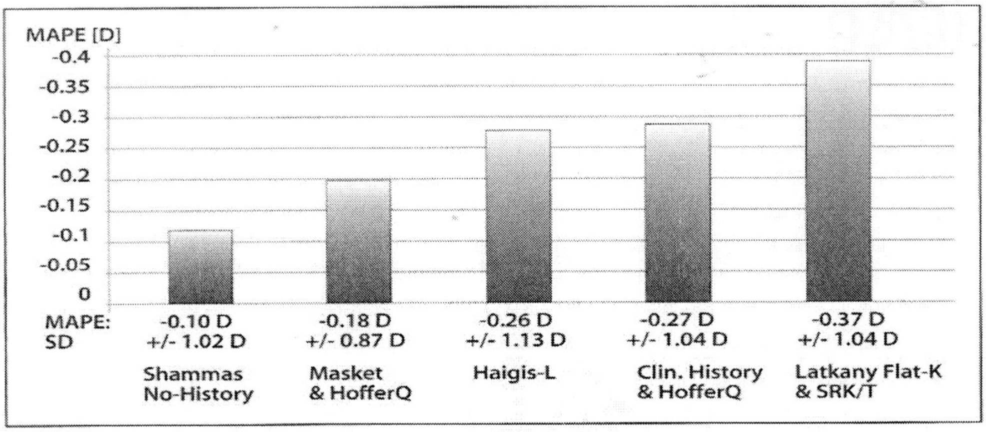

The mean arithmetic prediction errors and standard deviations in the top five most popular IOL calculation methodologies.[5]

McCarthy reported that using the methods in the table above 70% to 85% of eyes could achieve target refraction within 1.0D. [26]

Today biometry with the Lenstar LS 900 (Haag-Streit) incorporates the Shammas no-history method in its software. It is available for calculations post LASIK or PRK including both myopic and hyperopic laser treatments. This machine is an optical coherence biometry similar to the IOL Master (Carl Zeiss Meditec).

Conclusion

The calculation of IOL power in an eye with history of corneal refractive surgery has dramatically changed in recent years. A complex task, requiring arithmetic equations to obtain true corneal power, retrieval of past patient data and IOL formula selection has been simplified enormously. Literature and publications have provided many recommendations and several methods to assist surgeons in their quest to provide these patients with the desired post operative target refraction and remain spectacle free.

Advances in technology have helped eliminate errors of axial length, with the introduction of optical biometers. The development of IOL formulas that do not employ keratometry readings to predict the estimated lens position (ELP) have benefited the process. Formula alterations such as the Aramberri double-K correction initially and more recently the Haigis L and Shammas PL and have contributed enormously.

Manufacturers have combined the advances in technology with software that amalgamates the adapted formulas. This allows biometry to be preformed in minutes providing reliable IOL power estimation, irrespective of available historical data or whether laser treatment was myopic or hyperopic in nature. Biometry takes the same amount of time for post refractive surgery patients as for virgin corneas.

Equipment however is expensive and many models use different methods. Lenstar LS 900 (Haag-Streit) uses the Shammas PL formula, IOL Master (Carl Zeiss Medtec) incorporates the Haigis L formula and the BESSt2 works with the Pentacam (Oculus Opikgerate GmbH). The ASCRS calculator is available on line to all practices and does not incur any cost as is necessary when acquiring some of the more expensive newer equipment.

The challenges surrounding IOL power calculation for post refractive surgery patients have been addressed from many different aspects. The practicality of generating results during a busy clinic for these patients has been solved. However it remains as with all measurements that the data extracted is only as reliable as the accuracy of the data entered. Results are still user dependant even though optical biometers have replaced contact ultrasound biometry. Measurements outside the norm must be queried, final figures should be evaluated and post operative audits are essential. The educated mind must prevail despite advancing methods, techniques and technology.

References

[1] Hill W.E. Accurate keratometry readings. *Cataract and Refractive Surgery Today*.2009 June 2009,09(06):32-34.

[2] Haigis W. Basic error sources in IOL calculation after refractive surgery. *Cataract and Refractive Surgery Today*. May 2012, 07(5):31-32.

[3] Holladay JT, Prager TC, Chandler TY, et al. A three-part system for refining intraocular lens power calculations. *J. Cataract Refract. Surg.* 1988;14(1):17-24.

[4] Hoffer KJ. The Creator's Forum: IOL power calculations for post refractive surgery eyes. *Cataract and Refractive Surgery Today*. May 2012,07(5):35.

[5] Aristodemou P, Knox Cartwright NE, Sparrow JM, Johnston RL. Formula choice: HofferQ, Holladay 1, or SRKT and refractive outcomes in 8108 eyes after cataract surgery with biometry by partial coherence interferometry. *J. Cataract Refract. Surg.* 2011; 37:63-71.

[6] Carl Zeiss Meditec AG, 2010, p.74. *User manual IOLMaster with Advanced Technology*. Jena, Germany.

[7] IOLMaster - Carl Zeiss Meditec, accessed 10th January 2013, *www.meditec.zeiss.com/ .../TrainingIOLMforallversions/.../IOLMaster_Training_Slides.pdf* - Cached

[8] Holladay JT. IOL calculations following radial keratotomy surgery. *Refract. Corneal. Surgery*. 1989; 5:3.

[9] Hoffer KJ. Intraocular lens power calculation for eyes after refractive keratotomy. *J. Refract. Surg.* 1995;11:490-493.

[10] Gimbel HV, Sun R.J Accuracy and predictability of intraocular lens power calculation after laser in situ keratomileusis. *Cataract. Refract. Surg.* 2001 Apr;27(4):571-6.

[11] Aramberri J. Intraocular lens power calculation after corneal refractive surgery: double-K method. *J. Cataract. Refract. Surg.* 2003 Nov;29(11):2063

[12] Koch DD, Wang L. Calculating IOL power in eyes that have had refractive surgery. *J. Cataract Refract. Surg*. 2003 Nov;29(11):2039-42.

[13] Feiz V, Moshirfar M, Mannis MJ, Reilly CD, Garcia-Ferrer F, Caspar JJ, Lim MC. Nomogram-based intraocular lens power adjustment after myopic photorefractive keratectomy and LASIK: a new approach. *Ophthalmology*. 2005 Aug;112(8):1381-7.

[14] Masket S, Masket SE. Simple regression formula for intraocular lens power adjustment in eyes requiring cataract surgery after excimer laser photoablation. *J. Cataract Refract. Surg*. 2006 32 (3) 430 - 434.

[15] Hasson M. ASCRS IOL calculator power predictions depend on accurate input. *Ocular Surgery News*, US Edition, October 25, 2010.

[16] Warren Hill, M.D. Li Wang, M.D., Ph.D. Douglas D. Koch, M.D. American Society of Cataract and Refractive Surgeons IOL Calculator Version 4.3, accessed 10th January 2013, http://iolcalc.org/

[17] Wang L, Hill WE, Koch DD. Evaluation of intraocular lens power prediction methods using the American Society of Cataract and Refractive Surgeons Post-Keratorefractive Intraocular Lens Power Calculator. *J. Cataract Refract. Surg*. 2010 Sep;36(9):1466-73.

[18] Huang D. OCT enhances IOL power calculations in post-LASIK eyes. *Ocular Surgery News*, U.S. Edition, August 25, 2012.

[19] Goldsberry D.H, Achieving better outcomes using free online post –LASIK IOL calculators. *Cataract and Refractive Surgery Today*. May 2012,07(5):50-52.

[20] Olsen T. The Creator's Forum: IOL power calculations for postrefractive surgery eyes. *Cataract and Refractive Surgery Today*. May 2012,07(5):36-40.

[21] American Academy of Ophthalmology, (2008-2009). *Refractive Surgery*. San Francisco, CA :American Academy of Ophthalmology.

[22] Borasio E, Stevens J, Smith GT .Estimation of true corneal power after keratorefractive surgery in eyes requiring cataract surgery: BESSt formula. *J. Cataract Refract. Surg*. 2006 Dec;32(12):2004-14.

[23] Haigis W. The Creator's Forum: IOL power calculations for postrefractive surgery eyes. *Cataract and Refractive Surgery Today*. May 2012,07(5):34-35.

[24] Shammas HJ, Shammas MC, Garabet A, Kim JH, Shammas A, LaBree L.Correcting the corneal power measurements for intraocular lens power calculations after myopic laser in situ keratomileusis. *Am. J. Ophthalmol*. 2003 Sep;136(3):426-32.

[25] Shammas HJ, Shammas MC.No-history method of intraocular lens power calculation for cataract surgery after myopic laser in situ keratomileusis. *J. Cataract Refract. Surg*. 2007 Jan;33(1):31-6.

[26] http://www.haag-streit.com/products/biometry/lenstar-ls-900r/the-solution-for-demanding-cases/shammas-no-history-for-post-refractive-cases.html. Accessed 20th January 2013.

In: Current Understanding and New Techniques …
Editor: Michael O'Keefe
ISBN: 978-1-62808-748-2

Chapter 8

High Order Aberrations

Caitriona Kirwan*
Mater Private Hospital, Dublin, Ireland

Abstract

Higher order aberrations are refractive errors that cannot be corrected by conventional optical methods. Overall, they account for approximately 10% of the refractive error of the eye. Laser refractive surgery has been largely responsible for raising awareness of these aberrations, mainly due to their deleterious effect on retinal image quality. Spherical aberration and coma are the most important higher order aberrations and give rise to symptoms such as glare and haloes. Major technological advances have made measurement and treatment of these aberrations possible. Wavefront treatments and aspheric ablation profiles aim to treat and reduce post laser higher order aberrations. Aspheric intraocular lenses aim to manipulate spherical aberration in pseudophakic eyes.

Introduction

Light travels in waves spreading out in all directions in a spherical pattern from a point source. As light emanates from a source it forms a wavefront, which is defined as the shape of the light waves that are in phase with one another. In an aberration free optical system or 'ideal' eye, a perfect wavefront is formed. In normal eyes however, disturbances or aberrations of this perfect wavefront occur. The wavefront aberration is the degree to which the actual wavefront deviates from the ideal wavefront in the plane of the eyes exit pupil (figure 1) and is quantified by calculating the root mean square (RMS) in microns of the deviation.

The wavefront aberration is the sum of an infinite number of fundamental shapes. These shapes are commonly expressed as Zernike terms or polynomials. Zernike terms are grouped

* caitrionakirwan@eircom.net

into various orders (figures 2, 3) and are numbered starting at zero. Zero order aberrations consist of one term, the 1st order has 2 terms, the 3rd has 4 terms and so on.

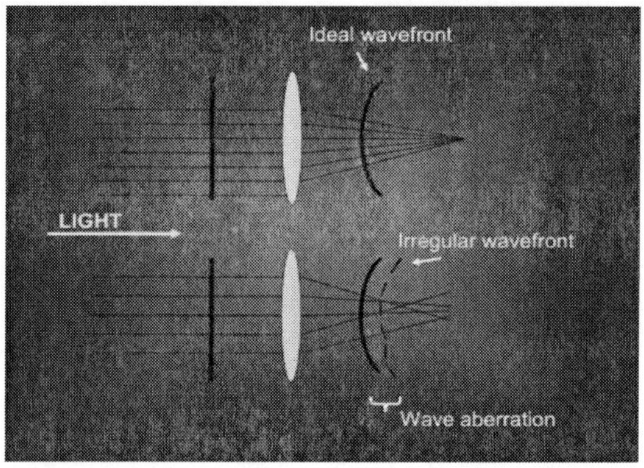

Figure 1. Ideal and aberrated wavefronts.

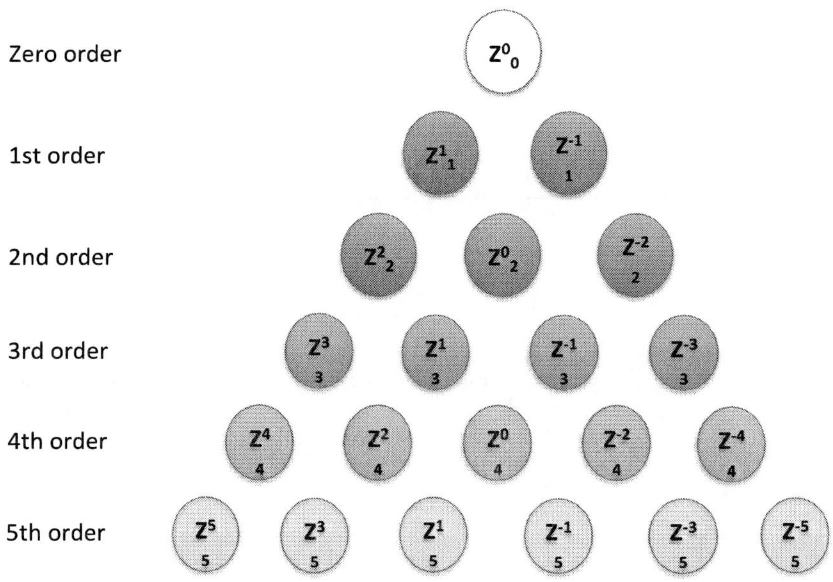

Figure 2. Zernike Pyramid: lower order aberrations: zero, 1st & 2nd order terms. Higher order aberrations: 3rd, 4th, 5th orders shown (higher orders not shown in this figure).

Lower order aberrations	Order	Zernike Polynomial	Zernike Term
	Zero	Z^0_0	Piston
	1st	Z^1_1, Z^{-1}_1	Tilt (prism)
	2nd	Z^2_2, Z^0_2, Z^{-2}_2	Astigmatism, Defocus
Higher order aberrations	3rd	$Z^3_3, Z^1_3, Z^{-1}_3, Z^{-3}_3$	Trefoil, Coma
	4th	$Z^4_4, Z^2_4, Z^0_4, Z^{-2}_4, Z^{-4}_4$	Tetrafoil, Secondary astigmatism, Spherical aberration
	5th	$Z^5_5, Z^3_5, Z^1_5, Z^{-1}_5, Z^{-3}_5, Z^{-5}_5$	Pentafoil, Trefoil, Coma

Figure 3. Zernike polynomials and corresponding terms. (Orders zero to 5th shown).

Aberrations are classed as lower order or higher order aberrations. The first three orders: zero (piston), first (tilt/prism) and second order (defocus, regular astigmatism) aberrations constitute lower order aberrations (LOA's). Zero and first order terms are not visually significant. Second order terms - defocus (positive - myopia, negative – hyperopia) and regular astigmatism can be corrected by standard optical methods such as glasses and contact lenses. The subsequent orders; 3rd and above, constitute what are collectively known as higher order aberrations (HOA's) and account for approximately 10% of total ocular aberrations [1]. HOA's are the subject of intense research as they are thought to degrade retinal image quality and act as an impediment to 'eagle vision'. They have been shown to reduce contrast sensitivity and cause glare and haloes. Conventional optical devices cannot correct these aberrations but technological advances mean that they may be amenable to correction by laser refractive surgery.

The first fifteen terms are the most visually significant and provide sufficient information to determine image quality. Zernike terms are expressed in the form $Z^m{}_n$ where n denotes the order of the aberration and m its angular frequency. Each term may be positive or negative in value. Zernike terms are based on aberrations that demonstrate radial symmetry. Irregular corneas such as those with keratoconus do not have sufficient radial symmetry and calculation of the wavefront using Zernike polynomials may not be possible in this setting [2]. Fourier analysis is an alternate method used to calculate wavefront aberration and is capable of calculating highly aberrated wavefronts from irregular corneas [3]. Unlike Zernike polynomials, Fourier analysis requires the sum of multiple Fourier terms to represent the wavefront aberration.

The Point Spread Function (PSF) may be defined as the image a distant point of light forms on the retina and as such is indicative of retinal image quality. Each aberration or Zernike term has a predictable effect on the PSF and image quality. The PSF image can be calculated using mathematical equations. This involves specifying the Zernike term in question by means of n (order of aberration) and m (angular frequency), pupil diameter (up to 8 mm), the RMS of the wavefront error (μm) and the wavelength of light (nm).[4]

The majority of HOA's arise from the anterior corneal surface and the lens, with a minority arising from the posterior corneal surface and the retina. They are significant in infancy [5] and early childhood and decrease with age to adulthood [6]. It has been suggested that this change takes place as part of normal emmetropisation [6]. Thereafter they increase gradually again to old age [7-10].

HOA's fluctuate constantly as they are affected by pupil size and by the accommodative state of the eye. Unsurprisingly, they are affected significantly by corneal [11-13] and lenticular pathology [14-17] and have been found at greater levels in patients with macular disease relative to controls [18]. It has been hypothesized that multiple reflections from the diseased macula may be responsible. Spherical aberration and coma are the most visually significant aberrations.

Spherical Aberration

Spherical aberration arises due to differences in the refraction of light rays travelling parallel to the optical axis, striking a lens at varying positions. Light rays entering the periphery of the lens are refracted differently to those entering more centrally with the result that they fail to converge on the same point. In an oblate cornea (flatter centrally), the peripheral rays are bent to a greater degree than central rays (positive spherical aberration) (figure 4) whereas in a prolate cornea (steeper centrally), the peripheral rays are bent to a greater extent (negative spherical aberration) (figure 5).

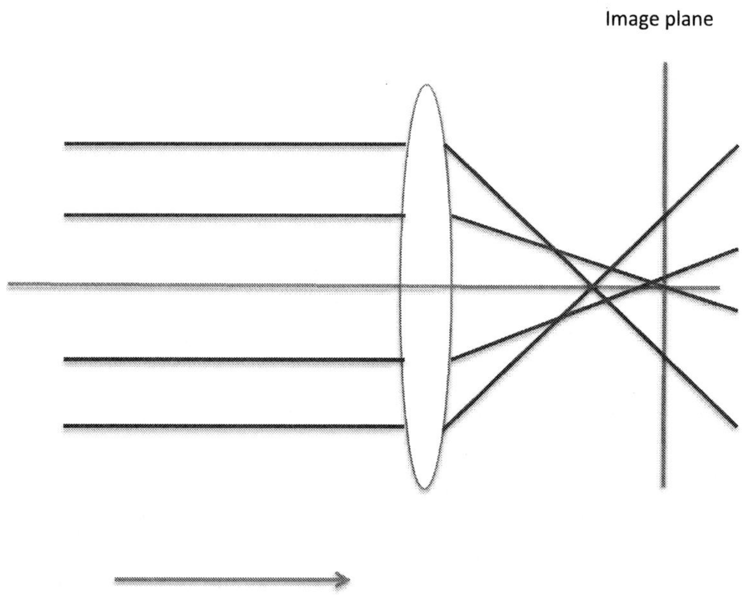

Figure 4. Positive spherical aberration: the peripheral rays are refracted to a greater degree than those entering more centrally.

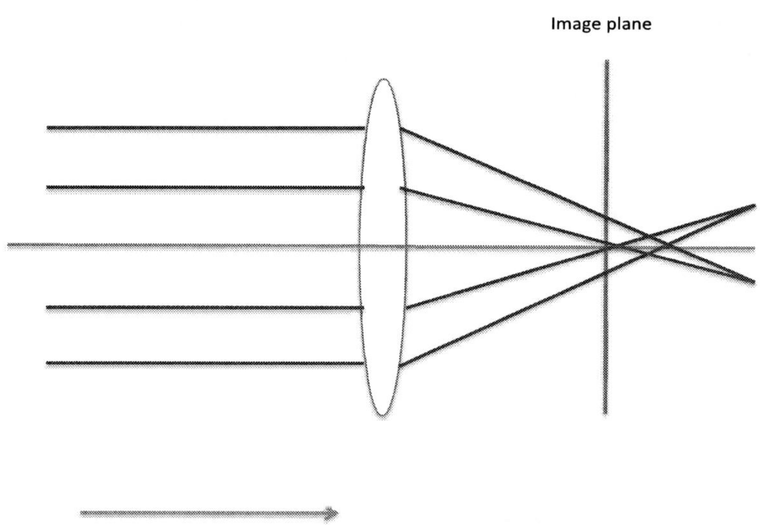

Figure 5. Negative spherical aberration: the peripheral rays are refracted to a lesser degree than those entering more centrally.

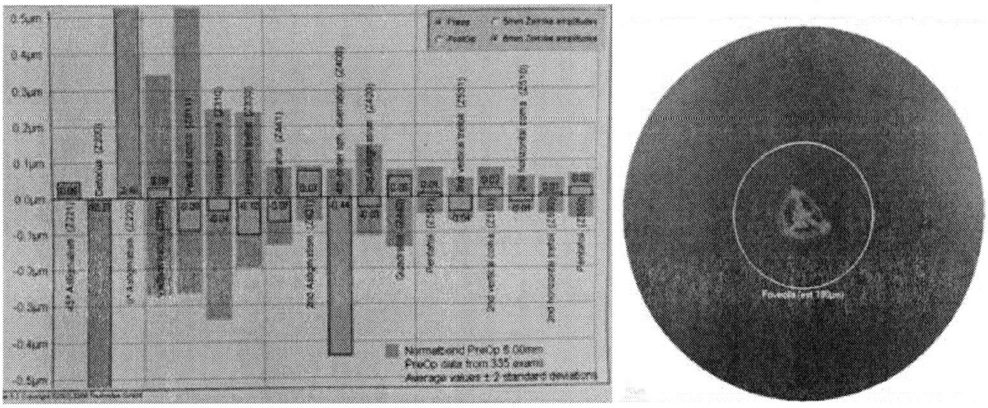

Figure 6. (a) Aberrometry (Zywave, Bausch & Lomb, Surrey, UK) of a myopic male (-7D spherical equivalent) demonstrating significant negative spherical aberration; (b) point spread function of the same eye demonstrating peripheral ring or halo.

Spherical aberration results in blurring of images and complaints of glare and haloes. The effect of spherical aberration on the retinal image can be predicted and demonstrated by the point spread function (figure 6) {see point spread function later in chapter}. A compensatory affect for spherical aberration has been described in young eyes [19]. Spherical aberration of the cornea is usually positive. In contrast the spherical aberration of the young crystalline lens is usually negative thus counteracting to a large extent corneal spherical aberration. However, with age, various changes occur within the lens including hardening of the nucleus, an increase in refractive index and change in shape [20]. As a result, lenticular spherical aberration increases and becomes positive around the age of 40 years, thus adding to total ocular spherical aberration [21]. This has been shown to have a deleterious affect on visual acuity [22] and contrast sensitivity [23].

Accommodative state influences the entire wavefront error but has a significant affect on spherical aberration. As the eye accommodates, spherical aberration increases and becomes more negative. This change occurs predominantly in younger individuals. In presbyopes, only minor changes occur due to the limited available amplitude of accommodation [24].

Spherical aberration is the most important aberration implicated in night-time myopia. Under photopic conditions, the pupil constricts preventing light rays from entering through the periphery of the lens thus minimizing spherical aberration. In dim lighting condition, the pupil enlarges; rays enter through the periphery and the focal point moves forward with the effect of inducing a myopic shift.

Pupil size has a strong influence over spherical aberration. It has been shown to increase with the 4th power of the pupil diameter. Doubling of pupil size brings about a 16-fold increase in spherical aberration [25].

Spherical aberration does have some benefits most notably providing increased depth of focus, which has a beneficial effect on near vision. Rocha et al. demonstrated an increase in depth of focus to a maximum of 2 D by inducing spherical aberration – both positive and negative, by means of an adaptive optics simulator [26]. Best results were achieved by inducing 0.6 μm's of spherical aberration with decrements in depth of field observed with induction of 0.9 μm's. Induction of trefoil and coma did not affect depth of focus.

Coma

Coma or *comatic aberration* arises from light entering the eye off axis. The incident or incoming rays strike the lens at differing angles and on passing through the various lens zones are refracted differently. The resultant asymmetric image formed has a tail or comet like blur which is directed away from the optical axis (figure 7).

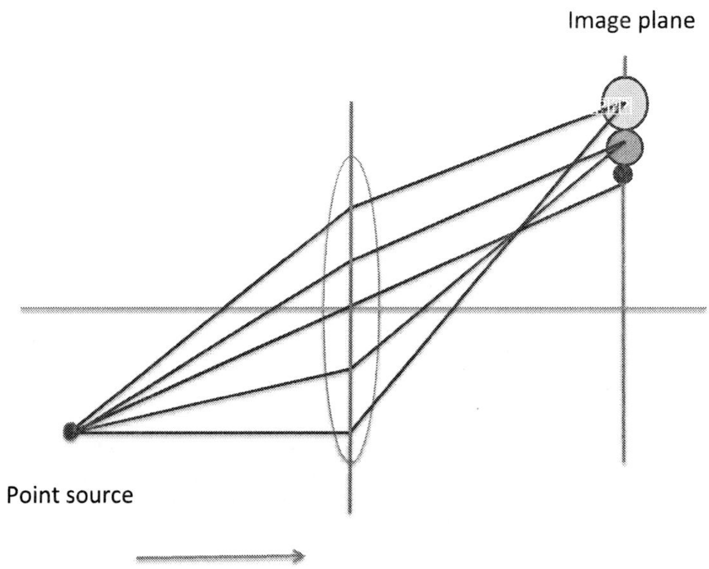

Figure 7. Ray diagram of coma. Light entering the eye off axis gives rise to a blurred image that is comet like or tail shaped.

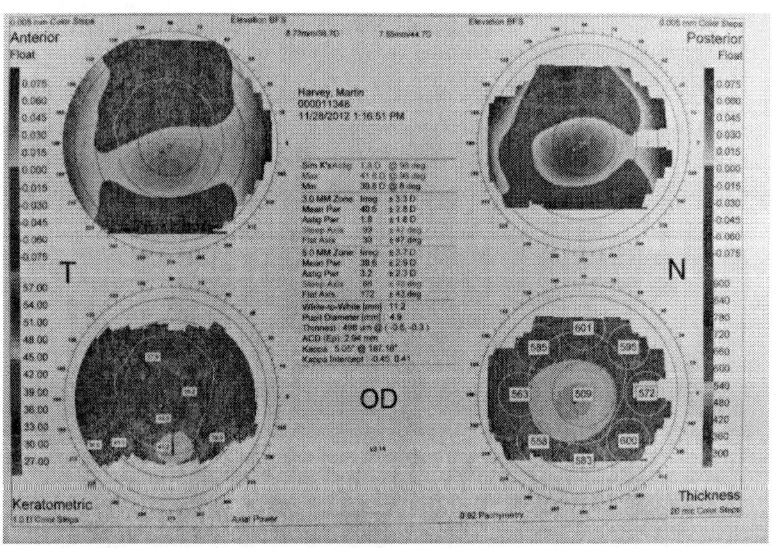

(a)

Figure 8. (Continued).

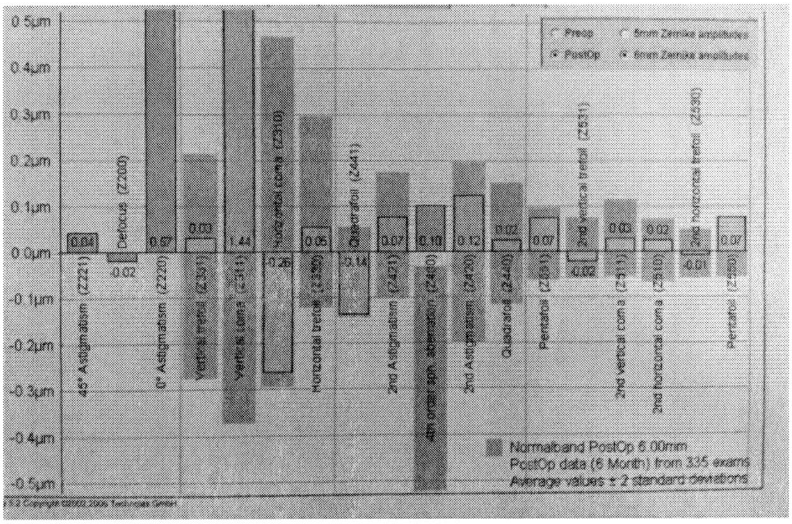

(b)

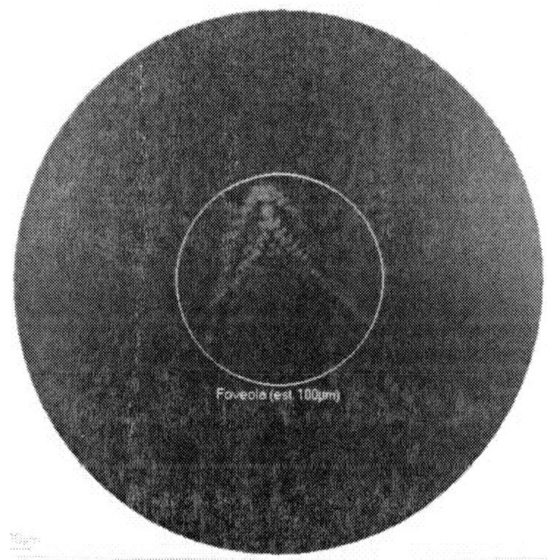

(c)

Figure 8. (a) Corneal topography (Orbscan, Bausch & Lomb) demonstrating forme fruste keratoconus in a patient undergoing assessment for refractive surgery; (b) aberrometry (Zywave) from the same eye demonstrating significant vertical coma; (c) point spread function showing typical comet shape.

Coma is commonly encountered in patients with clinical or subclinical (forme fruste) keratoconus (figure 8) and it is the most common higher order aberration encountered in eyes with this condition [11-12]. The detection of increased amounts of vertical coma in patients is an important indicator of possible keratoconus [27-29]. It prompts very careful analysis of corneal topography and curvature maps, particularly in those patients undergoing assessment for laser refractive surgery. Coma is also commonly observed in eyes post penetrating keratoplasty and following decentered laser ablation (figure 9) in keratorefractive surgery [30-32]. Dry eye may also induce significant levels of coma. Tear film irregularity associated with dry eye has been found to increase HOA's and coma in particular thus impacting on visual performance [33, 34]. Artificial tears have been shown to decrease tear film irregularity and reduce higher order aberrations [35].

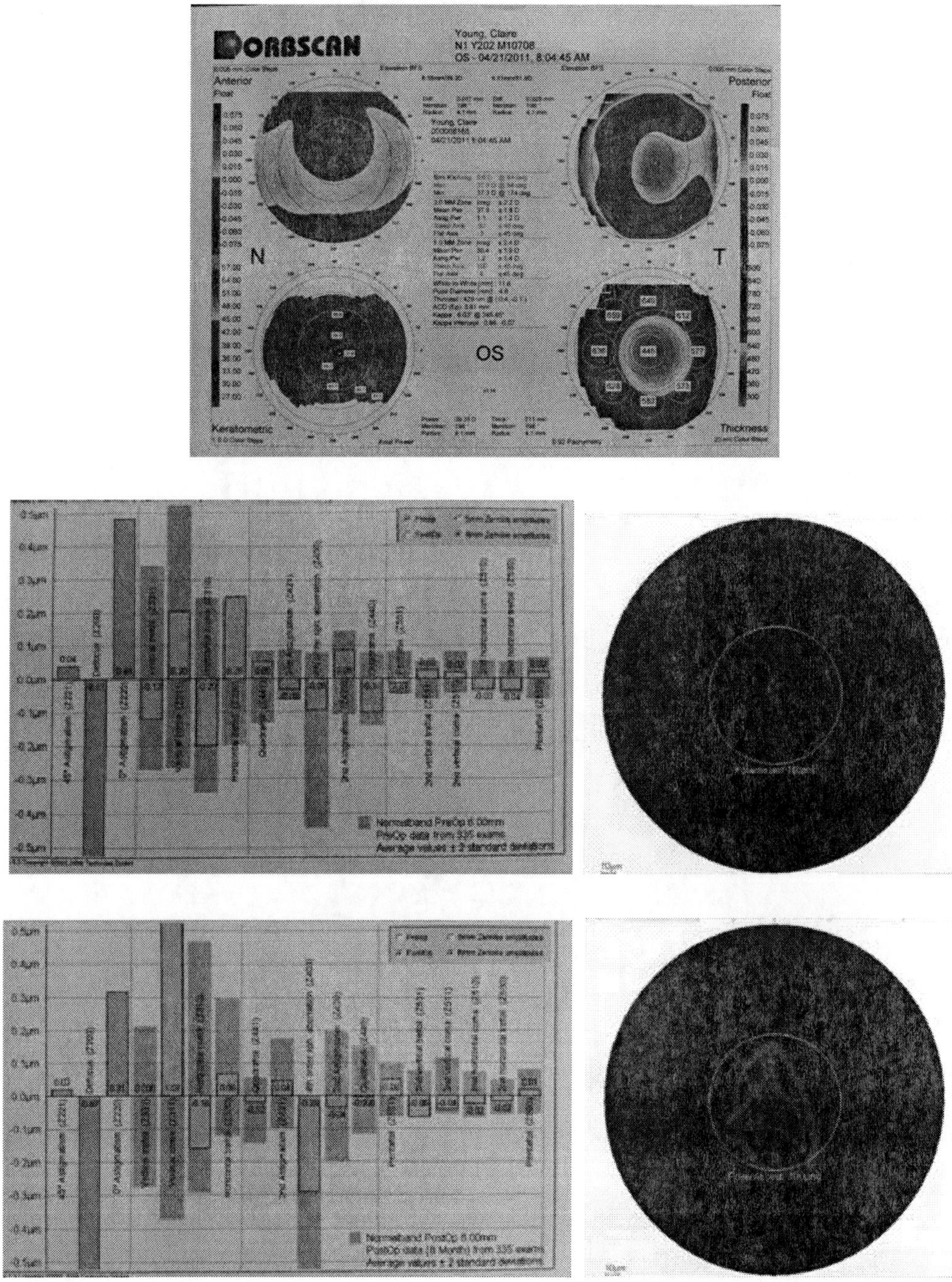

Figure 9. (a) Corneal topography of a patient post LASIK for 5D of myopia, demonstrating slightly decentered ablation; (b) aberrometry and point spread function prior to LASIK surgery; (c) aberrometry post LASIK demonstrating significant induced vertical coma due to ablation decentration and altered point spread function.

Patients with significant coma may complain of images appearing sharp centrally but blurred peripherally or of having a 'tail'. Using purpose designed soft contact lenses, Fernandez-Sanchez et al. investigated the effect of varying degrees of 3rd order coma and trefoil on high and low contrast visual acuities and contrast sensitivity [36].

They found a significant reduction in each of these parameters at high levels (1 micron approximately) of coma and trefoil. All higher order aberrations have been found to increase with increasing pupil size. However, coma increases to a lesser extent than spherical aberration [37].

Wavefront Sensors/Aberrometers

Wavefront sensors are devices with the capability to measure the wavefront aberration of an optical system. Numerous sensors or 'aberrometers' based on different underlying principles are in clinical use today. Whereas the majority of instruments measure total ocular aberrations, some have the capacity to record corneal topography simultaneously, permitting differentiation between corneal and total ocular aberrations.

Hartmann Shack Aberrometry

The principles of Hartmann-Shack aberrometry underlie the most commonly used aberrometers in clinical practice. This technique involves projection of light into the eye and measurement of the distortion in a wavefront of light emitted from the eye after it has passed through the eye's optics.

The reflected light passes through a series of tiny lenses or 'lenslets' and is broken up into multiple beams. In an aberration free optical system, the reflected waves will be focused to form a perfectly aligned lattice or grid of images, each falling on the optical axis of the lenslet through which it has passed. In a human eye, aberrations result in formation of a more disorganized grid, the extent of which depends on the level of aberrations encountered (figure 10). The displacement of each spot from the corresponding lenslet optical axis is calculated and the wavefront aberration is determined.

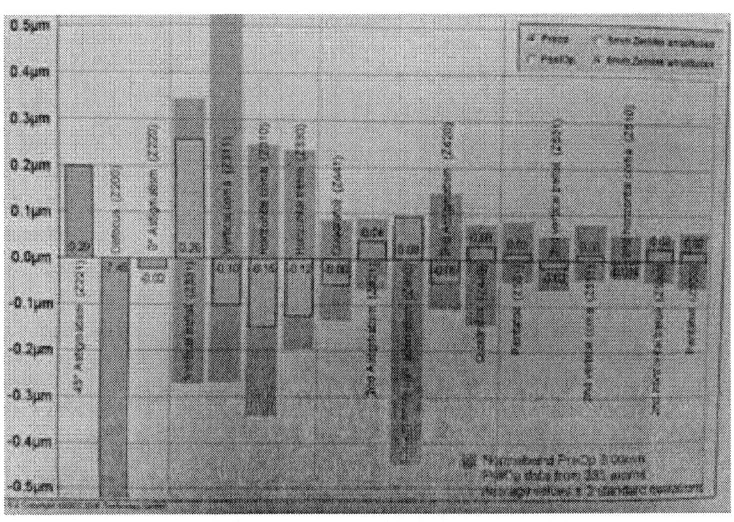

Figure 10. (Continued).

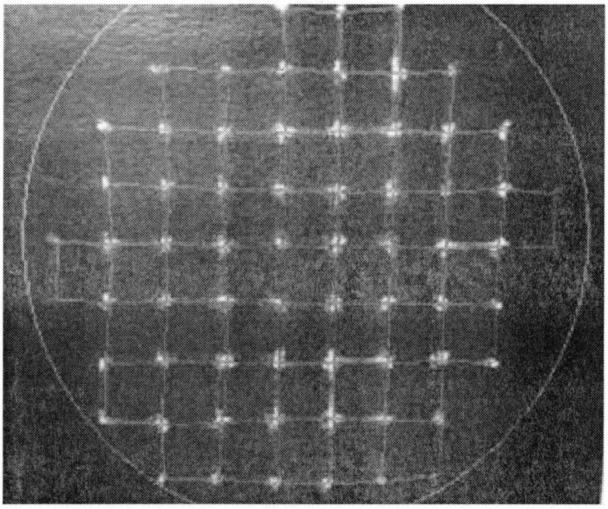

(a)

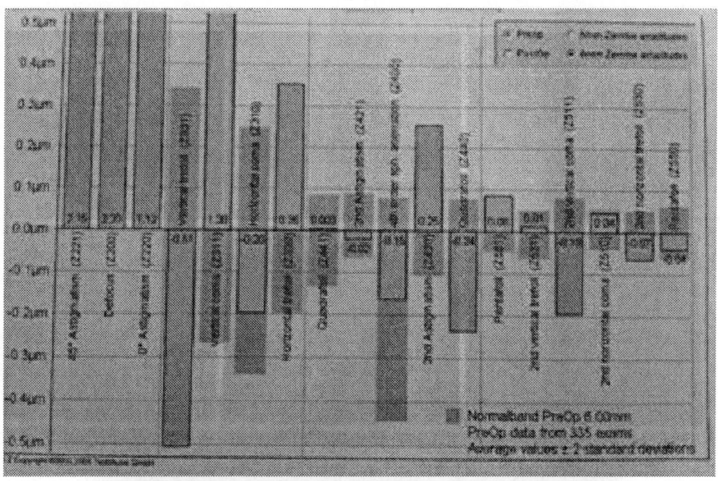

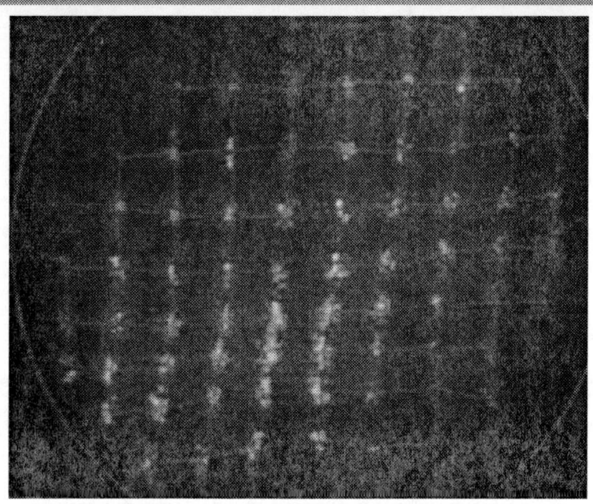

(b)

Figure 10. (a) Aberrometry demonstrating a low level of HOA's and corresponding raw data depicting excellent uniformity of grid formation; (b) Some grid distortion is evident from an eye with a greater amount of HOA's.

Tscherning Aberrometry

This form of aberrometry is named after Marius Tscherning who published his work on optical aberrations of the eye in 1894 [38]. This technique involves illumination of a mask consisting of 168 pinholes with a collimated Nd:YAG (532nm) laser beam. Upon passing through the disc, a bundle of thin parallel leaser beams are formed which are projected onto the retina. The pattern formed on the retina is determined by the optical errors of the eye. This pattern is imaged onto the sensor of a low light charge coupled device (CCD) camera [39]. Deviations in the retinal pattern from the ideal location are calculated in the form of Zernike polynomials. The Allegretto Wave Analyser (Alcon, Fort Worth, Texas, USA) is an example of this form of aberrometer in clinical use. Similar to H-S aberrometers, Tscherning aberrometers provide accurate wavefront data but may be considered by some to be somewhat less user-friendly than Hartmann-Shack aberrometers.

Ray Tracing Aberrometry

This technique is similar to the Tscherning aberrometer in that a thin infrared laser beam is projected onto the retina. However, the beams enter in succession rather than simultaneously thus reduces the risk of light rays intersecting enabling measurement of greater degrees of aberrations. These aberrometers have the ability to detect larger magnitude errors (such as those found in patients with keratoconus) than Hartmann Shack or Tscherning aberrometers. The iTrace Visual Function Analyzer (Tracey Technologies, Houston, Texas, USA) is a ray tracing aberrometer in widespread clinical use.

Skiascopy/Dynamic Retinoscopy

As the name suggests this technique is based on the principle of retinoscopy but uses an infrared laser beam instead of visible light. The retina is scanned with a slit beam and the reflected light is captured by an array of rotating photodetectors. The time lag to detection of the reflected light is converted into refractive power maps from which the wavefront profile is derived. The NIDEK OPD-Scan (Gamagori, Japan) aberrometer utilizes this technology.

Much work has been done comparing measurements of HOA's recorded using various instruments. In general, results obtained by different aberrometers are not comparable even when based on the same underlying principles [40-42].

HOA's, Cataract & IOL's

Lenticular pathology such as cataract induces higher order aberrations. These changes have been proposed to account for complaints of poor subjective vision in patients with mild opacities but good high contrast Snellen acuity [14]. Coma-like aberration dominates in eyes with cortical opacities whereas spherical aberration is more prevalent in eyes with nuclear cataracts [14, 15]. Posterior capsule opacification post cataract surgery is also associated with the development of higher order aberrations and Nd:YAG laser capsulotomy has been shown to reduce these significantly [16].

As previously discussed, the healthy cornea gives rise to positive spherical aberration. Standard spherical intraocular lenses (IOL's) due to their shape introduce further positive spherical aberration to the eye [43]. Due to the known affect of spherical aberration on retinal image quality, intraocular lenses have been developed to manipulate spherical aberration in pseudophakic eyes. Specific alterations in surface curvature give rise to these 'aspheric' lenses. They may be designed to eliminate, reduce or to have no additive affect on corneal spherical aberration.

The average cornea has been shown to generate approximately 0.27 microns of positive spherical aberration [8, 44]. The Tecnis Z900 (AMO) was one of the first aspheric IOL's to be developed. This IOL has 0.27 microns of negative spherical aberration at the 6mm optical zone and aims to largely counteract corneal spherical aberration. The Acrysof IQ (Alcon) has 0.20 microns of negative spherical aberration that aims to reduce but not eliminate spherical aberration within the average eye. Other aspheric lenses such as the Crystalens (Bausch & Lomb), Sofport AO (Bausch & Lomb) and Akreos AO (Bausch & Lomb) do not have any inherent spherical aberration and are described as 'aberration free'. As such they do not introduce further spherical aberration but do not negate that of the cornea [45, 46].

Many studies have confirmed lower levels of spherical aberration in eyes implanted with aspheric compared with spherical IOL's. A number of these studies reported better visual acuity and contrast sensitivity with aspheric IOL's [47-50] but in many the results have been equivocal [51-53]. A number of factors may be responsible. Spherical aberration increases depth of focus and its elimination may lead to problems with near vision and ability to read. [49, 50]. IOL decentration of more than 0.5mm may negate the benefits of the aspheric IOL [43, 54]. IOL tilt can also strongly influence optical performance. Holladay et al. showed benefit of aspheric over spherical lenses provided IOL tilt did not exceed 7 degrees [44]. Small pupil diameter may also limit the benefits of lens asphericity [55, 56]. Another important factor is patient selection. Corneal spherical aberration is not uniform throughout the population and therefore preoperative aberrometry has been advocated to facilitate selection of the most appropriate IOL to meet the patients needs [57-59]. This is particularly important in patients with a history of laser refractive surgery. Myopic ablation produces an oblate cornea, increasing positive spherical aberration. A high negative spherical aberration IOL may be considered for these patients. Conversely, hyperopic ablation produces a prolate cornea and negative spherical aberration. Implantation of a traditional spherical IOL may be the most appropriate in these cases.

HOA's and Refractive Surgery

Our current knowledge and understanding of higher order aberrations has been driven largely by the development of laser refractive surgery. In its infancy, good refractive outcomes were tempered by subjective problems of monocular diplopia, glare and haloes. Following the introduction of aberrometry to clinical practice it became evident that these problems arose from the induction of higher order aberration. Large pupils, small treatment optical zones (more importantly the relationship between these two parameters) [60-63] and greater ablation depths [64] were found to be important causative factors. Technological advances led to the introduction of wavefront treatments whereby patients total ocular aberrations – lower and higher order could be targeted and treated. These advances together with rotational tracking devices have led to significant improvements in quality vision outcomes for refractive surgery patients. However, HOA's can still be induced by laser refractive surgery. Oshika et al. published an important paper examining the influence of pupil size on the relationship between HOA's and contrast sensitivity post LASIK [63]. They found that in eyes with photopic pupil diameter below 4mm, contrast sensitivity was affected most by induced coma. At pupil sizes above 4mm however, it was most affected most by induced spherical aberration and not coma. The authors concluded that those patients with larger pupils would benefit most from wavefront guided treatments in order to minimize induced spherical aberration whereas those with small pupils may benefit most from eye tracking to minimize treatment decentration and induced coma.

Laser refractive surgery results in changes in corneal curvature towards oblateness or prolateness. These changes have been associated with the induction of HOA's [65]. Aspheric ablation profiles or 'wavefront optimized' have been developed in an effort to minimize this. They act by pre-compensating for expected induced spherical aberration and by attempting to maintain the pre-existing corneal asphericity. [66-67] Aspheric ablation profiles have been shown to induce less spherical aberration with improved visual outcomes compared with non-aspheric treatments [68-69]. Buhren et al. found that induced spherical aberration, while reduced remained significant but the aspheric ablation profiles increased tolerance of decentered ablations [66].

Conclusion

Excimer laser refractive error correction has opened up a new world of optics to the ophthalmologist. In our efforts to improve quality visual outcome for our patients, refractive surgery has changed dramatically from the early days of correcting spherical and cylindrical errors. Through increased knowledge and understanding of higher order aberrations, means of treating and preventing their development have evolved. This knowledge is now also being applied to IOL selection in cataract surgery where it seems that tailored selection of an aspheric lens may give the best visual outcome. However, as we strive to manipulate higher order aberrations it must be remembered that accurate correction of lower order sphere and cylinder must be achieved if the patient is to appreciate the visual benefits.

References

[1] MA Lawless. Wavefronts role in corneal refractive surgery. *Clin. Exp. Ophthalmol.* 2005;33(2):199-209.

[2] Klyce SD, Karon MD, Smolek MK. Advantages and disadvantages of the Zernike expansion for representing wave aberration of the normal and aberrated eye. *J. Refract. Surg.* 2004;20(5):S537-41.

[3] Dai GM. Comparison of wavefront reconstructions with Zernike polynomials and Fourier transforms. *J. Refract. Surg*. 2006;22(9):943-8.
[4] Fisher RE. 2000 Optical System Design. New York, McGraw Hill.
[5] Wang J, Candy TR. Higher order monochromatic aberrations of the human infant eye. *J. Vis*. 2005;23;5(6):543-55.
[6] Brunette I, Bueno JM, Parent M, Hamam H, Simonet P. Monochromatic aberrations as a function of age, from childhood to advanced age. *Invest Ophthalmol. Vis. Sci.* 2003;44(12):5438-46.
[7] McLellan JS, Marcos S, Burns SA. Age-related changes in monochromatic wave aberrations of the human eye. *Invest Ophthalmol. Vis. Sci*. 2001;42(6):1390-5.
[8] Wang L, Dai E, Koch DD, Nathoo A. Optical aberrations of the human anterior cornea. *J. Cataract Refract. Surg*. 2003;29(8):1514-21.
[9] Wang L, Koch DD. Ocular higher order aberrations in individuals screened for refractive surgery. *J. Cataract Refract. Surg*. 2003;29(8):1896-1903.
[10] Amano S, Amano Y, Yamagami S, Miyai T, Miyata K, Samejima T, Oshika T. Age-related changes in corneal and ocular higher-order wavefront aberrations. *Am. J. Ophthalmol*. 2004;137(6):988-92.
[11] Maeda N, Fujikado T, Kuroda T, Mihashi T, Hirohara Y, Nishida K, Watanabe H, Tano Y. Wavefront aberrations measured with Hartmann-Shack sensor in patients with keratoconus. *Ophthalmology*. 2002;109(11):1996-2003.
[12] Pantanelli S, MacRae S, Jeong TM, Yoon G. Characterizing the wave aberration in eyes with keratoconus or penetrating keratoplasty using a high-dynamic range wavefront sensor. *Ophthalmology*. 2007;114(11):2013-21.
[13] McCormick GJ, Porter J, Cox IG, MacRae S. Higher-order aberrations in eyes with irregular corneas after laser refractive surgery. *Ophthalmology*. 2005;112(10):1699-709.
[14] Lee J, Kim MJ, Tchah H. Higher-order aberrations induced by nuclear cataract. *J. Cataract Refract Surg*. 2008;34(12):2104-9.
[15] Sachdev N, Ormonde SE, Sherwin T, McGhee CN. Higher-order aberrations of lenticular opacities. *J. Cataract Refract. Surg*. 2004;30(8):1642-8.
[16] Rocha KM, Nosé W, Bottós K, Bottós J, Morimoto L, Soriano E. Higher-order aberrations of age-related cataract. *J. Cataract Refract. Surg*. 2007;33(8):1442-6.
[17] Levy J, Lifshitz T, Klemperer I, Knyazer B, Ashkenazy Z, Kratz A, Belfair N. The effect of Nd:YAG laser posterior capsulotomy on ocular wave front aberrations. *Can. J. Ophthalmol*. 2009;44(5):529-33.
[18] Bessho K, Bartsch DU, Gomez L, Cheng L, Koh HJ, Freeman WR. Ocular wavefront aberrations in patients with macular diseases. *Retina*. 2009;29(9):1356-63.
[19] Smith G, Cox MJ, Calver R, Garner LF. The spherical aberration of the crystalline lens of the human eye. *Vision Res*. 2001;41(2):235-43.
[20] Dubbelman M, Van der Heijde GL. The shape of the aging human lens: curvature, equivalent refractive index and the lens paradox. *Vision Res*. 2001;41(14):1867-77.
[21] Glasser A, Campbell MC. Vision Res. Biometric, optical and physical changes in the isolated human crystalline lens with age in relation to presbyopia. *Vision Res.* 1999;39(11):1991-2015.
[22] Marcos S. Aberrations and visual performance following standard laser vision correction. *J. Refract Surg*. 2001;17(5):S596-601.

[23] Hemenger RP, Tomlinson A, Caroline PJ.Role of spherical aberration in contrast sensitivity loss with radial keratotomy. *Invest Ophthalmol. Vis. Sci.* 1989;30(9):1997-2001.

[24] Radhakrishnan H, Charman WN. Age-related changes in ocular aberrations with accommodation. *J. Vis.* 2007;7(7):11.1-21.

[25] Basic & Clinical Science Course Section 3: Clinical Optics (2011-2012). *American Academy of Ophthalmology* 2011-2012 pp 100.

[26] Rocha KM, Vabre L, Chateau N, Krueger RR. Expanding depth of focus by m.odifying higher-order aberrations induced by an adaptive optics visual simulator. *J. Cataract Refract. Surg.* 2009;35(11):1885-92.

[27] Gordon-Shaag A, Millodot M, Ifrah R, Shneor E. Aberrations and topography in normal, keratoconus-suspect, and keratoconic eyes. *Optom. Vis. Sci.* 2012;89(4):411-8.

[28] Jafri B, Li X, Yang H, Rabinowitz YS. Higher order wavefront aberrations and topography in early and suspected keratoconus. *J. Refract. Surg.* 2007;23(8):774-81.

[29] Alió JL, Shabayek MH. Corneal higher order aberrations: a method to grade keratoconus. *J. Refract. Surg.* 2006;22(6):539-45.

[30] Lee SB, Hwang BS, Lee J. Effects of decentration of photorefractive keratectomy on the induction of higher order wavefront aberrations. *J. Refract. Surg.* 2010;26(10):731-43.

[31] Padmanabhan P, Mrochen M, Viswanathan D, Basuthkar S. Wavefront aberrations in eyes with decentered ablations. *J. Cataract Refract. Surg.* 2009;35(4):695-702.

[32] Bühren J, Yoon G, Kenner S, MacRae S, Huxlin K. The effect of optical zone decentration on lower- and higher-order aberrations after photorefractive keratectomy in a cat model. *Invest Ophthalmol. Vis. Sci.* 2007;48(12):5806-14.

[33] Koh S, Maeda N, Hirohara Y, Mihashi T, Ninomiya S, Bessho K, Watanabe H, Fujikado T, Tano Y. Serial measurements of higher-order aberrations after blinking in normal subjects. *Invest Ophthalmol. Vis. Sci.* 2006;47(8):3318-24.

[34] Montés-Micó R. Role of the tear film in the optical quality of the human eye. *J. Cataract Refract. Surg.* 2007;33(9):1631-5.

[35] Montés-Micó R, Cerviño A, Ferrer-Blasco T, García-Lázaro S, Ortí-Navarro S. Optical quality after instillation of eyedrops in dry-eye syndrome. *J. Cataract Refract. Surg.* 2010 ;36(6):935-40.

[36] Fernández-Sánchez V, Ponce ME, Lara F, Montés-Micó R, Castejón-Mochón JF, López-Gil N. Effect of 3rd-order aberrations on human vision. *J. Cataract Refract. Surg.* 2008;34:1339-44.

[37] Wang Y, Zhao K, Jin Y, Niu Y, Zuo T. Changes of higher order aberration with various pupil sizes in the myopic eye. *J. Refract. Surg.* 2003;19:S270-4.

[38] Norn M, Jensen OA. Marius Tscherning (1854-1939): his life and work in optical physiology. *Acta Ophthalmol. Scand.* 2004;82(5):501-8.

[39] Mrochen M, Kaemmerer M, Mierdel P, Krinke HE, Seiler T. Principles of Tscherning aberrometry. *J. Refract. Surg.* 2000;16(5):S570-1.

[40] Cerviño A, Hosking SL, Montés-Micó R. Comparison of higher order aberrations measured by NIDEK OPD-Scan dynamic skiascopy and Zeiss WASCA Hartmann-Shack aberrometers. *J. Refract. Surg.* 2008;24(8):790-6.

[41] Kim DS, Narváez J, Krassin J, Bahjri K. Comparison of the VISX wavescan and NIDEK OPD-scan aberrometers. *J. Refract. Surg.* 2009;25(5):429-34.

[42] Visser N, Berendschot TT, Verbakel F, Tan AN, de Brabander J, Nuijts RM. Evaluation of the comparability and repeatability of four wavefront aberrometers. *Invest Ophthalmol. Vis. Sci.* 2011;52(3):1302-11.

[43] Atchison DA. Design of aspheric intraocular lenses. *Ophthalmic Physiol. Opt.* 1991;11:137-146.

[44] Holladay JT, Piers PA, Koranyi G, Van der Mooren M, Sverker Norrby NE. A New Intraocular Lens Design to Reduce Spherical Aberration of Pseudophakic Eyes. *J. Refract. Surg* 2002;18:683-691

[45] Packer, MI, Fine H, Hoffman RS. Aspheric intraocular lens selection: the evolution of refractive cataract surgery. *Curr. Opin Ophthalmol.* 2008,19:1–4.

[46] Beiko GH, Haigis W, Steinmueller A. Distribution of corneal spherical aberration in a comprehensive ophthalmology practice and whether keratometry can predict aberration values. *J. Cataract Refract. Surg* 2007;33:848-858.

[47] Caporossi A, Martone G, Casprini F, Rapisarda L. Prospective randomized study of clinical performance of 3 asperic and 2 spherical intraocular lenses in 250 eyes. *J. Refract. Surg.* 2007;23:639-648.

[48] Morales EL, Rocha KM, Chalita MR, Nosé W, Avila MP. Comparison of optical aberrations and contrast sensitivity between aspheric and spherical intraocular lenses. *J. Refract. Surg.* 2011;27(10):723-8.

[49] Nanavaty MA, Spalton DJ, Boyce J, Saha S, Marshall J. Wavefront aberrations, depth of focus, and contrast sensitivity with aspheric and spherical intraocular lenses: fellow-eye study. *J. Cataract Refract. Surg* 2009;35:663-71.

[50] Nochez Y, Majzoub S, Pisella PJ. Effect of residual ocular spherical aberration on objective and subjective quality of vision in pseudophakic eyes. *J. Cataract Refract. Surg.* 2011;37:1076-81.

[51] Landers J, Goggin M. Ocular preference following implantation of aspheric and spherical intraocular lenses; an intra-individual comparison. *Clin. Exp. Optom.* 2010;93(6):419-25.

[52] Johansson B, Sundelin S, Wikberg-Matsson A, Unsbo P, Behndig A. Visual and optical performance of the Akreos Adapt Advanced Optics and Tecnis Z9000 intraocular lenses: Swedish multicenter study. *J. Cataract Refract. Surg.* 2007;33:1565-72.

[53] Moorfields IOL Study Group, Allan B. Binocular implantation of the Tecnis Z9000 or AcrySof MA60AC intraocular lens in routine cataract surgery: prospective randomized controlled trial comparing VF-14 scores. *J. Cataract Refract. Surg.* 2007;33:1559-64.

[54] Altmann GE, Nichamin LD, Lane SS, Pepose JS. Optical performance of 3 intraocular lens designs in the presence of decentration. *J. Cataract Refract. Surg* 2005;31:574-585.

[55] Belluci R, Morselli S. Optimizing higher0order aberrations with intraocular lens technology. *Curr. Opin. Ophthalmol* 2007;18:67-73.

[56] Eom Y, Yoo E, Kang SY, Kim HM, Song JS. Change in efficiency of aspheric intraocular lenses based on pupil diameter. *Am. J. Ophthalmol.* 2013;155:492-498.

[57] Montés-Micó R, Ferrer-Blasco T, Cervino A. Analysis of the possible benefits of aspheric intraocular lenses: review of the literature. *J. Cataract Refract. Surg* 2009;35:172-181.

[58] Packer M, Fine IH, Hoffman RS. Aspheric intraocular lens selection based on corneal wavefront. *J. Refract. Surg.* 2009;25(1):12-20.

[59] Mester U, Kaymak H. The aspheric blue light filter IOL AcrySof IQ compared to the AcrySof SA60AT : influence of IOL power, pupil diameter, and corneal asphericity on postoperative spherical aberration. *Ophthalmologe*. 2008;105:1029-35.

[60] Bühren J, Kühne C, Kohnen T. Influence of pupil and optical zone diameter on higher-order aberrations after wavefront-guided myopic LASIK. *J. Cataract Refract. Surg.* 2005;31:2272-80.

[61] Mok KH, Lee VW. Effect of optical zone ablation diameter on LASIK-induced higher order optical aberrations. *J. Refract. Surg*. 2005;21:141-3.

[62] Cheng ZY, Chu RY, Zhou XT. Zhonghua Yan Ke Za Zhi. Influence of diameter of optical zone ablation on LASIK-induced higher order optical aberrations in myopia. *Zhonghua Yan Ke Za Zhi*. 2006;42:772-6.

[63] Oshika T, Tokunaga T, Samejima T, Miyata K, Kawana K, Kaji Y. Influence of Pupil Diameter on the Relation between Ocular Higher-Order Aberration and Contrast Sensitivity after Laser In Situ Keratomileusis. *Invest Ophthalmol. Vis. Sci.* 2006;47:1334-1338.

[64] Bühren J, Kohnen T. Factors affecting the change in lower-order and higher-order aberrations after wavefront-guided laser in situ keratomileusis for myopia with the Zyoptix 3.1 system. *J. Cataract Refract. Surg*. 2006;32:1166-74.

[65] Holladay JT, Janes JA. Topographic changes in corneal asphericity and effective optical zone after laser in situ keratomileusis. *J. Cataract Refract. Surg*. 2002;28:942–947.

[66] Bühren J, Nagy L, Yoon G, MacRae S, Kohnen T, Huxlin KR. The effect of the asphericity of myopic laser ablation profiles on the induction of wavefront aberrations. *Invest Ophthalmol. Vis. Sci*. 2010;51:2805-12.

[67] Mrochen M, Donitzky C, Wüllner C, Löffler J. Wavefront-optimized ablation profiles: theoretical background. *J. Cataract Refract. Surg*. 2004;30:775-85.

[68] Srivannaboon S, Reinstein DZ, Archer TJ, Chansue E. Spherical aberration from myopic excimer laser ablation for aspheric and non-aspheric profiles. *Optom. Vis. Sci.* 2012;89:1211-8.

[69] Taneri S, Oehler S, Macrae SM. Aspheric wavefront-guided versus wavefront-guided LASIK for myopic astigmatism with the Technolas 217z100 excimer laser. *Graefes Arch. Clin. Exp. Ophthalmol*. 2013;251:609-16.

In: Current Understanding and New Techniques …
Editor: Michael O'Keefe
ISBN: 978-1-62808-748-2

Chapter 9

Medical Legal Issues

*Marc B. Guerin**
Moorfields Eye Hospital, London, UK

"We are all exceptional cases; we all want to appeal against something.
Each of us insists on being innocent at all costs, even if he has
to accuse the whole human race and heaven itself"
Albert Camus, The Fall

1. Introduction

In an age of increasing patient expectations and aggressive marketing, costly and acrimonious medicolegal disputes are becoming more frequent. Doctors may bitterly resent an allegation of negligence made by a patient whose legal representation is determined to extract a significant financial settlement. Whilst it is true that the ultimate *raison d'etre* of medical law is to enforce the principle of *primum non noceredo*, this is easily overlooked amidst the adversarial nature of medicolegal disputes. [1] It is a common occurrence that a spurious claim is settled in favour of the plaintiff at the steps of the courthouse simply to avert further expense. Refractive surgery is a unique subspecialty where an error of millimetres can result in devastating and irreversible consequences. It involves an elective lifestyle motivated procedure on a normal eye in often highly motivated, self-paying perfectionists. One of the easiest ways for a surgeon to prevent dissatisfaction in this cohort of patients is compliance with the relevant medical law. This chapter will address the current basics of medical law, outline common reasons for claims of medical malpractice and offer some guidelines for evolving a system that offers a good outcome for the patient while preventing litigation.

* Consultant Ophthalmologist and Barrister at Law; e-mail: marcguerin@hotmail.com

2. The Law

Medical malpractice can lead to an action in criminal, contractual or negligence law. As far back as 1914, the New York Court of Appeals stated that "Every human, of adult years and of sound mind, has a right to determine what shall be done with his own body: and a surgeon who performs an operation without the patients consent commits an assault". [2] In 1957 in California, the term 'informed consent' was introduced to judicial parlance for first time and in 1972 'informed consent' was enshrined as a legal principle in the US case of Canterbury v. Spence. [3, 4] The most common legal conduit for a malpractice claim today is in the tort of negligence, and to make a successful claim the plaintiff must negotiate 5 legal hurdles. The patient must firstly prove the existence of a legal duty of due care by the surgeon to the plaintiff, that a breach of this duty occurred, cause and effect occurred, the patient suffered injury or damage and finally that this damage is recognised in law. Any missing step negates the claim. The duty of care is usually self-evident but not always. For example an ophthalmologist creates a duty of care, if while covering for a colleague he gives medical advice to a patient over the phone, having never met the patient before. Furthermore, a question of vicarious liability and resultant duty of care may arise if the surgeon's employees have committed an act of negligence in the performance of their duties. The standard applicable in England and Wales to an alleged breach of the surgeon's duty is outlined in the case Bolam v Friern Hospital Management Committee. [5] This case held that, providing a doctor follows a course of action that a reasonable body of doctors would pursue, negligence will not ensue. This appears a generous test, and it does not matter if the body of doctors in question is a minority group. This reasoning is similar to a recent US case where a $4,000,000 award was made to a commercial airline pilot who suffered adverse night-time visual symptoms because pupillometry was not properly performed preoperatively as would have been done by other doctors. [6] However there is a limitation on this "body of doctors" test if the court concludes that the body in question is entirely unreasonable. With regard to causation, this can be either direct or proximate. An exception to this is the doctrine of *res ipsa loquitur*, whereby the negligence can be directly inferred from the facts. Finally the patient must prove injury (financial/physical/psychological) and this damage must be recognised by the court. The award of damages in the civil law is intended to compensate the claimant for the loss and damage caused by the defendant. Of course the difficulty in ophthalmic cases is that it can be difficult to disprove a patient's claimed loss of subjective vision as objective assessments of visual function are often easily manipulated.

Negligence may be alleged at any or all of the 3 stages of the doctor/patient relationship in refractive surgery including preoperatively, postoperatively or during the refractive procedure itself. Preoperatively, there are 2 areas crucial to avoiding pitfalls, namely, patient selection and informed consent. With regard to patient selection, the Bolam test as outlined above applies.

As to what precisely needs to be disclosed in the consenting process is jurisdiction dependent. The consenting process is not simply an opportunity to divest legal duties, but should be viewed as an opportunity to create a relationship of trust with the patient. It is always incumbent upon the surgeon to advise and educate patients preoperatively about their treatment options, potential complications and to seek to identify, and moderate, unrealistic expectations. The difficulty lies in striking a balance between the interests of the surgeon and those who rely on them. In this author's jurisdiction of the Republic of Ireland, the Supreme Court recently upheld the view that the medical defendant is obliged to give a warning to the plaintiff of any material risk according to what a reasonable patient would want disclosed and which is a known or foreseeable complication of an operation patient's knowledge, understanding and expectations.[7,8]

In Ireland, the courts distinguish between elective and emergency procedures, in that for elective procedures "there is an obligation wherever there is a risk- however exceptional or remote- of grave consequence involving severe pain stretching for an appreciable time into the future and involving the possibility of further operative procedures, to warn of that risk in the clearest possible language".[9] However, in cases not involving a risk of on-going severe pain, such as laser eye surgery, the obligation to warn is lessened to a "significant risk which would affect the judgement of a reasonable patient".

As to whether a risk was significant, both the statistical frequency of the risk and the severity of its consequences must first be ascertained. [10] The UK law of informed consent is based on a House of Lords case called *Sidaway v. Board of Governors of the Bethlem Royal Hospital* which is in turn based on the aforementioned Bolam case. [11] In essence a doctor should disclose what a reasonable relevant body of the profession would outline in a consenting process. The governing and advisory clinical bodies in the UK also give guidance. The National Institute for Health and Clinical Excellence (NICE) demands that surgeons ensure "that patients fully understand the benefits and potential risks of the procedure, and provide them with clear written information, such as that published by NICE". [12] The General Medical Council advises ''if you are the doctor providing treatment or undertaking an investigation, it is your responsibility to discuss it with the patient and obtain consent as you will have a comprehensive understanding of the procedure or treatment. How it is carried out and the risks attached to it. Where this is not practicable, you may delegate these tasks provided you ensure that the person to whom you delegate is suitably trained and qualified, has sufficient knowledge of the proposed investigation or treatment and understands the risks involved, and acts in accordance with the guidance in this booklet.'' [13]

The timing of the consent process is also important. The UK Department of Health proclaims that ''If a patient is not asked to signify their consent until just before the procedure is due to start, at a time when they may be feeling particularly vulnerable, there may be real doubt as to its validity.''[14] This is reiterated by Irish Supreme Court, which specifically noted in a case involving slippage of an extraocular muscle post strabismus repair, that informed consent immediately prior to surgery is not the preferred course of action. [15] In that case the judge noted "There are obvious reasons why, in the context of elective surgery, a warning given only shortly before an operation is undesirable. A patient may be stressed, medicated or in pain in this period and may be less likely for one or more of these reasons to make a calm and reasoned decision in such circumstances....While I have noted the views of a number of the experts to the effect that this practice of warning day patients on the day of their operation had its advantages, it seems to me that the disadvantages were far greater, including the possibility of an embittered patient later asserting that he was too stressed or in too much pain to understand what was said or to make a free decision and that he was thus effectively deprived of any choice."

A recent 2011 UK case has led to an interesting development with regard to potential negligence of expert witnesses. In Jones versus Kaney, the UK Supreme Court removed immunity from expert witnesses. [16] This has received a mixed reaction, perhaps ensuring proper preparation and consideration from witnesses in the future, but preventing other experts providing opinions if it leaves them open to claims from dissatisfied litigants.

3. Medical Negligence Trends

The Medical Protection Society (MPS), a medical indemnifier, noted that between 2007 to 2011in Ireland, the number of medicolegal claims against doctors handled by them increased by 20% with an increase in award size of 37%. [17] During the same period, the frequency of claims in UK rose by 47%, with claim pay-outs increasing by 26%, while in South Africa there was a 25% increase with a phenomenal 111% rise in monetary awards. Although no tangible evidence exists, there may be a correlation with the economic recession associated with that period. Interestingly, and reflective of a general finding among many of the medical insurers, only 2% of cases reached actually trial in court.

The National Health Service Litigation Authority (NHSLA) is a not for profit Special Health Authority established in 1995 in the UK that provides indemnity cover for legal claims against the NHS. It has noticed a significant increase in claims in recent times. Over the last five years the annual number of claims of clinical negligence notified to the NHSLA has risen by 52%. [18] Claims rose by over 30% between 2009/2010 to 2020/2011 with a 12% increase in payments made in the same period.

Another UK indemnity society, the Medical Defence Union (MDU) noted that "Laser eye surgery….. became a significant source of claims against MDU members around the year 2000 when we began to receive increasing numbers of claims with a166% increase in negligence claims related to laser refractive surgery between 1997 and 2003 and by 2006 accounted for a third of all ophthalmology claims on the MDU's files." [19] Many of their cases involved dissatisfaction with vision postoperatively and corneal scarring.

Ophalmic Mutual Insurance Company, (OMIC), a prominent US ophthalmic indemnifier, found a peak of LASIK claims against their members in 2000 which have been reducing in frequency since then, although a subsequent spike in 2006 and 2007 was noted. [20] By 2008, refractive surgery was their third most litigious subspeciality behind cataract surgery and general ophthalmology. Between 1989 and August 2008, OMIC made indemnity payments on 65 of 231 closed refractive claims, with an average payment of just under $145,000. 85% of all refractive claims made were secondary to LASIK

4. Common Causes of Negligence

Abbott in 2003 produced the first published study that identified and correlated significant predictors and risk factors with malpractice liability claims in the US following PRK and LASIK. High patient volume, prior claims against the surgeon, male gender, aggressive advertising, less time spent with patients, and comanagement with optometrists were all found to be associated with a higher level of claims [21].

Bailey and Bailey have published an excellent article identifying specifics central to claims of negligence in refractive surgery in the UK. [22] One hundred and one closed cases of claims were reviewed with a single expert witness assessing all cases. Their findings can be divided into preoperative, intraoperative and postoperative categories. Informed consent, a fundamental part of the preoperative routine, was noted to be important in 65% of the total number of claims, involving in all cases a failure to warn. In 97% of these cases, there was no contemporaneous written evidence of any discussion of risk or outcome. In the majority of cases the patient claimed to have seen the informed consent for the first time on the day of surgery. The author of this chapter has published on the understanding and recall of patients who were consented prior to LASIK and LASEK. [32] Attitudes, understanding and recall of our informed consenting process of 102 patients undergoing first time refractive surgery were examined. Only 2 patients remembered all 5 risks outlined preoperatively, while 11 remembered no risks at all. 65% of patients consulted the internet to learn more about the operationconclusion, our study indicates that patients understanding and recall of the consent process is poor.

Thus it is imperative for the surgeon to outline laboriously and in detail the procedure and all potential risks. Our analysis demonstrates that, despite a lengthy and detailed consenting process, patient understanding and recall of the procedures and risks remained poor. This is similar to the findings of Cheung et al. who noted that, despite repetitive explicit counselling, only 39% of patient undergoing cataract surgery knew what a cataract was, 28% knew what surgery entailed and 43% misunderstood that surgery was completely risk free. [24] Informed consent must be a process rather than simply signing a form, and should include a detailed outline by the doctor to the patient, setting out treatment options, risks involved and expected outcomes.

Further preoperative issues occurred in 29% of the cases analysed by Bailey, comprising contraindications and risk factors including "high refractive error, particularly hyperopia, presence of amblyopia, pre-existing dry eye, keratoconus, corneal endothelial dysfunction, cataract, and personality disorder". The authors note that insufficient emphasis was placed on explaining to the patients the relevance of these preoperative findings. Missed preoperative ectasia is a significant cause of claims of negligence, with 12.7% of the laser refractive cases in Baileys study demonstrating post-operative keratectasia. In the US case of Schiffer versus Speaker, a multimillion dollar award was made on the basis of missed preoperative ectasia. [25] This award included $750,000 awarded to the plaintiff for conscious pain and suffering $2,000,000 for future pain and suffering (10 years). $500,000 for lost earnings, and $4,000,000 awarded to Plaintiff for future lost earnings (7 years). In a separate 2009 case, a New York jury awarded $5.6 million to the plaintiff, $3.1 million of which was for the pain and suffering element, for undetected preoperative forme fruste keratoconus. [26] Twenty four percent of claims in Bailey's study concerned intraoperative surgical error, such as proceeding with laser ablation in the presence of a full or partial thickness buttonhole, or a short flap where the bed was insufficient to receive the ablation. With regard to postoperative care, 23% of cases involved the patient being unable to contact the clinic or was advised inappropriately by a non-medically qualified member of staff and the resulting delay in management adversely affected the outcome.

Clear, honest and timely communication is central to avoiding malpractice claims. Hickson et al. suggested that the physician's ability to establish rapport with, provide access to and communicate effectively with the patients is as important as technical competence in protecting against litigation. [27] Abbott reported that many claims and lawsuits centred on poor physician relationship and lack of communication with the patient [28].

The correct information and warnings must be given beforehand, and acknowledgement with a properly worded apology should be proffered if a complication does occur. It has been suggested that a five-step process should contribute to making a meaningful apology to a patient. [27] These steps include (1) recognition; (2) regret; (3) responsibility; (4) remedy; and (5) re-alignment.

It is undoubtedly true that patients will seek legal redress if they feel their doctor is hiding something, has not acknowledged a mistake or is being overtly defensive. To encourage better doctor/patient relations and perhaps reduce malpractice claims, several US states have enacted legislation to make apologies from doctors for their medical mistakes inadmissible in court. The phraseology 'I regret that you have had a bad experience with your refractive surgery. Neither one of us expected you to have these problems. I am very sorry this has happened' has been suggested. [27]

6. Recommendations

The below is a guide based on case law, analysis of reasons for claims and also takes into account the OMIC, Royal College of Ophthalmologists (RCOphth) and the American Academy of Ophthalmology (AAO) guidelines [30, 31, 32].

i) The Surgeon

The surgeon should be appropriately trained with certified completion of relevant residency, fellowships, and courses (e.g. RCOphth Certificate in Laser Refractive Surgery). They must be registered with the relevant governing body, maintain professional insurance, undertake frequent and regular audits, undergo continuing medical education in refractive surgery, and be a member of a national or international refractive surgery association e.g. American and/or European Societies for Cataract and Refractive Surgery or United Kingdom and Ireland Society of Cataract and Refractive Surgeons.

ii) Preoperative History and Examination

Prior to surgery, the surgeon performing the surgery must perform and document a comprehensive history and examination, including a medical history looking for relevant medical conditions such as rheumatoid arthritis, connective tissue disorders, diabetes and herpes. He should also perform a slit lamp exam, cycloplegic refraction, objective tear measurement and review tomography, pachymetry, pupil size (and refractive stability and specular microscopy for phakic implants and RLE). Corneal tomography is often a stumbling block. Whilst it remains uncertain as to where the cut-off for safety is in respect of a laser-assisted treatment on any particular cornea, overt signs are simply indefensible. Extra care and time should be taken with presbyopic patients.

iii. Patient Age

In this author's practice, patients should be at least 20 years old, with a stable refraction for at least 12 months previously.

iv. Informed Consent

The operating surgeon must seek informed consent and document in the medical records the risks, benefits, alternatives discussed. Each patient should be offered a copy of the consent form prior to the day of surgery, ideally at the time of first consultation.

All patients should be provided with information leaflets and many patients like the option to watch an explanatory video. These media should reinforce the oral information provided to a patient, including prognosis, purpose of the proposed procedure, benefits and risks (especially specific to that patient), alternatives, whether the procedure is experimental, contact telephone number and costs. Audio recording the consent is a further option, although in this author's opinion is unwarranted if the above is performed.

v. Equipment

The surgeon should ensure a system whereby treatment parameters entered are double checked with a third party. In Oliver v Abell, $1,750,000 was awarded to the plaintiff due to an incorrect treatment entered into the laser system resulting in the surgeon performing surgery on the wrong axis of plaintiff's eye. [33] Furthermore the surgeon then performed an enhancement treatment inappropriately early within one month of the initial surgery. (Of note this verdict was later overturned because of the fact, undisclosed to the litigants prior to trial, that the trial judge's husband occasionally worked on cases with the law firm that represented the plaintiff.).

Laser facilities must be appropriately registered and equipment should be properly maintained and calibrated with appropriate documentation. A back-up power supply for the laser is required. Lasers should be used as per FDA requirements and surgeons should inform the patient if this is not the case.

vi. The Surgery

The first 5 cases performed by a surgeon should be surface treatments and done sequentially with 1-7 intervening days. Surgeons must enrol on continuous medical education courses.

vii. Postoperatively

The surgeon or a designated ophthalmologist must perform the first postoperative exam. The patient should have access to a fully qualified member of the surgical team at all times.

Clinical enquiries must be passed to an experienced physician without unreasonable delay.

vii. Clinical and Information Governance

Surgeons must undertake clinical audits and regularly review the results. They must also investigate, record, and collate all adverse events and report and discuss them with the appropriate advisory committee. There should be documented clinical protocols for all surgical procedures performed. All entries in patients' notes should be clearly readable, signed, and dated and all computer entered patient data encrypted appropriately.

ix. Marketing

All advertising must not be misleading or guarantee results. Surgeon must follow relevant guidelines e.g. FDA and FTC or UK Advertising Standards Agency advertising guidelines.

x. Communication

The surgeon must be open and honest and forthright both before and after the surgery. If there has been a complication, patients should be made aware of same as soon as practical and an apology can be made with the appropriate wording. Waiving surgical fees where an adverse event has occurred may aid in preventing a claim.

Conclusion

If refractive surgeons want to satisfy their patients and avoid a complaint or lawsuit, they must take every precaution in choosing appropriate patients, providing the best information, and performing the best techniques with appropriate equipment. Case law indicates the importance of the preoperative stage in particular – screening patients comprehensively and consenting them with reference to outcomes relevant to their preoperative assessment is crucial. Communication, good clinical and information governance and common sense are the edifices on which medical law is built, and the surgeon should implement relevant protocols in an effort to avoid costly and distressing litigation.

References

[1] "*Primum non noceredo*" translates to "first do no harm", part of The Hippocratic Oath taken by physicians swearing to practice medicine ethically and honestly.
[2] Schloendorff v. Society of New York Hospital, 211 N.Y. 125, 105 N.E. 92 (1914).

[3] Salgo v Leland Stanford, Jr., University Board of Trustees, 154 Cal.App.2d 560, 317 P.2d 170 (1957).
[4] Canterbury v. Spence, 464 F.2d 772 (D.C. Cir. 1972)
[5] Bolam v Friern Hospital Management Committee [1957] 1 WLR 582.
[6] Post v. University Physicians, Inc., 2002 WL 32832041 (Ariz. Super. 2002).
[7] Geoghan v Harris [2000] 3IR536.
[8] Fitzpatrick V Whyte (2005) IEHC 479, and (2007) IEHC 479.
[9] Walsh v. Irish Family Planning Ltd [1992] 1 IR 496 510 Flaherty J.
[10] Fitzpatrick V Whyte (2005) IEHC 479, and (2007) IEHC 479.
[11] Sidaway v. Board of Governors of the Bethlem Royal Hospital Governors [1985] AC 871.
[12] www.nice.org.uk
[13] Seeking patient's consent: the ethical considerations. General Medical Council, November 1998.
[14] Reference Guide to Consent for Examination or Treatment. Department of Health, March 2001, section 10.
[15] Fitzpatrick V Whyte (2005) IEHC 479, and (2007) IEHC 479.
[16] Jones v Kaney [2011] UKSC 13
[17] https://www.medicalprotection.org/uk/podcasts/claims-experience-in-ireland.
[18] www.nhsla.com
[19] Tomkins C. Over 120 years of defending ophthalmologists *Br J Ophthalmol* 2006;90:1084-5
[20] OMICDIGEST Volume 18 Number 4 Fall 2008.
[21] Abbott RL, Ou RJ, Bird M. Medical malpractice predictors and risk factors for ophthalmologists performing LASIK and photorefractive keratectomy surgery. *Ophthalmology* 2003;110:2137–46.
[22] Bailey CS, Bailey JA. Claims of alleged medical negligence in refractive surgery: causes and avoidance. *Cont Lens Anterior Eye*. 2007;30:144-147.
[23] Guerin M, O'Keeffe M Informed consent in refractive eye surgery: learning from patients and the courts. *Ir Med J.* 2012 Sep;105(8):282-3.
[24] Cheung D, Sandramouli S The consent and counselling of patients for cataract surgery: a prospective audit *Eye (Lond)*. 2005 Sep;19(9):963-71.
[25] Schiffer v. Speaker, Index No.101191/03 (Supreme Court New York County 2005).
[26] Devadas v. Niksarli, Index No. 107637/07 (Supreme Court New York County)
[27] Hickson GB and Jenkins AD. Identifying and addressing communication failures as a means of reducing unnecessary malpractice claims *NCMedJ* 2007 68:362-4.
[28] Abbott RL. Informed Consent in Refractive surgery. *Cur Opin Ophth* 9: 29-34.
[29] Potter, John W. (2008) "Implementation of dispute resolution in refractive surgery," *ADR Bulletin*: Vol. 10: No. 7, Article 4.
[30] http://www.omic.com/wp-content/uploads/2012/12/Guide-to-Refractive-Surgery-6-3-10.pdf
[31] Royal College of Ophthalmologists, London "Standards for Laser Refractive Surgery" published April 2012.
[32] http://one.aao.org/CE/PracticeGuidelines/PPP_Content.aspx?cid=0bc8c7ce-26df-46da-bf2b-7e908bedaf64
[33] Oliver v. Abell, No. 99-CI-1816 (Ky. Cir. Ct. Nov. 1, 2001).

In: Current Understanding and New Techniques ...
Editor: Michael O'Keefe
ISBN: 978-1-62808-748-2

Chapter 10

Long-Term Refractive Changes after Refractive Surgery

Andrea Ryan[1,*] and Michael O'Keefe[2,†]

[1]Cork University Hospital, Cork, Ireland

[2]Mater Private Hospital, Dublin, Ireland

Abstract

Long-term stability of the refractive correction following excimer laser refractive surgical intervention is a highly desirable outcome for both patients and surgeons and is to the forefront of patient expectations. Refractive changes over time will be influenced by many factors both surgical (laser systems, ablation zone diameters, magnitude of attempted corrections etc.) and non-surgical (physiological changes in refraction with ageing, variations in corneal wound healing responses etc.). Rapidly evolving technological advancements and greater understanding of the corneal response to excimer laser ablation has led to significant changes in surgical practice in the last 2 decades. Extrapolating the results of long-term studies that date from procedures employed more than a decade ago to modern techniques is a significant limitation to our ability to inform patients about the potential long-term stability of currently employed procedures. Loss of patients to long-term follow-up is a hindrance to reliable data collection on regression. Notwithstanding these limitations, the news for prospective laser refractive surgical patients is generally very good, especially in low-moderate levels of ametropia. Once an initial stable refraction is obtained following surgery in the first postoperative 6 months to 1 year, it tends to remain quite stable over time. Regression is more significant and outcomes more unpredictable in high ametropia. High degrees of myopia and hyperopia are no longer corrected by excimer laser ablation and phakic intraocular lens implantation in such patients provides a more stable refractive solution.

* andrearyan11@gmail.com.
† mokeefe@materprivate.ie.

Introduction

One of the most frequently posed questions by patients considering laser refractive surgery is "How long will it last?"

The long-term stability of the refractive correction is an issue of significant importance to patients and surgeons alike. The question is not easy to answer and will depend on many variables.

In this chapter, we will discuss long-term refractive changes following hyperopic and myopic excimer laser refractive procedures in the form of surface ablation and laser in situ keratomileusis (LASIK), the factors that are important in post-surgical regression and the incidence and outcome of re-treatments.

Physiologic Change in Refraction with Ageing

When considering long-term refractive stability after refractive surgery, it is important to take into account the normal physiologic change in refraction with ageing. Two large population-based studies have confirmed a hyperopic change in refraction over time in persons younger than 65 years of age and a myopic change in those older than 65 years of age, which is related to the degree of nuclear sclerosis.[1, 2] In the Beaver Dam Eye Study, the five year change in spherical equivalent (SE) refraction of persons aged 45, 55, 65, and 75 years of age was +0.15, +0.18, +0.10 and -0.07 dioptres (D) respectively.[1] In the Blue Mountains Eye Study, the mean change in SE refraction over 5 years of persons aged 49 to 54, 55 to 64, 65 to 74, and 75 years or older at baseline was +0.41D, +0.30D, +0.05D, and -0.22D, respectively.[2]

A myopic population will differ from the normal adult population. Ellingsen et al. showed that in simple myopes with low to moderate myopia (-1 to -6D) a myopic shift tends to occur until the 6th decade when a hyperopic shift occurs.[3] The mean change per patient age-decade was: 20s, -0.60D; 30s, -0.39D; 40s, -0.29D; 50s, +0.28D; 60s, +0.41D. Ellingsen also demonstrated that a myopic population shows a subgroup that remains relatively stable and a subgroup that experiences significant refractive shift over time.

High myopes may experience more significant myopic progression than low-moderate myopes. It has been shown that highly myopic eyes (>6D) often continue to undergo axial length (AL) elongation even in later life, with 31% of eyes undergoing elongation of more than 1mm in AL over a mean period of 8 years.[4, 5] A 1mm elongation in AL is equivalent to a myopic shift of 2 to 2.5D. [6] In a long-term follow-up study of photorefractive keratectomy (PRK) for myopia, Rajan et al. found that 33% of patients who had unilateral PRK experienced late myopic progression in both the un-operated and operated eyes of magnitude 1 to 3.2D between the ages of 28 and 36 years.[7] All were high myopes (6 to 10D). Late myopic progression could therefore be mistaken for post-surgical myopic regression in such patients and pre-surgical counselling should make patients aware of the possibility of late progression of their myopia.

Long-term Stability of Refraction following Excimer Laser Refractive Surgery

In addition to considering the long-term physiological changes in refraction that occur with ageing and the natural history of ametropia of various degrees, it is also important to emphasise that our ability to draw conclusions about the potential long-term stability of modern refractive surgical procedures is limited by our dependence on studies that stem from techniques and procedures that have undergone significant modification over the years. Due to the constant improvement and evolution of technology and of technique, long-term data of a decade or more will inevitably be derived from the use of equipment and techniques that are now somewhat obsolete. Most notably, older excimer laser systems were of the broad beam type as opposed to today's flying spot or scanning spot lasers. The use of small optical zones has been abandoned due to the recognition of night visual disturbances and regression. It is not yet known if modern advancements such as wavefront-guided ablation, topography-guided ablation or femtosecond-laser assisted LASIK will provide more predictable and stable results in the long-term compared to conventional treatment.

Many long-term studies are hindered by difficulty in recalling patients for re-evaluation many years after surgery. Most of the published long-term studies reassess only a portion of the original cohorts after 10 years making the data prone to potential bias.

With these provisos, it is still useful to utilise the data from published long-term studies to try to extrapolate information on the potential long-term stability of currently employed refractive procedures.

Hyperopia

Prior to the advent of excimer laser refractive surgery, numerous procedures were tried for the correction of hyperopia with limited predictability and progressive regression following treatment. These procedures included keratophakia, cryolathe keratomileusis, thermokeratoplasty, hexagonal keratotomy and automated lamellar keratoplasty.

The excimer laser led to the development of hyperopic PRK and hyperopic LASIK. Short-term studies of these techniques demonstrated acceptable efficacy for corrections up to +4.0D, with less predictability for higher corrections. [8-13]

Surface Ablation for Hyperopia

In general, surface ablation for hyperopia, either by PRK or by modern variations on the technique such as laser epithelial keratomileusis (LASEK), is characterized by initial overcorrection towards myopia followed by hyperopic regression towards emmetropia over 3 to 6 months and then a more gradual hyperopic regression over time. [14-16] There are very few published long-term studies on hyperopic surface ablation, with a maximum follow-up of 1-2 years in most studies. A single study reports outcomes up to 7.5 years. A summary of long-term studies with at least 2 years follow-up of hyperopic surface ablation is provided in Table 1.

The longest follow-up study in the literature of hyperopic PRK is that by O'Brart et al. and reports outcomes at 7.5 years.[15] The authors report that stability was not achieved until the 12th postoperative month but remained stable thereafter. An initial myopic overshoot occurred, followed by hyperopic regression to emmetropia over 3 to 6 months then a more gradual hyperopic regression from 6 to 12 months of mean +0.48D (range -0.88 to +2.50D). Between 12 months and mean 7.5 years, a mean hyperopic shift of +0.28D occurred, which the authors felt was consistent with the physiological hyperopic shift in refraction with ageing. Ten percent of eyes showed a change in SE refraction of >+1.0D and 14% a change of >+0.50D.

LASIK for Hyperopia

Long-term data on the stability of hyperopic LASIK corrections are also limited with the longest reported follow-up in the literature being 5 years. Therefore, the long-term stability is uncertain. Most studies show a degree of hyperopic regression at the last visit with the magnitude increasing with higher attempted degrees of hyperopia correction. For this reason, laser vision correction for hyperopia has been described as a 'semi-permanent' solution.[17]

A summary of long-term studies on hyperopic LASIK is provided in Table 2.

The studies with 5 years of follow-up show predictability within 1D of the target refraction of 82% for attempted corrections up to +2.0D, 71-74% for attempted corrections up to +3.0D and 33-67% for attempted corrections above +3.5-4.0 D and up to +6.0D depending on the magnitude. [18-20]

Mean hyperopic regression from 1 to 5 years ranges from +0.18D to +1.85 depending on the magnitude of baseline attempted hyperopia correction. [18-20] For lower degrees of hyperopia (up to +4.0D), the mean change is most commonly <+0.50D and would appear to be within the limits of normal physiological change in refraction with ageing. For higher degrees of hyperopia, the change exceeds that of normal ageing.

Hyperopic regression of >+1D occurred in 5% of eyes from 6 months to 4 years in Kezirian's study in which only 11% of eyes had an attempted correction of >+4.0D. [21] Regression of ≥+0.50D occurred in 51% and >+1D in 28% of eyes from 1 to 5 years in Jaycock's study in which 34% had an attempted correction ≥+3.50D. [20] Esquenazi concluded that long-term stability was poor for attempted correction of hyperopia greater than +3.0D. [19]

Factors Influencing Hyperopic Regression

Degree of Hyperopia

The single greatest factor influencing hyperopic regression is the magnitude of attempted correction. Long-term predictability and stability is much greater with lower attempted hyperopic corrections of ≤+3.50 D. Attempted correction of higher degrees of hyperopia, especially >+4.0D, results in less predictable results and greater hyperopic regression over time. [13, 18, 19, 22]. Attempted correction of high hyperopic astigmatism (>2D) is also associated with undercorrection. [23]

Age

There is some evidence that hyperopic regression may be greater in younger persons, possibly related to more aggressive wound healing responses or to the unmasking of latent hyperopia with development of presbyopia over time. O'Brart et al. found that following hyperopic PRK, patients older than 50 years at the time of initial surgery remained much closer to emmetropia and experienced less hyperopic drift over mean 7.5 years than those <50 years at the time of surgery. [15] Following LASIK, Jaycock found that the hyperopic shift from 1 to 5 years was +0.67D for patients younger than 40 years of age and +0.44D for patients 43-55 years of age. [20]

Ablation Diameter/Optical Zone

While it can be a challenge to perform larger ablations (which require the cutting of larger LASIK flaps) in small hyperopic eyes, there is some evidence that larger diameter optical zones (≥6mm) are associated with greater predictability and stability of refraction. [24-26]

PRK versus LASIK

A systematic review of PRK versus LASIK for hyperopia correction revealed only non-randomised studies that appear to agree that the techniques are of comparable efficacy in the short-term. [27] In general, a greater initial myopic overshoot is observed after PRK followed by a hyperopic regression, whereas a faster stability of refraction is achieved with LASIK. [28, 29] There are no long-term studies directly comparing the outcome of the 2 procedures.

Two long-term studies – one of hyperopic PRK by O'Brart et al. and one of hyperopic LASIK by Jaycock et al. - were performed by the same authors on eyes with a similar preoperative range of hyperopia using the same laser delivery system, treatment nomograms and 6mm optical zone size. The long-term results of PRK for hyperopia reported by O'Brart showed good refractive stability from 1 to 7.5 years with mean hyperopic drift of +0.28D and hyperopic shift of >0.50D in 40% and >1D in 10%. However, the long-term results of hyperopic LASIK in the similar population of patients reported by Jaycock did not show stability from 1 to 5 years with mean hyperopic shift +0.53D and 50% experiencing more than 0.50D of hyperopic drift and 28% more than 1D. The authors suggested that there may be a difference in the long-term stability between LASIK and PRK.

Table 1. Summary of Long-term Studies of Hyperopic Surface Ablation

Study*	Laser System	Technique	OZ (mm)	FU (yrs)	Baseline Group (SE) (D)	No. of Eyes	Preoperative SE	Postoperative SE at Last Visit	Mean SE Regression (D)	% Eyes within 0.50 or 1D of Target at Last Visit		UCVA at last visit (% eyes)	
							Mean +/- SD (D)			0.50D	1.0D	6/6 or better	6/12 or better
O'Brart 2005	Summit SVS Apex Plus	PRK	6	7.5	All Eyes +1.50 and +3.00 +4.50 and +6.00	40	+4.70 +1.50 and+3.00 +4.50 and+6.00	+0.83 … …	+0.28 (1 to 7.5yrs) … …	28 27 24	53 67 40	15 … …	58 … …
Spadea 2006	Zeiss Meditec Mel 70G	PRK	6	2	All Eyes	100	+2.85+/-1.10	+0.34+/-0.92	+0.53 change in mean SE 6-24mths	36	78	46	98
Autrata 2003	Nidek EC-5000	LASEK PRK	5.5 5.5	2 2	+2 to +5 +2 to +5	108 108	+3.76 +/-1.38 +3.58 +/-1.29	+0.32 +/-0.29 +0.74 +/-0.35	… …	78 57	92 86	67 73	91 81
O'Brart 2007	Schwind ESIRIS	LASEK	7	1-2	All Eyes 0 to +2.50 +2.63 to +5	70 47 23	+2.32	+0.13 +/-0.43	Not significant	86 94 70	100 100 96	78	98 ≥6/9
Stevens 2002	Visx Star	PRK	..	1-2	All Eyes (astigmatism) 0 to +1.75 Sphere Up to -2.5 Cylinder	27	+2.90	+0.40	…			70	93

* First Author and Year, OZ= optical zone, FU=follow-up, yrs=years, No.=number, SE=spherical equivalent, SD=standard deviation, D=diopters, UCVA=uncorrected visual acuity, PRK=photorefractive keratectomy, LASEK=laser epithelial keratectomy.

Table 2. Summary of the Long-term studies of Hyperopic LASIK

Study*	Laser System	FU (yrs)	Baseline Group (SE) (D)	No. of Eyes	Preoperative SE (D)	Postoperative SE (D) at Last Visit	Mean SE Regression (D) +/- SD	% Eyes within 0.50 or 1D of Target at Last Visit		UCVA at last visit (% eyes)	
					Mean +/- SD			0.50D	1.0D	6/6 or better	6/12 or better
Desai 2008	Visx Star S2	5	All Eyes	41	+2.53 +/-1.25	+0.53 +/-0.81	+0.40 +/-0.79 (1-5yrs)	43	69	34	88
			<+2.0	17	+1.34 +/-0.36	+0.44 +/-0.69	+0.18 +/-0.50	53	82	41	100
			+2.0 to +4.0	12	+2.66 +/-0.28	+0.58 +/-0.56	+0.30 +/-0.75	50	75	42	92
			>+4.0 up to +5.25	12	+4.10 +/-0.69	+0.59 +/-1.18	+0.55 +/-1.07	33	67	17	67
Kezirian 2008	Wavelight Allegretto Wave	4	All Eyes	127	+2.2 +/-1.41	…	+0.19 +/-0.53 (6mo-4yrs)	…	94	…	…
			≤+2	58%							
			>+2 to ≤+4	31%							
			>+4 to +6.12	11%							
Esquenazi 2004	Technolas Keracor 117C	5	All Eyes	125	+3.84 +/-1.13	…	…	67	82	50	66
			+1.00 to +2.75		+2.03 +/-0.87	+0.48 +/-0.79	+0.35	63	74	72	93
			+3.00 to +4.25		+3.34 +/-0.92	+1.52 +/-1.45	+0.73	42	46	49	68
			+4.50 to +6.50		+5.25 +/-1.17	+3.39 +/-1.98	+1.85	22	33	12	43
Jaycock 2005	Summit SVS Apex Plus	4-5	All Eyes (+0.75 to +7.00)	47	+3.58 +/-1.48	+0.89 +/-0.94	+0.92 (3-55mo) +0.53 (12-54mo) (range +0.125 to +3.13)	32	60	43	87
			Attempted Correction:								
			+1.00 to +3.00D	31				…	71	…	…
			+3.50 to +6.00D	16				…	37.5	…	…

*First Author and Year, FU=follow-up, yrs=years, SE=spherical equivalent, D=diopters, No.=number, SD=standard deviation, UCVA=uncorrected visual acuity, mo=months.

In terms of variations on surface ablation techniques, Autrata reported that refractive stability was achieved earlier and maintained better at 2 years following hyperopic LASEK compared to hyperopic PRK. [16] Stability was achieved at 6 months following LASEK and at 12 months following PRK.

Newer Technologies (Wavefront-Guided, Wavefront-optimised, Topography-Guided, Femtosecond Laser Assisted LASIK)

There are no long-term studies greater than 2 years reporting the results of newer advancements in excimer laser surgery such as wavefront-guided or topography-guided ablations for the correction of hyperopia. It is not yet known if there will be long-term differences in refractive stability with such ablations or with other advancements such as the thinner and more predictable LASIK flaps that have been made possible by the femtosecond laser.

A short-term comparison of conventional versus wavefront-optimised hyperopic LASIK showed no significant difference in the SE refractive outcome at 6 months but the residual cylinder was less in the wavefront-optimised group. [30] Nagy et al. reported better results with wavefront-guided PRK versus conventional treatment for hyperopia correction at 6 months. [31]

A 2 year prospective study utilising topography-guided LASIK for correction of hyperopia +/- astigmatism of up to +7.25D sphere and up to -4.75 cylinder, found that 76% of eyes were within 0.50 D and 94% within 1.0D of the refractive target at 2 years.[32] The authors suggest that using the topographic approach to compensate for the angle kappa in hyperopes may be the key to producing more reliable results rather than centring the ablation over the pupil in standard LASIK hyperopic corrections.

A non-randomised study of femtosecond laser assisted LASIK versus microkeratome LASIK for hyperopia, found that the femtosecond group achieved slightly better refractive results at 3 months with mean residual error of +0.44 ± 0.6D in the femtosecond laser group versus +0.72 ± 0.8 D in the microkeratome group (p=0.02). [33]

Dry Eye

Esquenazi et al. noted that eyes with chronic dry eye symptoms showed a greater hyperopic regression at 5 years than eyes that did not –the mean difference in SE refraction from target refraction was +1.43 D for eyes with dry eye symptoms compared to +0.84 D for eyes without dry eye symptoms.[19]

Re-treatment Following Hyperopia Excimer Laser Surgery

Hersh et al. reported a 6% re-treatment rate within the first year for eyes treated by hyperopic LASIK of mean initial attempted SE +3.38 +/-0.80 D and range +2.50 to +4.50D.

[34] In terms of variables associated with the need for re-treatment, these eyes did not significantly differ from the main cohort of eyes treated for hyperopia but the number of cases was small (6 re-treatments out of 163 eyes). Most were re-treated for overcorrection.

There is no good long-term data on re-treatment rates after the first year following hyperopic LASIK or PRK.

The efficacy of re-treatment when it is performed appears to be satisfactory. A study by Ortega-Usobiaga et al. found that the efficacy of re-treatment of hyperopia after primary hyperopic LASIK was greater when the primary attempted SE refraction was <+3.0D and the safety of re-treatment was lower when the attempted SE re-treatment was >+1.0D and when the attempted SE refraction correction of both procedures combined was >+4.0D. [35] Alio found that following hyperopic LASIK re-treatment, eyes with preoperative SE refraction ≤+3.9 D showed 70% predictability within 0.50D of emmetropia at 1 year versus 46% for eyes with preoperative SE ≥+4.0D. [36] A study of wavefront-guided re-treatment of primary wavefront-guided hyperopic LASIK showed 88% within 0.50D and 100% within 1D of emmetropia at mean 15 months but the authors reported that the refractive results were not as good as re-treatments on primary myopic LASIK eyes.[37]

Saeed [38]and Aslanides[39] reported good stability of refraction up to 4 years following LASIK re-treatment by flap lift in which a minority of eyes were initially hyperopic.

Spadea reported very good results re-treating hyperopic PRK by transepithelial topography guided surface ablation.[40] Mean re-treatment of +2.23+/-0.65D (range +1.25 to +3.25D) resulted in mean SE refraction +0.03+/-0.29D at 3 years and 100% within 1D of target. No eye developed haze greater than grade 1 and no loss of CDVA occurred.

Myopia

Compared to hyperopic excimer laser surgery, there are significantly more long-term data (up to 10 years or more) on myopic surface ablation and LASIK. Many studies, however, include levels of attempted myopia correction that would be considered a contraindication to laser refractive surgical correction today. Studies that pool all preoperative levels of myopia may underestimate the stability of lower attempted corrections.

It is now well recognized that significant regression develops in the long-term following both PRK and LASIK for high and extreme high myopia, especially that of >10D magnitude. Post LASIK ectasia was reported in 1998 and high attempted myopia correction was recognized as a risk factor. Studies evaluating the long-term outcome of excimer laser procedures for high and extreme high myopia are less relevant to modern refractive surgical practice as such high degrees of myopia are now most commonly corrected by phakic intraocular lens implantation or refractive lens exchange.

In this section, we will address the following questions on long-term refractive changes post myopic surface ablation and LASIK-

- What is the likelihood of the refraction being within 1D of the target 10 years after surgery (predictability)?
- By how much, on average, will the refraction change after the initial stabilization (mean regression)? How will this vary for different levels of myopia?

- What are the predictors or factors that determine greater myopic regression?
- Is there a difference in the long-term stability of myopia correction by PRK versus LASIK?
- What is the likelihood of needing a re-treatment? How stable is the refraction following re-treatment?

Long-term Predictability of Myopic Excimer Laser Sugery

PRK

Table 3 shows the reported long-term predictability of PRK for various degrees of myopia. It can be seen that for low-moderate myopia, the predictability within 1D of emmetropia is 80% at 10 years (and even up to 16 years) with good consistency between studies. For myopia >6D, predictability within 1D is 66-70% at 10 years but a significant variability and decline in predictability occurs for myopia >10D (29-40%).

Table 3. Long-term Predictability of Myopic Photorefractive Keratectomy

Level of Preoperative Myopia	Eyes Within 1D of Target Refraction in Long-term Studies of PRK by Author					
	Postoperative Time					
	8years		10-13 years		16 years	
<6D	78% 83%	Pietila [41]Shojaei [42]	75% 87.5% 81% 50-75% 57%	Alio [43] Dirani [44] O'Connor* [45] Rajan [7] Koshimizu [46]	80%	Guerin *[47]
>6D (range)	69% 78%	Pietila (6-10D) [41] Shojaei (610D) [42]	66% 67% 75%	Alio (6-18D) [48] Dirani (6-18D) [44] Koshimizu (6-10D) [46]		
>10D to extreme	57% 72%	Pietila [41] Shojaei [42]	29% 41%	Koshimizu [46] Rosman [49]		

* Includes myopia up to 7.25D.

LASIK

Approximating the long-term predictability of LASIK from the published literature is more difficult as the studies vary highly in the magnitude of attempted myopia correction, the categorization of low-moderate myopia (<6D in some studies and ≤10D in others) and the inclusion of retreated eyes in several studies. A summary is provided in Table 4.

For myopia <6D, the predictability within 1D is approximately 70% at 6-9 years and in studies that include retreatments, is 95% or more at 10 years. For myopia up to 10D, predictability within 1D is approximately 65% at 10 years. In extreme high myopia >10D, the predictability within 1D decreases significantly and varies between 0 to 55% at 10 years.

Table 4. Long-term Predictability of Myopic LASIK

Level of Preoperative Myopia	Eyes Within 1D of Target Refraction in Long-term Studies of LASIK by Author					
	Postoperative Time					
	5-6years		6-9 years		10-11 years	
<6D	91-96%	O'Doherty [50] (1.4% RT)	69% 42%	Dirani [44] Zalentein* [51]	93-100% 64%	D'Arcy (11% RT) [52] Alio** [53]
>6D (range)	50%	O'Doherty (6-13D) [50] (14% RT)	65%	Dirani (6-18.5D) [44]	72% 88%	D'Arcy (6-13D) (39% RT)[52] Alio (6-10D) (18% RT) [54]
>10D to extreme	46%	Sekundo [55]			42% 55% 0%	Alio [56] Kymionis [57] Orucoglu[58](10% within 2D)

* Includes myopia up to 11.5D **Includes myopia up to 10D, D=diopters, RT=re-treated.

Long-term Regression following Myopic Excimer Laser Surgery

Most long-term studies of both PRK and LASIK show that the refraction stabilizes in the first postoperative year and remains quite stable thereafter with a small myopic drift occurring over 10 years. The regression in highly myopic eyes, especially in myopia >10D, is less predictable.

PRK

Several long-term studies have shown that in eyes with myopia <10D, mean myopic regression from 1 to 10 years or more following PRK is 0.50D or less. Some studies show a similar stability even in high myopes but in this group, a higher magnitude of regression is more common and may exceed 1D or more in 10 years.

A summary of long-term studies of PRK for the correction of myopia with an emphasis on postoperative regression is provided in Table 5.

In terms of the regression pattern, the trend most commonly reported was of initial hyperopic overcorrection that increased with the magnitude of attempted myopia correction, followed by a sharp myopic regression which usually stabilized within the first postoperative year. This was then followed by a much slower gradual myopic shift over the subsequent decade.

Table 5. Summary of long-term studies of Myopic Photorefractive Keratectomy

Study*	Laser System	OZ (mm)	FU (yrs)	Preoperative SE Myopia Range (D)	No. of Eyes	No. of Eyes at Latest FU	Preoperative SE (D)	Postoperative SE (D) at Last Visit	SE Regression (D)
							Mean +/- SD		
Guerin 2012	Summit UV200	5	16	1.75 to 7.25	120	39 (33%)	-4.36+/-1.58	-0.69+/-0.79	<0.50 myopic shift in the mean SE refraction for the total cohort from 2 to 16 yrs (-0.27 to -0.69) and -0.75 from 1 to 16 yrs (+0.06 to -0.69).
Bricola 2009	Summit UV200	4-5	14	<6 ≥6 (-6 to -13)	31 18		-3.37 +/-2.1 -7.68 +/-1.4	-0.17+/-0.80 -0.67+/-1.40	No significant change from 6 mo to 14 yrs in any group.
Dirani 2010		…	2-13 10-13 2-13 10-13	<6 ≥6 to 18.25	85 40	16 (19%) 9 (23%)	-4.05+/-1.17 -7.97+/-2.00	-0.64+/-0.83 -0.59+/-0.49 -1.06+/-1.71 -0.40+/-1.4	Change in mean SE <0.50 from 6mo to 10-13 yrs (-0.25 to -0.59) No change in mean SE from -0.40 at 6mo to -0.40 at 10-13yrs
O'Connor 2006	Summit UV200	5	12	1.75 to 7.25	120	58 (48%)	-4.4 +/-1.58	-0.58+/-0.72	<0.50 myopic shift in the cohort mean SE from 2 to 12 yrs (-0.27 to -0.58) or -0.64 from 1 to 12 yrs.
Rajan 2004		4	12	-2 Treatment -7 Treatment (SE up to 17.5)				-0.30+/-1.0 -4.47+/-1.16	-0.30+/-0.14 from 1 to 12 yrs -0.90+/-0.30 from1 to 12 yrs
Alio 2009	Visx 20/20	5.5-6	10	6-10	34		-8.42+/-1.34	…	-0.75+/-0.98 from1 to 10 yrs
Alio 2008	Visx 20/20	5.5-6	10	≥6 to 17.75	267		-8.87+/-2.25	…	-1.20+/-1.89 from 1 to 10 yrs
Alio 2008	Visx 20/20	6	10	<6	225		-3.81+/-1.29	…	-0.46+/-0.87 from 1 to 10 yrs
Koshimizu 2010	Visx 20/20-B	6	10	2.25 to 14.13	42		-8.91+/-3.03	-1.13+/-1.41	-0.51+/-0.78 in 10 yrs

Study*	Laser System	OZ (mm)	FU (yrs)	Preoperative SE Myopia Range (D)	No. of Eyes	No. of Eyes at Latest FU	Preoperative SE (D)	Postoperative SE (D) at Last Visit	SE Regression (D)
							Mean +/- SD		
				3.25 to 6 6.25 to 10 >10.25	7 20 14		-5.25+/-0.36 -8.02+/-0.89 -12.52+/-1.3	-0.91+/-0.85 -1.20+/-1.37 -1.17+/-1.79	No significant change in eyes with preoperative myopia <6
De Benito-Llopis 2009		6	10	2 to 14 CCT <500um			-6.12+/-2.67	-0.65+/-0.80 Sph -0.63+/-0.78 Cyl	<0.50 change in mean sphere from 1 to 10 yrs (-0.27 to -0.65). Includes 19% RT eyes for late regression, 12% for early undercorrection and 9% both.
Rosman 2010	Visx 20/20	4.5,5,6 multizone	10	>10 to 17.75	51		-12.44 +/-1.5	-1.81 +/-1.79	-1.28 +/-1.78 from 1 to 10 yrs. (includes 50% RT eyes)
Shojaei 2009	Nidek EC-5000	5.5-6	8	≤6 6.1 to 10 >10 to 14.5	112 36 46		-4.00 +/-1.84 -6.80 +/-1.74 -11.0 +/-3.74	-0.23 +/-0.19 (2% RT) -0.84 +/-0.48 (17% RT) -1.21 +/-0.95 (17% RT)	<0.50 in all groups from 3-8 years after a period of stabilisation in all eyes in first 2 yrs. Overall 16% developed regression. 8% RT for 'significant regression' and 3% for undercorrection in first 2 yrs – 2% in low myopes, 17% in both high myope groups (6-10 and >10).
Pietila 2004	Aesculap-Meditec MEL 60	5	8	≤6.0 6.1 to 10 >10	69 16 7		-4.07 +/-1.06 -7.78 +/-1.05 -11.4+/-1.04	… … …	-0.42+/-0.48 from 2-8 yrs -0.37+/-0.34 from 2-8 yrs -0.41+/-0.50 from 2-8 yrs

* First Author and Year, FU=follow-up, yrs=years, SE=spherical equivalent, D=diopters, No.=number, mo=months, CCT=central corneal thickness, Sph=sphere, Cyl=cylinder, RT=re-treated.

Table 6. Long-term Studies of Myopic LASIK

Study*	Laser System	FU (yrs)	Preoperative SE Myopia Range (D)	No. of Eyes	No. of Eyes At Final FU	Preoperative SE (D)	Postoperative SE (D) at Last Visit	Mean SE Regression (D) +/- SD
						Mean +/- SD		
Kymionis 2007	Aesculap Meditec MEL 60	11	10 to 19	11	11	-12.96 +/-3.17	-1.14 +/-1.67	No significant change in SE refraction from 6 mo to 11 yrs.
D'Arcy 2012 and O'Doherty 2006	Bausch and Lomb 217 Technolas	10	Up to 13 Subgroups: <3.0 3.0 to 6.0 >6.0 to 13	94 23 49 22	54 (57%) 7 (30%) 29 (59%) 18 (82%)	-4.85+/-2.35 -2.42+/-0.45 -4.45+/-0.84 -8.29+/-1.84	-1.6 -1.15 -0.93 -1.94	Change in the mean SE from 2 mo to 10 yrs: -1.24 (20% RT) -1 (14% RT) -0.76 (10% RT) -0.96 (39% RT)
Condon 2007	Summit, Ciron-Technolas and Meditec 60	1-11 5-6 7-8 9-11	10 to 35	107	 78 (73%) 68 (63%) 15 (14%)	-15.71 +/-6.8	… -2.41 -2.71 -2.91	Change in the mean SE of -0.50 from 5-6 yrs to 9-11 yrs postoperatively (33% RT)
Zalentein 2009	Visx Star and Star 2	7-8	3.8 to 11.5	38		-6.8 +/-1.7	-1.38 +/-1.03	Change in mean SE -0.97 from 2 mo to 7 yrs.
Liu 2008	Summit Apex Plus	7	3 to 15.25 3.12 to 6 >6.12 to 15.25	104 44 60	59 (79%)	-6.28 +/-2.52 -4.59 +/-0.75 -8.57 +/-2.25	+0.25 +/-0.71 +0.35 +/-0.62 +0.09 +/-0.8	No significant change from 1 to 7 yrs in any group.
Sekundo 2003	Schwind Keratom 1	6	All Eyes High	33		-13.65	-0.88	Change in mean SE -0.63 from 1-6 yrs
Rosman 2010	Visx 20/20	10	>10 to 17.75			-12.81 +/-1.64	-1.48 +/-1.99	-1.49 +/-2.17(27.6% RT eyes)
Alio 2009	Visx 20/20	10	6 to 10	34		-8.30+/-1.21	…	-0.80+/-1.14 from 1-10yrs
Alio 2008	Visx 20/20	10	<10	97		-7.27+/-1.9	…	-0.90+/-1.31 from 1-10yrs
Alio 2008	Visx 20/20	10	>10 to 24.5	196		-13.95+/-2.79	…	-1.76+/-1.79 from 1-10yrs
Dirani 2010		2-9 6-9	<6	162	 13 (8%)	-3.98+/-1.27	-0.33+/-0.59 -0.62 +/-0.72	Change in mean SE of -0.43 from 6 mo to 6-9 yrs (-0.19 at 6 mo (n=85) to -0.62 at 6-9 yrs (n=13))
		2-9 6-9	≥6.00 to 18.25	102	 31 (30%)	-7.64+/-1.66	-0.63+/-0.90 -0.54 +/-0.95	Change in mean SE of -0.3 from 6 mo to 6-9 yrs (from -0.24 at 6 mo (n=59)to -0.54 (n=31) at 6-9 yrs)
Orucoglu 2012		12.5	≥14 to 38	39		-21.70+/-5.86	-6.09+/-3.35	-6.1+2.2 from1mo to 10yrs

* First Author and Year, FU=follow-up, yrs=years, SE=spherical equivalent, D=diopters, No.=number, mo=months, RT=re-treated.

Pietila found that myopic regression stabilized at 1 year (all levels) and only a slight myopic shift occurred thereafter up to 8 years (<0.50D from 2 to 8 years).[41] Similarly, Guerin et al. (myopia up to 7.25D) showed that initial overcorrection regressed rapidly toward emmetropia at 1 year and only a mild myopic regression occurred thereafter up to 16 years. [47] Similarly, Rajan (all levels of myopia) found initial hyperopic overcorrection followed by regression to 12 months and stability at 12 years.[7] Bricola (all levels up to 13D) reported that refractive stability was achieved at 6 months and maintained at 14 years following myopic PRK. [59]

Shojaei found that, in all groups of myopia, regression stabilized by 2 years postoperatively. [42]Regression in the first 18 months correlated to the preoperative refraction but regression between 3 to 8 years did not correlate with preoperative refraction, age or to the change in the first postoperative year. Regression was less than 0.50 D in all myopic groups between 3-8 years. The authors concluded that if a good result is obtained initially then it remains relatively stable over time.

LASIK

The long-term studies of LASIK for myopia correction have generally focused on higher degrees of myopia, often into the extreme myopia range that would nowadays be considered unsuitable for treatment by LASIK. Despite the millions of procedures performed worldwide, there are little reliable data on the long-term stability of low myopia correction by LASIK in the published literature.

A summary of the long-term studies of myopia correction by LASIK is provided in Table 6.

Three studies provide long-term data on the correction of myopia <6D. In the range 3-6D, Liu found no significant change in refraction from 1 to 7 years.[60] For the same range, the combined studies of O'Doherty and D'Arcy (who followed the same cohort of patients at 5 years and 10 years respectively), reveal a change in the mean SE refraction of -0.76D from 2 months to 10 years postoperatively (59% follow-up).[50, 52] This includes 10% re-treated eyes.

A study by Dirani found that the change in the mean SE refraction for eyes with preoperative myopia <6D was -0.47D from 3 months to mean 6-9 years but only 8% of eyes were evaluated at 6-9 years.[44]

For myopia >6D, the reported long-term regression is very variable. Some studies show excellent stability despite high attempted magnitudes of myopia correction. Liu found no significant change in refraction from 1 to 7 years for a treated range 6 to 15D.[60] Kymionis found no significant change in refraction from 6 months to 11 years for myopia >10 to 19D. [57] Dirani showed a change in the mean SE of -0.25D from 3 months to 6-9 years for myopia 6 to 18D (30% follow-up at 6 to 9 years). [44] Condon reported that with deliberate undercorrection in many eyes with extreme high myopia (10 to 35D), the refraction remained quite stable up to 9-11 years postoperatively. [61]

Other studies show regression of approximately 1D from 1 to 10 years for myopia up to 10-13D and significantly more regression in more extreme myopia. Alio found mean regression from 1 to 10 years of -0.90 +/-1.31D for myopia up to 10D, -0.80 +/-1.14D for myopia 6-10D and -1.76 +/-1.79D for myopia >10D. [53, 54, 56] O'Doherty and D'Arcy's results show a change in the mean SE of -0.96D from 2 months to 10 years for myopia 6-13D (82% follow-up) but includes 39% re-treated eyes.[50, 52] Zalentein reported a change in the mean SE refraction of -0.97D between 2 months and 7.5 years for myopia up to 11.5D. [51] At 7 years postoperatively, 46% of patients were wearing corrective spectacles full or part time. Sekundo showed a change in the mean SE of -0.63D from 1 to 6 years in high myopes (attempted corrections 8-19D) with gross regression of 3D occurring in 9% of eyes. [55] A severe and relentless regression of mean -6.1 +/-3.35D from 1 month to mean 12.5 years was found by Orucoglu for eyes treated for extreme myopia >14 to 38D. [58]

Most studies found that the rate of myopic regression slowed with time. Alio reported that the rate of myopic regression in high myopes >10D stabilized between 2-5 years postoperatively. [56]

The mean regression was -0.25+/-0.18 D per year from 3 months to ten years. However, this rate gradually decreased from -0.93+/-0.20 D per year between three months and one year to -0.13 +/-0.32 D per year between five and ten years.

Factors Influencing Myopic Regression

Myopic regression may be due to corneal or non-corneal causes. As has been discussed earlier, a subset of myopic persons will continue to undergo progressive myopic shift over time due to axial length elongation. This can cause progressive myopia independent of biomechanical changes in the cornea post excimer laser surgery. Regression rates will be impacted by the age of subjects at the time of follow-up as natural hyperopic shifts with ageing may offset myopic regression. In older persons, lenticular changes can also induce myopic shift.[62] It is only possible to distinguish corneal biomechanical change from other factors if these are directly measured. None of the long-term studies measured axial length changes. It is also difficult to interpret the refractive change induced by changes in keratometry as it has been shown that changes in topographic corneal power may underestimate changes in subjective refraction following PRK and LASIK. [63] Alio et al. demonstrated a small increase in corneal power between 3 months and 10 years after PRK and LASIK in low and high myopia which the authors felt may explain some but not all of the observed myopic regression.[43, 48, 53, 56] Alio also concluded that similar factors appear to affect regression after PRK and LASIK. [54]

Regression has been found to be correlated with preoperative SE refraction, attempted correction and ablation depth. [64, 65] Pietila and Shojaei found that regression following PRK was correlated to the preoperative refraction in the first postoperative year to 18 months but not thereafter. [41, 42] Alio found significant correlation between myopic regression and the achieved correction following both PRK and LASIK for all levels of myopia. [43, 48, 53, 56]

Zalentein found that regression post LASIK was significantly greater in myopes >6D and in patients younger than 30 years. [51]

Long-term Stability of LASIK versus PRK for Myopia

There are no long-term prospective studies directly comparing the stability of the 2 types of surgery and it is difficult to draw comparisons between studies due to differences in technique, laser machines, baseline levels of myopia corrected and ablation diameters.

Alio et al. performed a retrospective, non-randomised matched comparison of the long-term results of LASIK and PRK in high myopes (6 to 10D) at 10 years postoperatively. [54] They found mean regression from 1 to 10 years in eyes that had no re-treatment of -0.80+/-1.14D in LASIK eyes and -0.75+/-0.98D in PRK eyes with mean regression per year of -0.09+/-0.13D in LASIK eyes and -0.08+/-0.11D in PRK eyes. Their findings showed no significant difference in regression between the 2 modalities at any time point with regression stabilizing between 2-5 years postoperatively. There was a lower re-treatment rate for LASIK (18% versus 35%) and overall higher predictability following LASIK (88% versus 62% within 1D at 10 years). However, they commented that the newer techniques in surface ablation such as increased optical zone sizes may affect the predictability results for PRK. Rosman et al. also found that LASIK and PRK had similar long-term efficacy for high myopia (>10D) at 10 years postoperatively but haze was a significant problem in PRK eyes. [49]

By contrast, Miyai et al. performed a retrospective comparison of the results of LASIK and PRK for myopia of mean 6D over a 4 year period and found a short-term superiority of LASIK in terms of efficacy which was not maintained at 4 years. [66] Indeed, SE refraction remained stable during 4 year follow-up in the PRK group but showed a gradual myopic shift in the LASIK group and became significantly more myopic than the PRK group at 4 years leading the authors to suggest that the stability of the LASIK procedure is less than that of PRK.

In terms of variations in surface ablation technique, Cui et al. performed a meta-analysis to compare results of LASEK and PRK for treatment of myopia up to 9D and found no advantage to LASEK over PRK up to 1 year postoperatively.[67]

Re-treatment following Myopic Excimer Laser Surgery

While the long-term studies discussed heretofore do give us valuable information about refractive change and regression over time in eyes that have had excimer laser surgery, many of the studies exclude eyes that had re-treatments performed at any time point following the initial surgery. Clearly, this is important to calculate refractive change following a single treatment unaltered by enhancement. However, this will exclude eyes that most likely had the greatest refractive change over time and will select more stable patients by definition. It is therefore important to examine re-treatment rates also.

Early postoperative undercorrections and overcorrections occur and are often enhanced by a re-treatment procedure between 3-6 months postoperatively once the refraction appears to have stabilized. Enhancement may also be required for induced astigmatism, decentred ablations or induced higher order aberrations. Such initial enhancement rates will vary from centre to centre. When considering long-term stability and regression, these initial enhancements are probably not directly relevant. The rate of re-treatment for regression after such time as an initial stable refraction is achieved is more relevant.

Reported re-treatment rates vary significantly between studies due to differences in the laser equipment employed, the upper limits of ametropia treated, ablation zone diameters, individual surgeon thresholds for performing re-treatment and duration of follow-up. Not all studies distinguish between re-treatments performed for regression and those performed for other reasons.

Re-treatment Rate following Myopic Surface Ablation

The reported re-treatment rates over a ten year period following PRK for myopia are variable. An approximate risk for requiring a re-treatment after the first postoperative year following PRK is 10% for low-moderate myopia and 20% for high myopia up to 10 years.

Guerin found a re-treatment rate of 7.5% at 16 years post PRK for myopia up to 7.25D. [47] Shojaei found a low rate of 1.8% at 8 years following PRK for myopia <6D. [42] Alio, on the contrary, found a 42% re-treatment rate at 10 years following PRK for myopia <6D. [43] This was largely due to a high percentage of re-treatments in the first year (30%), predominantly for primary undercorrection. The rate after 1 year was 12%. Regression (myopic change in SE refraction of 0.50 or more between visits) occurred in 10% of eyes. Both undercorrection and regression occurred in 6%.

DeBenito-Llopis also found a 40% re-treatment rate for all levels of myopia up to 14D treated by PRK at 10 years. [68] Again, the rate was nearly 30% in the first year. The rate decreased to 3% between 5 and 10 years. Koshimizu reported a 32% retreatment rate for myopia up to 14D at 10 years.[46]

In high myopia, the re-treatment rate has been reported to be 46-50% at 10 years.[48, 49] In these studies a rate of 25% occurred in the first year predominantly for undercorrection and reduced thereafter to 5% between 5 and 10 years. Shojaei found a 17% rate at 8 years.[42]

Re-treatment Rate following Myopic LASIK

The approximate re-treatment rate following LASIK for myopia after the first postoperative year is 10% at 10 years for myopia <10D and 10-20% for high myopia.

D'Arcy found an 11% rate at 10 years for myopia <6D and Alio found a 20.6% rate at 10 years for myopia up to 10D. [52, 53] After the first year, the rate was 8-9% in both studies.

Following LASIK for high myopia, the reported ten year re-treatment rate is 30-40% with a high percentage in the first postoperative year. Alio found a 28% rate at 10 years for myopia >10D and D'Arcy found a 39% rate at 10 years for myopia >6D.[52, 56] Both studies found a 17% rate in the first postoperative year. D'Arcy found late regression in 22% after 5 years while Alio found the rate decreased to 3% after 5 years.

It is important to bear in mind that the re-treatment rate may not provide the full picture of refractive regression. Myopia may regress but be unsuitable for re-treatment due to insufficient corneal parameters. In Orucoglu's study of extreme high myopia, all eyes regressed by >1D between 1 month and 10 years postoperatively but only one eye underwent re-treatment due to inadequate residual corneal thickness in the remainder. [58] Equally, patients may choose optical correction in the form of spectacles or be satisfied with the increase in near ability afforded by myopic regression, especially if unilateral. Most studies do not report the percentage of patients using optical correction. In addition to the 20% re-treatment rate for the entire cohort (myopia up to 13D) in the study by D'Arcy et al., an additional 7.4% of patients who were not re-treated were using monovision or spectacles for distance correction at 10 years.[52] In high myopes, Alio reported that only 40% avoided the use of spectacles at 10 years following LASIK. [56] Zalentein reported that 46% of patients were wearing full or part-time spectacles at 7.5 years post LASIK for myopia up to 11.5D. [51]

Factors Associated with Re-treatment

It is clear that higher attempted myopic corrections are associated with a higher re-treatment rate. Some studies have also shown a higher re-treatment rate in older persons.

Netto and Wilson reported a significantly higher rate of re-treatment (for any reason) in older patients, especially those more than 40 years following LASIK for myopia (14% in patients >40 years vs 5-8.5% in those <40 years). [69] No difference in re-treatment rates was noted for different degrees of myopia less than 10D but was significantly higher for myopia >10D. Other studies have found no significant difference in terms of age between those requiring enhancement and those not. [38, 70]

Randleman reported that following wavefront optimized LASIK and PRK, the re-treatment rate was not influenced by age or the preoperative degree of myopia. [71] In most studies re-treatment was required in only one eye but one study showed similar regression tended to occur in both eyes. [70]

Stability of Re-treatment Following Myopic Excimer Laser Surgery

The stability of the refraction following re-treatment is also a concern. Do re-treated eyes have a higher natural tendency for regression or does the re-treatment itself alter the regression rate? What is the chance that multiple re-treatments will be required?

The long-term studies providing detailed information about re-treated eyes are those by Alio.

Alio examined the rate of regression following re-treatment of PRK and LASIK and compared it to the rate of regression following primary PRK and primary LASIK for eyes that did not have a re-treatment. [43, 48, 53, 56]

For PRK correction of myopia <6D, the rate of myopic regression per year was statistically significantly less following re-treatment in the first postoperative year compared to non-retreated eyes but was not significantly different per year thereafter. [43] Overall, mean regression was -0.46 +/-0.87 D in non-retreated eyes from 1-10 years following primary PRK and was -0.02 +/-0.96 D from 1-10 years following re-treatment PRK. Similarly, for high myopia >6D, re-treatment did not increase the rate of regression.[48] These studies involved eyes that predominantly had early re-treatments for undercorrection and less for late regression. For myopia <6D, the rate of multiple re-treatment in the entire cohort was 9.3% with no eye re-treated more than twice. For myopia >6D, the rate of multiple re-treatment was 11% for re-treatment twice and 2% for re-treatment 3 times.

Following LASIK for myopia <10D, re-treatment did not increase the rate of regression compared to primary LASIK. [53] The rate of regression was very similar in both groups after 5 years (-0.05 +/-0.21D per year in non-retreated eyes and -0.03 +/-0.24 D per year in re-treated eyes between 5 and 10 years). In the first postoperative year, the mean change in refraction was hyperopic in re-treated eyes, followed by a greater myopic regression in the second year, then stabilization and a gradual myopic drift from 5 to 10 years similar in rate to non-retreated eyes. Similarly following LASIK for myopia >10D, the regression rate was not higher following re-treatment and after a greater hyperopic change in the first year in re-treated eyes, the rate of myopic regression per year was not different between the groups after the first year (-0.18 +/-0.32 D per year versus -0.19 +/-0.43 D per year from 2 to 5 years).[56]

These are the only long-term studies that compare the regression rates between re-treated and non-retreated eyes. As already stated, most of these re-treatments were for early undercorrection. It is not known if eyes that undergo later regression differ in regression rate following re-treatment that eyes that do not regress.

Multiple studies have examined the short-term visual and refractive outcome of eyes having re-treatments alone but most do not have long-term follow-up of more than 2 years. The outcome of re-treatment varies by the re-treatment method, magnitude of attempted re-treatment and duration of follow-up.

There are several options for performing re-treatments. Primary LASIK can be retreated by flap lift, flap re-cut or by surface ablation. Primary surface ablation can be re-treated by repeat surface ablation or by LASIK.

Re-treatment of Primary Myopic LASIK

Flap Lift

In studies of re-treatments by flap lift following LASIK for myopia, regression following re-treatment was insignificant up to 1 year in most studies. [65, 69, 70, 72] A few studies found a small 0.25D to 0.50D myopic regression at 1 year in re-treated eyes.[64, 73] Saeed [38]and Aslanides [39] reported outcomes up to 4 years and showed mild (-0.25D) and non-significant regression respectively. Multiple re-treatment rates are in the range of 3-9% of all re-treated eyes or 0.3-0.7% of all eyes. [38, 64, 65, 69, 72] Loss of 1 line of corrected distance visual acuity (CDVA) occurs in 3-26% and loss of 2 or more lines of CDVA occurs in 0-4% of re-treated eyes. [38, 39, 64, 65, 69, 70, 72-76]

Complications of flap lift include epithelial ingrowth, flap striae, diffuse lamellar keratitis and dry eye.

Epithelial ingrowth under the flap is reported to occur in up to 31% of cases following flap lift depending on the technique used (cutting the epithelium prior to flap lift appears to be associated with a lower rate than abrading it). [64] Minor degrees are very common and occurred in 100% of eyes in one series. [70] In one large series, clinically significant epithelial ingrowth affecting vision occurred in none of 3866 cases of primary LASIK and in

2.3% of 646 cases of flap lift re-treatment cases. [70] The risk was greater if flap-lift re-treatment was performed ≥3 years after primary LASIK (7.7% versus 1%). Treatment of epithelial ingrowth by flap lift and scraping is associated with a relatively high risk of recurrence (36% at 1 year) but overall good visual acuity outcomes. [77]

Alio et al. reported that wavefront guided treatment was slightly superior to conventional treatment for re-treatment of LASIK at 6 months. [78]

Surface Ablation to Retreat Primary LASIK

Surface ablation can be performed to enhance previous LASIK if the flap cannot be lifted or recut or if the residual stromal thickness is deemed insufficient to lift the flap.

The purported advantages of surface laser re-treatment are that it spares stroma under the flap, reduces microstriae, reduces the risk of dry eye, is not associated with epithelial ingrowth and has the potential to treat flap-induced higher order aberrations using wavefront-guided technology. The main limitation of PRK re-treatment of LASIK is haze formation.

The generation of haze involves a complex cascade of wound healing responses following injury by photoablation. Re-treatment over a previously ablated area is more likely to generate haze from repeated injury to an area with residual activated keratocytes. Deeper ablations that reach the area of apoptotic keratocytes around the flap interface are more likely to result in dense haze formation. The corneal sensory nerves may have an important role in modulating corneal wound healing and the delayed recovery of the nerves following LASIK may be a factor in aggressive wound healing if re-treatment PRK is performed too early.[79]

It has been reported that attempted SE correction of -2.0D or greater or an ablation depth of more than 40 microns is associated with significant haze following PRK re-treatment of primary LASIK. [80-82] A pivotal study by Carones et al. published in 2001 of PRK re-treatment of myopic regression following primary LASIK for high myopia showed that while the refractive outcome was good at 1 month postoperatively, significant myopic regression developed in all eyes by 1 year (often greater than the level prior to PRK re-treatment) with dense haze in 82% of eyes and loss of CDVA of 2 or more lines in 65%.[80] Following this study, re-treating LASIK by PRK was widely considered to be inadvisable and "Don't zap the flap" was a belief held for several years among refractive surgeons.

With an increased understanding of factors involved in haze formation and interventions that can reduce it, surface ablation re-treatment of LASIK has more recently regained acceptance as a reasonable therapeutic option in certain circumstances.

The prophylactic use of intraoperative topical mitomycin C to reduce haze formation has been successful in reducing rates and density of haze formation and producing improved outcomes for PRK re-treatment of primary LASIK. [83-85]

It is thought that the time interval between the original LASIK procedure and the re-treatment surface ablation is important in reducing haze formation as this will affect the amount of residual activated keratocytes and the recovery of the corneal nerve plexus following the original surgery. Less haze and better visual results have been reported by studies with an extended time interval between the two procedures. [38, 79]

Beerthuizen et al. reported successful re-treatment of small amounts of ametropia (range -2 to +1.38) by LASEK and PRK surface ablation following primary LASIK with good visual outcome and stability at 1 year (8% of eyes had a change in SE refraction of >0.50 between 6 and 12 months).[81] The magnitude of attempted SE correction was much lower in this study than that of Carones et al. and severe late onset haze (after 8 months) occurred in 11% of eyes. Beerthuizen found that reduction in microstriae under the flap (even though not visible in most cases preoperatively) by surface ablation of Bowman's membrane was beneficial to visual acuity outcomes. Shaikh et al. achieved good results using PRK to re-treat eyes that had flap complications during attempted primary LASIK. [84] Saeed et al. also achieved good results with LASEK re-treatment of primary LASIK for myopia and hyperopia with no eye developing haze greater than grade 1. [86] In this study, 29% were originally treated for high myopia and 14% had a re-treatment of ≥2D of myopia and 4.5% ≥2D of hyperopia.

Guell et al. proposed a method of intraepithelial PRK for re-treatment after LASIK avoiding ablation depths of more than 50 microns so as not to disrupt Bowman's membrane but this method failed to significantly affect the refractive status in 48% of eyes. [87]

Re-treatment of Primary Myopic Surface Ablation

Surface Ablation Re-treatment of Primary Surface Ablation

PRK can be used to re-treat eyes that had a primary PRK procedure. Haze formation is again a limiting factor. Eyes with original high myopia, significant regression (especially >3.50D myopia) and with pre-existing significant haze following the primary procedure (especially if grade ≥2) have a high risk of further haze, regression and loss of CDVA if re-treated by PRK. [88-90]

In a study by Gartry of re-treatment PRK, the SE refraction at 18months post-retreatment was -0.41+/-0.69D in the group with minimal haze prior to re-treatment but had regressed back to pre-retreatment levels at -4.14+/-2.34D in the group with significant haze.[88] Chatterjee et al. found better predictability re-treating eyes with <2D myopia versus eyes with ≥4D. [89] Pop et al. also showed a significant difference in the predictability of PRK re-treatment in eyes with and without preoperative haze (84% versus 50% within 1D of target at 6 months postoperatively). [90]

Studies from the 1990s on PRK re-treatment by PRK show 50-96% (average about 75%) predictability within 1D, 21-24% loss of ≥1 lines of CDVA and 67-100% uncorrected visual acuity (UCVA) 6/12 Snellen or better (average about 82%). [25, 88, 90-93] Results vary highly according to the degree of pre-retreatment myopia and presence or absence of haze.

Spadea reported very good results re-treating myopic PRK by transepithelial topography guided surface ablation.[40] Re-treatment of mean -2.54 +/-2.60D (range -0.5 to -6D) resulted in mean SE refraction of -0.05 +/-0.66D at 3 years and 100% of eyes within 0.75D of target. No eye developed haze greater than grade 1 and no loss of BCVA occurred.

The use of topical mitomycin C 0.02% at the time of re-treatment has also been shown to reduce the incidence of postoperative haze formation. [94]

Retreatment of Primary Surface Ablation by LASIK

Primary surface ablation can also be re-treated by LASIK if there is sufficient corneal thickness.

Aslanides reported excellent long-term stability of refraction at 4 years postoperatively following LASIK re-treatment of PRK using a wavefront-customised and aspheric ablation. [39]

Ozdamer et al. retreated myopia 1.5 to 12.5D with LASIK following primary PRK and found 80% within 1D of emmetropia, 69% 6/12 Snellen or better UCVA, no difference in haze pre and postoperatively and 4% loss of ≥2 lines CDVA at 6 months. [95] Similarly, Comaish reported 70% predictability within 1D and 73% UCVA of 6/12 Snellem or better at 6 months post LASIK re-treatment of surface ablation with poorer predictability in eyes with greater preoperative haze. [96] Lazaro reported good visual and refractive results 1 year post LASIK re-treatment of primary PRK but significant preoperative haze did not reduce. [97]

Ectasia

One particular rare complication of LASIK surgery and, very rarely, of surface ablation that causes significant refractive shift and loss of uncorrected and corrected visual acuity is iatrogenic keratectasia. This is a progressive corneal steepening, usually inferiorly, causing increasing myopia and astigmatism that can present days to years following LASIK. [98] The true incidence is undetermined but estimates range from 0.04% [98] to 0.2% [99] to 0.66%. [100] In long-term follow-up studies of high to extreme myopia >10D treated by LASIK, the incidence of ectasia was 0.9% and 1% in the studies of Condon and Alio, respectively. [56, 61]

Many of the reported ectasia cases in the literature had preoperative characteristics that would exclude them from having LASIK treatment today. Two major risk factors for the development of post-LASIK ectasia are pre-existing disposition to ectasia (keratoconus or forme fruste keratoconus) and removing excessive amounts of corneal tissue at the time of laser ablation, particularly leaving a residual stromal thickness less than 250 microns. This can happen because of flap creation that is thicker than expected or because of too high an attempted correction. Rare cases of ectasia in patients with no identifiable preoperative risk factors have been reported. [101] Ectasia has also rarely occurred following surface ablation but can occur if preoperative risk factors such as keratoconus are present. [102, 103]

Phakic Intraocular Lenses

Nowadays, phakic intraocular lenses (pIOLs) are the preferred refractive surgical option for high myopia for many surgeons.

These lens implants show good stability of refraction over medium term follow-up of 4-5 years in high myopes. One potential long-term concern with regard to pIOLs that does not apply to excimer laser surgery is endothelial cell loss.

A 5 year follow-up of a posterior chamber pIOL for high myopia revealed good stability of refraction with a small but statistically significant myopic shift of less than 0.25D in the SE refraction between 6 months postoperatively and the final visit. [104] A retrospective study of an iris-fixated pIOL in high myopes in Asian-Indian eyes, showed stability of the mean SE refraction over 4 years. [105] In that study, 73% of eyes were within 1D of the attempted correction at 4 years but only 37% within 1D of emmetropia (undercorrected) and cumulative endothelial cell loss at 4 years was 12.5%.

One long-term study has demonstrated no significant change in mean SE refraction between 1, 6 and 10 years post iris-fixated pIOL implantation in moderate to high myopes

(3.75 to 25D) with 69% within 1D of the intended correction at 10 years and a mean decrease of 9 +/-16% in endothelial cell density. [106]

A Cochrane review of pIOLs versus excimer laser surgery for high myopia >6D concluded that pIOLs are safer with less loss of CDVA at 1 year postoperatively, better contrast sensitivity and higher patient satisfaction. [107]

Rosman et al. found better predictability and stability with an angle-supported pIOL at 10 years versus LASIK in eyes with myopia >10D. [108]

A short-term follow-up of 1 year comparing LASIK to a foldable iris-fixated pIOL for myopia 6 to 9D showed no difference between the 2 in terms of refraction or UDVA but better CDVA and better contrast sensitivity at high spatial frequencies in the pIOL group. The pIOL group had lower endothelial cell count. [109]

Conclusion

Long-term refractive stability is excellent following laser refractive surgical correction in the form of surface ablation and LASIK for low to moderate ametropia at least up to 5 years postoperatively for hyperopia <4D and up to 10 years or more for myopia <10D. Higher attempted corrections are associated with less predictable outcomes and higher regression of the refractive correction over time.

The likelihood of needing a re-treatment in the first postoperative year following excimer laser surgery will be very dependent on local practice and will vary significantly from centre to centre. The rate after the first year up to 10 years is approximately 10% in low-moderate myopia and up to 20% in high myopia. If a re-treatment is performed, the refraction will usually remain stable over time and not regress more than if a re-treatment was not required. A minority of all eyes (<1%) will require more than 1 re-treatment. If a re-treatment is not required, the mean change in refraction is usually less than 0.50 D over the subsequent decade in low-moderate myopes and can be a 1D or more in high myopes. Even some high to extreme high myopes, though often undercorrected, will remain quite stable over time. High ametropia is now preferably corrected by pIOL implantation for which good refractive stability has been demonstrated up to 10 years postoperatively.

References

[1] Lee, KE; Klein, BE; Klein, R. Changes in refractive error over a 5-year interval in the Beaver Dam Eye Study. *Invest Ophthalmol Vis Sci* 1999; 40: 1645-9.

[2] Guzowski, M; Wang, JJ; Rochtchina, E; Rose, KA; Mitchell, P. Five-year refractive changes in an older population: the Blue Mountains Eye Study. *Ophthalmology* 2003; 110: 1364-70.

[3] Ellingsen, KL; Nizam, A; Ellingsen, BA; Lynn, MJ. Age-related refractive shifts in simple myopia. *J Refract Surg* 1997; 13: 223-8.

[4] Saka, N; Ohno-Matsui, K; Shimada, N; Sueyoshi, S; Nagaoka, N; Hayashi, W , et al. Long-term changes in axial length in adult eyes with pathologic myopia. *Am J Ophthalmol* 2010; 150: 562-568 e1.

[5] Saka, N; Moriyama, M; Shimada, N; Nagaoka, N; Fukuda, K; Hayashi, K , et al. Changes of axial length measured by IOL master during 2 years in eyes of adults with pathologic myopia. *Graefes Arch Clin Exp Ophthalmol* 2012;

[6] Meng, W; Butterworth, J; Malecaze, F; Calvas, P. Axial length of myopia: a review of current research. *Ophthalmologica* 2011; 225: 127-34.

[7] Rajan, MS; Jaycock, P; O'Brart, D; Nystrom, HH; Marshall, J. A long-term study of photorefractive keratectomy; 12-year follow-up. *Ophthalmology* 2004; 111: 1813-24.

[8] Kanellopoulos, AJ; Conway, J; Pe, LH. LASIK for hyperopia with the WaveLight excimer laser. *J Refract Surg* 2006; 22: 43-7.

[9] Zadok, D; Raifkup, F; Landau, D; Frucht-Pery, J. Long-term evaluation of hyperopic laser in situ keratomileusis. *J Cataract Refract Surg* 2003; 29: 2181-8.

[10] Kohnen, T; Mirshahi, A; Cichocki, M; Buhren, J; Steinkamp, GW. [Laser in situ keratomileusis for correction of hyperopia and hyperopic astigmatism using a scanning spot excimer laser. Results of a prospective clinical study after 1 year]. *Ophthalmologe* 2003; 100: 1071-8.

[11] Jin, GJ; Lyle, WA; Merkley, KH. Laser in situ keratomileusis for primary hyperopia. *J Cataract Refract Surg* 2005; 31: 776-84.

[12] Varley, GA; Huang, D; Rapuano, CJ; Schallhorn, S; Boxer Wachler, BS; Sugar, A. LASIK for hyperopia, hyperopic astigmatism, and mixed astigmatism: a report by the American Academy of Ophthalmology. *Ophthalmology* 2004; 111: 1604-17.

[13] Cobo-Soriano, R; Llovet, F; Gonzalez-Lopez, F; Domingo, B; Gomez-Sanz, F; Baviera, J. Factors that influence outcomes of hyperopic laser in situ keratomileusis. *J Cataract Refract Surg* 2002; 28: 1530-8.

[14] Carones, F; Brancato, R; Morico, A; Vigo, L; Venturi, E; Gobbi, PG. Photorefractive keratectomy for hyperopia using an erodible disc and axicon lens: 2-year results. *J Refract Surg* 1998; 14: 504-11.

[15] O'Brart, DP; Patsoura, E; Jaycock, P; Rajan, M; Marshall, J. Excimer laser photorefractive keratectomy for hyperopia: 7.5-year follow-up. *J Cataract Refract Surg* 2005; 31: 1104-13.

[16] Autrata, R; Rehurek, J. Laser-assisted subepithelial keratectomy and photorefractive keratectomy for the correction of hyperopia. Results of a 2-year follow-up. *J Cataract Refract Surg* 2003; 29: 2105-14.

[17] Rosen, ES. Hyperopia--RLE, pIOL, or LVC? *J Cataract Refract Surg* 2008; 34: 175-6.

[18] Desai, RU; Jain, A; Manche, EE. Long-term follow-up of hyperopic laser in situ keratomileusis correction using the Star S2 excimer laser. *J Cataract Refract Surg* 2008; 34: 232-7.

[19] Esquenazi, S. Five-year follow-up of laser in situ keratomileusis for hyperopia using the Technolas Keracor 117C excimer laser. *J Refract Surg* 2004; 20: 356-63.

[20] Jaycock, PD; O'Brart, DP; Rajan, MS; Marshall, J. 5-year follow-up of LASIK for hyperopia. *Ophthalmology* 2005; 112: 191-9.

[21] Kezirian, GM; Moore, CR; Stonecipher, KG. Four-year postoperative results of the US ALLEGRETTO WAVE clinical trial for the treatment of hyperopia. *J Refract Surg* 2008; 24: S431-8.

[22] Nagy, ZZ; Krueger, RR; Hamberg-Nystrom, H; Fust, A; Kovacs, A; Kelemen, E , et al. Photorefractive keratectomy for hyperopia in 800 eyes with the Meditec MEL 60 laser. *J Refract Surg* 2001; 17: 525-33.

[23] Ivarsen, A; Naeser, K; Hjortdal, J. Laser in situ keratomileusis for high astigmatism in myopic and hyperopic eyes. *J Cataract Refract Surg* 2012;

[24] El-Helw, MA; Emarah, AM. Predictability and stability of refraction with increasing optical zone diameter in hyperopic LASIK. *Clin Ophthalmol* 2010; 4: 455-8.

[25] Argento, CJ; Cosentino, MJ. Comparison of optical zones in hyperopic laser in situ keratomileusis: 5.9 mm versus smaller optical zones. *J Cataract Refract Surg* 2000; 26: 1137-46.

[26] Esquenazi, S; Mendoza, A. Two-year follow-up of laser in situ keratomileusis for hyperopia. *J Refract Surg* 1999; 15: 648-52.

[27] Settas, G; Settas, C; Minos, E; Yeung, IY. Photorefractive keratectomy (PRK) versus laser assisted in situ keratomileusis (LASIK) for hyperopia correction. *Cochrane Database Syst Rev* 2012; 6: CD007112.

[28] Spadea, L; Sabetti, L; D'Alessandri, L; Balestrazzi, E. Photorefractive keratectomy and LASIK for the correction of hyperopia: 2-year follow-up. *J Refract Surg* 2006; 22: 131-6.

[29] El-Agha, MS; Johnston, EW; Bowman, RW; Cavanagh, HD; McCulley, JP. Photorefractive keratectomy versus laser in situ keratomileusis for the treatment of spherical hyperopia. *Eye Contact Lens* 2003; 29: 31-7.

[30] Durrie, DS; Smith, RT; Waring, GOt; Stahl, JE; Schwendeman, FJ. Comparing conventional and wavefront-optimized LASIK for the treatment of hyperopia. *J Refract Surg* 2010; 26: 356-63.

[31] Nagy, ZZ; Palagyi-Deak, I; Kovacs, A; Kelemen, E; Forster, W. First results with wavefront-guided photorefractive keratectomy for hyperopia. *J Refract Surg* 2002; 18: S620-3.

[32] Kanellopoulos, AJ. Topography-guided hyperopic and hyperopic astigmatism femtosecond laser-assisted LASIK: long-term experience with the 400 Hz eye-Q excimer platform. *Clin Ophthalmol* 2012; 6: 895-901.

[33] Gil-Cazorla, R; Teus, MA; de Benito-Llopis, L; Mikropoulos, DG. Femtosecond laser vs mechanical microkeratome for hyperopic laser in situ keratomileusis. *Am J Ophthalmol* 2011; 152: 16-21 e2.

[34] Hersh, PS; Fry, KL; Bishop, DS. Incidence and associations of retreatment after LASIK. *Ophthalmology* 2003; 110: 748-54.

[35] Ortega-Usobiaga, J; Cobo-Soriano, R; Llovet, F; Ramos, F; Beltran, J; Baviera-Sabater, J. Retreatment of hyperopia after primary hyperopic LASIK. *J Refract Surg* 2007; 23: 201-5.

[36] Alio, JL; Galal, A; Artola, A; Ayala, MJ; Merayo, J. Hyperopic LASIK retreatments with the Technolas laser. *J Refract Surg* 2006; 22: 596-603.

[37] Kashani, S; Rajan, M; Gartry, D. Wavefront-guided retreatment after primary wavefront-guided laser in situ keratomileusis in myopes and hyperopes: long-term follow-up. *Am J Ophthalmol* 2009; 147: 417-423 e2.

[38] Saeed, A; O'Doherty, M; O'Doherty, J; O'Keefe, M. Analysis of the visual and refractive outcome following laser in situ keratomileusis (LASIK) retreatment over a four-year follow-up period. *Int Ophthalmol* 2007; 27: 23-9.

[39] Aslanides, IM; Kolli, S; Padron, S; Arba Mosquera, S. Stability of therapeutic retreatment of corneal wavefront customized ablation with the SCHWIND CAM: 4-year data. *J Refract Surg* 2012; 28: 347-52.

[40] Spadea, L; Di Gregorio, A. Enhancement outcomes after photorefractive keratectomy and laser in situ keratomileusis using topographically guided excimer laser photoablation. *J Cataract Refract Surg* 2005; 31: 2306-12.

[41] Pietila, J; Makinen, P; Pajari, T; Suominen, S; Keski-Nisula, J; Sipila, K , et al. Eight-year follow-up of photorefractive keratectomy for myopia. *J Refract Surg* 2004; 20: 110-5.

[42] Shojaei, A; Mohammad-Rabei, H; Eslani, M; Elahi, B; Noorizadeh, F. Long-term evaluation of complications and results of photorefractive keratectomy in myopia: an 8-year follow-up. *Cornea* 2009; 28: 304-10.

[43] Alio, JL; Muftuoglu, O; Ortiz, D; Artola, A; Perez-Santonja, JJ; de Luna, GC , et al. Ten-year follow-up of photorefractive keratectomy for myopia of less than -6 diopters. *Am J Ophthalmol* 2008; 145: 29-36.

[44] Dirani, M; Couper, T; Yau, J; Ang, EK; Islam, FM; Snibson, GR , et al. Long-term refractive outcomes and stability after excimer laser surgery for myopia. *J Cataract Refract Surg* 2010; 36: 1709-17.

[45] O'Connor, J; O'Keeffe, M; Condon, PI. Twelve-year follow-up of photorefractive keratectomy for low to moderate myopia. *J Refract Surg* 2006; 22: 871-7.

[46] Koshimizu, J; Dhanuka, R; Yamaguchi, T. Ten-year follow-up of photorefractive keratectomy for myopia. *Graefes Arch Clin Exp Ophthalmol* 2010; 248: 1817-25.

[47] Guerin, MB; Darcy, F; O'Connor, J; O'Keeffe, M. Excimer laser photorefractive keratectomy for low to moderate myopia using a 5.0 mm treatment zone and no transitional zone: 16-year follow-up. *J Cataract Refract Surg* 2012; 38: 1246-50.

[48] Alio, JL; Muftuoglu, O; Ortiz, D; Artola, A; Perez-Santonja, JJ; de Luna, GC , et al. Ten-year follow-up of photorefractive keratectomy for myopia of more than -6 diopters. *Am J Ophthalmol* 2008; 145: 37-45.

[49] Rosman, M; Alio, JL; Ortiz, D; Perez-Santonja, JJ. Comparison of LASIK and photorefractive keratectomy for myopia from -10.00 to -18.00 diopters 10 years after surgery. *J Refract Surg* 2010; 26: 168-76.

[50] O'Doherty, M; O'Keeffe, M; Kelleher, C. Five year follow up of laser in situ keratomileusis for all levels of myopia. *Br J Ophthalmol* 2006; 90: 20-3.

[51] Zalentein, WN; Tervo, TM; Holopainen, JM. Seven-year follow-up of LASIK for myopia. *J Refract Surg* 2009; 25: 312-8.

[52] D'Arcy, FM; Kirwan, C; O'Keefe, M. Ten year follow up of laser in situ keratomileusis for all levels of myopia. *Acta Ophthalmol* 2012; 90: e335-6.

[53] Alio, JL; Muftuoglu, O; Ortiz, D; Perez-Santonja, JJ; Artola, A; Ayala, MJ , et al. Ten-year follow-up of laser in situ keratomileusis for myopia of up to -10 diopters. *Am J Ophthalmol* 2008; 145: 46-54.

[54] Alio, JL; Ortiz, D; Muftuoglu, O; Garcia, MJ. Ten years after photorefractive keratectomy (PRK) and laser in situ keratomileusis (LASIK) for moderate to high myopia (control-matched study). *Br J Ophthalmol* 2009; 93: 1313-8.

[55] Sekundo, W; Bonicke, K; Mattausch, P; Wiegand, W. Six-year follow-up of laser in situ keratomileusis for moderate and extreme myopia using a first-generation excimer laser and microkeratome. *J Cataract Refract Surg* 2003; 29: 1152-8.

[56] Alio, JL; Muftuoglu, O; Ortiz, D; Perez-Santonja, JJ; Artola, A; Ayala, MJ , et al. Ten-year follow-up of laser in situ keratomileusis for high myopia. *Am J Ophthalmol* 2008; 145: 55-64.

[57] Kymionis, GD; Tsiklis, NS; Astyrakakis, N; Pallikaris, AI; Panagopoulou, SI; Pallikaris, IG. Eleven-year follow-up of laser in situ keratomileusis. *J Cataract Refract Surg* 2007; 33: 191-6.

[58] Orucoglu, F; Kingham, JD; Kendusim, M; Ayoglu, B; Toksu, B; Goker, S. Laser in situ keratomileusis application for myopia over minus 14 diopter with long-term follow-up. *Int Ophthalmol* 2012; 32: 435-41.

[59] Bricola, G; Scotto, R; Mete, M; Cerruti, S; Traverso, CE. A 14-year follow-up of photorefractive keratectomy. *J Refract Surg* 2009; 25: 545-52.

[60] Liu, Z; Li, Y; Cheng, Z; Zhou, F; Jiang, H; Li, J. Seven-year follow-up of LASIK for moderate to severe myopia. *J Refract Surg* 2008; 24: 935-40.

[61] Condon, PI; O'Keefe, M; Binder, PS. Long-term results of laser in situ keratomileusis for high myopia: risk for ectasia. *J Cataract Refract Surg* 2007; 33: 583-90.

[62] Fotedar, R; Mitchell, P; Burlutsky, G; Wang, JJ. Relationship of 10-year change in refraction to nuclear cataract and axial length findings from an older population. *Ophthalmology* 2008; 115: 1273-8, 1278 e1.

[63] Rosa, N; Furgiuele, D; Lanza, M; Capasso, L; Romano, A. Correlation of changes in refraction and corneal topography after photorefractive keratectomy. *J Refract Surg* 2004; 20: 478-83.

[64] Bragheeth, MA; Fares, U; Dua, HS. Re-treatment after laser in situ keratomileusis for correction of myopia and myopic astigmatism. *Br J Ophthalmol* 2008; 92: 1506-10.

[65] Lyle, WA; Jin, GJ. Retreatment after initial laser in situ keratomileusis. *J Cataract Refract Surg* 2000; 26: 650-9.

[66] Miyai, T; Miyata, K; Nejima, R; Honbo, M; Minami, K; Amano, S. Comparison of laser in situ keratomileusis and photorefractive keratectomy results: long-term follow-up. *J Cataract Refract Surg* 2008; 34: 1527-31.

[67] Cui, M; Chen, XM; Lu, P. Comparison of laser epithelial keratomileusis and photorefractive keratectomy for the correction of myopia: a meta-analysis. *Chin Med J (Engl)* 2008; 121: 2331-5.

[68] de Benito-Llopis, L; Alio, JL; Ortiz, D; Teus, MA; Artola, A. Ten-year follow-up of excimer laser surface ablation for myopia in thin corneas. *Am J Ophthalmol* 2009; 147: 768-73, 773 e1-2.

[69] Netto, MV; Wilson, SE. Flap lift for LASIK retreatment in eyes with myopia. *Ophthalmology* 2004; 111: 1362-7.

[70] Brahma, A; McGhee, CN; Craig, JP; Brown, AD; Weed, KH; McGhee, J , et al. Safety and predictability of laser in situ keratomileusis enhancement by flap reelevation in high myopia. *J Cataract Refract Surg* 2001; 27: 593-603.

[71] Randleman, JB; White, AJ, Jr.; Lynn, MJ; Hu, MH; Stulting, RD. Incidence, outcomes, and risk factors for retreatment after wavefront-optimized ablations with PRK and LASIK. *J Refract Surg* 2009; 25: 273-6.

[72] Febbraro, JL; Buzard, KA; Friedlander, MH. Reoperations after myopic laser in situ keratomileusis. *J Cataract Refract Surg* 2000; 26: 41-8.

[73] Perez-Santonja, JJ; Ayala, MJ; Sakla, HF; Ruiz-Moreno, JM; Alio, JL. Retreatment after laser in situ keratomileusis. *Ophthalmology* 1999; 106: 21-8.

[74] Rashad, KM. Laser in situ keratomileusis retreatment for residual myopia and astigmatism. *J Refract Surg* 2000; 16: 170-6.

[75] Mulhern, MG; Condon, PI; O'Keefe, M. Myopic and hyperopic laser in situ keratomileusis retreatments: indications, techniques, limitations, and results. *J Cataract Refract Surg* 2001; 27: 1278-87.
[76] Jin, GJ; Merkley, KH. Retreatment after wavefront-guided and standard myopic LASIK. *Ophthalmology* 2006; 113: 1623-8.
[77] Henry, CR; Canto, AP; Galor, A; Vaddavalli, PK; Culbertson, WW; Yoo, SH. Epithelial ingrowth after LASIK: clinical characteristics, risk factors, and visual outcomes in patients requiring flap lift. *J Refract Surg* 2012; 28: 488-92.
[78] Alio, JL; Montes-Mico, R. Wavefront-guided versus standard LASIK enhancement for residual refractive errors. *Ophthalmology* 2006; 113: 191-7.
[79] Neira-Zalentein, W; Moilanen, JA; Tuisku, IS; Holopainen, JM; Tervo, TM. Photorefractive keratectomy retreatment after LASIK. *J Refract Surg* 2008; 24: 710-2.
[80] Carones, F; Vigo, L; Carones, AV; Brancato, R. Evaluation of photorefractive keratectomy retreatments after regressed myopic laser in situ keratomileusis. *Ophthalmology* 2001; 108: 1732-7.
[81] Beerthuizen, JJ; Siebelt, E. Surface ablation after laser in situ keratomileusis: retreatment on the flap. *J Cataract Refract Surg* 2007; 33: 1376-80.
[82] Cagil, N; Aydin, B; Ozturk, S; Hasiripi, H. Effectiveness of laser-assisted subepithelial keratectomy to treat residual refractive errors after laser in situ keratomileusis. *J Cataract Refract Surg* 2007; 33: 642-7.
[83] Majmudar, PA; Forstot, SL; Dennis, RF; Nirankari, VS; Damiano, RE; Brenart, R , et al. Topical mitomycin-C for subepithelial fibrosis after refractive corneal surgery. *Ophthalmology* 2000; 107: 89-94.
[84] Shaikh, NM; Wee, CE; Kaufman, SC. The safety and efficacy of photorefractive keratectomy after laser in situ keratomileusis. *J Refract Surg* 2005; 21: 353-8.
[85] Srinivasan, S; Drake, A; Herzig, S. Photorefractive keratectomy with 0.02% mitomycin C for treatment of residual refractive errors after LASIK. *J Refract Surg* 2008; 24: S64-7.
[86] Saeed, A; O'Doherty, M; O'Doherty, J; O'Keefe, M. Laser-assisted subepithelial keratectomy retreatment after laser in situ keratomileusis. *J Cataract Refract Surg* 2008; 34: 1736-41.
[87] Guell, JL; Lohmann, CP; Malecaze, FA; Junger, J; Muller, A; Deneuville, S. Intraepithelial photorefractive keratectomy for regression after laser in situ keratomileusis. *J Cataract Refract Surg* 1999; 25: 670-4.
[88] Gartry, DS; Larkin, DF; Hill, AR; Ficker, LA; Steele, AD. Retreatment for significant regression after excimer laser photorefractive keratectomy. A prospective, randomized, masked trial. *Ophthalmology* 1998; 105: 131-41.
[89] Chatterjee, A; Shah, S; Bessant, DA; Doyle, SJ. Results of excimer laser retreatment of residual myopia after previous photorefractive keratectomy. *Ophthalmology* 1997; 104: 1321-6.
[90] Pop, M; Aras, M. Photorefractive keratectomy retreatments for regression. One-year follow-up. *Ophthalmology* 1996; 103: 1979-84.
[91] Rozsival, P; Feuermannova, A. Retreatment after photorefractive keratectomy for low myopia. *Ophthalmology* 1998; 105: 1189-92; discussion 1192-3.

[92] Kapadia, MS; Meisler, DM; Wilson, SE. Epithelial removal with the excimer laser (laser-scrape) in photorefractive keratectomy retreatment. *Ophthalmology* 1999; 106: 29-34.
[93] George, SP; Johnson, DG. Photorefractive keratectomy retreatments: comparison of two methods of excimer laser epithelium removal. *Ophthalmology* 1999; 106: 1469-79; discussion 1479-80.
[94] de Benito-Llopis, L; Teus, MA. Efficacy of surface ablation retreatments using mitomycin C. *Am J Ophthalmol* 2010; 150: 376-380 e2.
[95] Ozdamar, A; Sener, B; Aras, C; Aktunc, R. Laser in situ keratomileusis after photorefractive keratectomy for myopic regression. *J Cataract Refract Surg* 1998; 24: 1208-11.
[96] Comaish, IF; Domniz, YY; Lawless, MA; Webber, SK; Rogers, CM; Sutton, GL. Laser in situ keratomileusis for residual myopia after photorefractive keratectomy. *J Cataract Refract Surg* 2002; 28: 775-81.
[97] Lazaro, C; Castillo, A; Hernandez-Matamoros, JL; Iradier, MT; Garcia-Feijoo, J; Benitez-del-Castillo, JM , et al. Laser in situ keratomileusis enhancement after photorefractive keratectomy. *Ophthalmology* 2001; 108: 1423-9.
[98] Randleman, JB; Russell, B; Ward, MA; Thompson, KP; Stulting, RD. Risk factors and prognosis for corneal ectasia after LASIK. *Ophthalmology* 2003; 110: 267-75.
[99] Rad, AS; Jabbarvand, M; Saifi, N. Progressive keratectasia after laser in situ keratomileusis. *J Refract Surg* 2004; 20: S718-22.
[100] Pallikaris, IG; Kymionis, GD; Astyrakakis, NI. Corneal ectasia induced by laser in situ keratomileusis. *J Cataract Refract Surg* 2001; 27: 1796-802.
[101] Klein, SR; Epstein, RJ; Randleman, JB; Stulting, RD. Corneal ectasia after laser in situ keratomileusis in patients without apparent preoperative risk factors. *Cornea* 2006; 25: 388-403.
[102] Randleman, JB; Caster, AI; Banning, CS; Stulting, RD. Corneal ectasia after photorefractive keratectomy. *J Cataract Refract Surg* 2006; 32: 1395-8.
[103] Leccisotti, A. Corneal ectasia after photorefractive keratectomy. *Graefes Arch Clin Exp Ophthalmol* 2007; 245: 869-75.
[104] Perez-Cambrodi, RJ; Pinero, DP; Madrid-Costa, D; Blanes-Mompo, FJ; Ferrer-Blasco, T; Cervino, A. Medium-term visual, refractive, and intraocular stability after implantation of a posterior chamber phakic intraocular lens to correct moderate to high myopia. *J Cataract Refract Surg* 2011; 37: 1791-8.
[105] Titiyal, JS; Sharma, N; Mannan, R; Pruthi, A; Vajpayee, RB. Iris-fixated intraocular lens implantation to correct moderate to high myopia in Asian-Indian eyes: five-year results. *J Cataract Refract Surg* 2012; 38: 1446-52.
[106] Tahzib, NG; Nuijts, RM; Wu, WY; Budo, CJ. Long-term study of Artisan phakic intraocular lens implantation for the correction of moderate to high myopia: ten-year follow-up results. *Ophthalmology* 2007; 114: 1133-42.
[107] Barsam, A; Allan, BD. Excimer laser refractive surgery versus phakic intraocular lenses for the correction of moderate to high myopia. *Cochrane Database Syst Rev* 2012; 1: CD007679.

[108] Rosman, M; Alio, JL; Ortiz, D; Perez-Santonja, JJ. Refractive stability of LASIK with the Visx 20/20 excimer laser vs ZB5m phakic iol implantation in patients with high myopia (>-10.00 d): a 10-year retrospective study. *J Refract Surg* 2011; 27: 279-86.
[109] Albarran-Diego, C; Munoz, G; Ferrer-Blasco, T; Garcia-Lazaro, S; Belda-Salmeron, L. Foldable iris-fixated phakic intraocular lens vs femtosecond laser-assisted LASIK for myopia between -6.00 and -9.00 diopters. *J Refract Surg* 2012; 28: 380-6.

In: Current Understanding and New Techniques ...
Editor: Michael O'Keefe
ISBN: 978-1-62808-748-2

Chapter 11

Corneal Topography

*Arthur Cummings**
Wellington Eye Clinic, Beacon Court, Dublin, Ireland

Abstract

This chapter is introduced with a brief history of corneal topography and how it has evolved to become an indispensable tool in the cataract and refractive surgeon's arsenal. The different types of topography are introduced and described. The chapter is further divided into diagnostic and therapeutic uses for corneal topography.

Introduction

Corneal topography has only been available since the early1980's in research laboratories [1] and in 1986 commercially yet it seems implausible now that we could ever do refractive surgery, especially laser refractive correction, without a pre-operative corneal topography. As the use of premium IOL's (toric, accommodating and multifocal IOL's) has grown, so has the need for more detailed corneal information rather than just keratometry. The cornea and in fact, the pre-corneal tear film is the first and most powerful refractive interface in the entire eye [2]. If the cornea is not regular, one needs to think twice about using a premium IOL as the results may be disappointing. Corneal topography is an important reason that the incidence of post-LASIK ectasia has decreased with time [3]. Excluding cases of forme fruste keratoconus or irregular astigmatism are important when determining LASIK suitability[4]. Corneal topography helps too with cataract surgery for determining the ideal incision when one wants to be on the steep axis or wants to determine if there are corneal irregularities present. If there are irregularities present, typically the best advice is to use a standard monofocal IOL. Corneal topography is also useful for detecting and classifying ectatic disease like keratoconus, pellucid marginal degeneration and post-LASIK ectasia [3]. It can

* abc@wellingtoneyeclinic.com

also be used to detect milder corneal issues like basement membrane dystrophy, tear insufficiency and the effect of corneal scarring. Lastly, topography clearly demonstrates small and or decentred ablation zones and can be used therapeutically to design and drive a topography-guided ablation to correct these issues.

History

Corneal videokeratoscopy has been extensively used to obtain information of the shape of the anterior cornea [4]. The first corneal topograph can be dated back to 1880, when the Portuguese ophthalmologist Antonio Placido viewed a painted disk of alternating black and white rings reflected in the cornea. The rings reflected as lines projected on the anterior corneal surface or more accurately, the pre-corneal tearfilm. In 1896, Gullstrand incorporated the placido disk in his ophthalmoscope and commented it could "give a resultant accuracy that previously could not be obtained in any other way" (Gullstrand, 1909). The Placido disk was flat while the cornea is curved and hence reduced the accuracy of the peripheral corneal data. To circumvent this problem, a curved bowl was used to reduce the field defects by the Wesley-Jessen company in the 1950's. Later on, in the 1980's, the digitized images of the rings were analysed, rather than the live corneal image. Over time the analysis was done by computer with analysis of a photograph from a digital camera (Busin, Wilmanns & Spitznas, 1989). In the 1990s, various topography systems became commercially available from a number of suppliers [2].

Prior to the availability of corneal topography, the suitability of the cornea to undergo refractive surgery, mostly in the form of radial keratotomy at the time, was based on the clinical examination, the keratometry using a keratometer measuring the central 3mm and the corneal pachymetry measured with ultrasound. As technology and knowledge improved, so multiple pachymetry measurements over different areas were used in order to better understand the pre-operative cornea and its specific risk for ectasia or unwanted surprise outcomes. The need for a better pre-operative screening tool was the main reason behind the development of corneal topography [2]. The major application of the technology was to screen patients before refractive surgery [5]. It was also developed to examine the precise changes of refractive surgery on the corneal surface. This information would allow a better understanding of what radial incisions and laser ablations were doing to the corneal shape and thereby to improve refractive surgical techniques. Steven Klyce is widely regarded as the father of modern corneal topography or computerized videokeratoscopy and in an interview following his ASCRS Innovator's Lecture in 1984 he said "Corneal topographers are exquisitely sensitive to small changes in curvature of cornea and, therefore, they are very adept at detecting corneal pathology, such as keratoconus, very early on" [6]. Klyce developed the color-coded contour map, a display of corneal surface powers that has become the international standard for corneal topography. From that time onward his research team have developed statistical indices, such as the surface regularity index in order to add measures of the optical quality of the cornea [7]. With these indices and the color-coded maps, they evaluated all refractive surgery modalities, such as photorefractive keratectomy (PRK) and laser in-situ keratomileusis (LASIK) as the clinical researchers around the world were developing these procedures. This work was first published in an abstract presented at the Association for Research in Vision and Ophthalmology (ARVO) meeting in 1984 [1].

Klyce worked with Computed Anatomy (now Tomey) to help the company incorporate the use of the color-coded corneal topography map with a computer device it had in development. In 1986, the first commercial topography machine was introduced to the market by Computed Anatomy. Today numerous companies are manufacturing devices that measure corneal topography and other corneal parameters.

Principles and Instruments of Corneal Topography

Corneal topography is the study of the anterior surface of the cornea. Corneal tomography is the study of the anterior corneal surface, the posterior corneal surface and the area between these 2 surfaces (the corneal thickness or pachymetry). Corneal tomography is therefore a 3-dimensional imaging system while topography remains a one-dimensional anterior corneal surface analyser.

A) Corneal topography
   a) Corneal topography can be based on the following:
   b) Placido disk images
   c) Corneal elevation or height data
   d) OCT based corneal data
   e) Combined corneal topography and wavefront sensing

Approximately 70% of the refractive power of the eye derives from the air–tear film interface that is found on the anterior corneal surface [2]. The importance of the refractive power of the cornea has been the driving force behind the development of instruments to measure the shape, thickness and power of the cornea. Corneal topography is the study of the surface of the cornea. It has been used to diagnose and follow up corneal pathology, plan refractive surgery, and evaluate post-operative results.

The keratometer and Placido disk are reflection-based methods [2]. An object is projected onto a central corneal zone of known diameter and distance from the light source. The corneal tear film acts like a convex mirror, reflecting light, and a virtual upright image is produced. The relationship between the image and object size is used to estimate the radius of curvature along a particular meridian.

With the keratometer, only four data points are generated [2]. Two lie on the steepest axis, and the other two are on the flat axis, 90 degrees away. The keratometer (Von Helmholtz, Javal-Schiotz) reflects the four points over a central zone of 3 mm (2.88 to 4 mm depending on the radius of curvature of the cornea). The keratometer is very accurate for regular surfaces such as the central cornea of a normal eye but is not very useful for irregular surfaces or corneas. There is no data inside or outside of the central zone's 4 reference points. In addition, the keratometer has less accuracy for corneal powers below 36 D and above 50 D, although it can theoretically measure corneas from 30 to 60 D.

The Placido disk reflects a series of concentric rings (mires) off the cornea [2]. Each mire produces an upright virtual image in the anterior chamber of the subject's eye. The distance between each mire to the corneal apex is compared to the image's distance to the corneal apex; the ratio of image distance to mire distance determines the anterior corneal curvature along any particular meridian. Placido devices include photokeratoscopes (Corneoscope) and computerized videokeratoscopes (modern day topographers like the Oculus Keratograph or WaveLight Topolyzer). Placido disk devices can measure much larger areas than the keratometer. The computerized videokeratoscope can measure 15 to 38 mires over 95% of the corneal surface and has a theoretical range of 8 to 110 D.

Videokeratoscopes display topographical information using different maps [2]. A photograph of the cornea is provided as a raw image. Distortions of the tear film can be detected by the physician and can be used to determine the quality of the scan. The data is then presented as a color map with either an absolute or a normalized (relative) scale. On color maps, the warmer colours (red, orange, and yellow) represent the steeper areas while the cooler colours (blue and green) represent the flatter regions.

The absolute scale is a fixed system in which each color is consistently assigned to a particular curvature or power. This facilitates the comparison of topographies between patients and over time in the same patient to assess the long-term effect of a procedure for example. Each videokeratoscope has its own absolute color map with fixed dioptric intervals covering the range of corneal powers. The normalized (relative) scale maximizes the utilization of all possible colours to evaluate a specific cornea. The color map with a normalized scale has narrower intervals between the assigned colours, possibly 0.25 or 0.5D increments. Although the normalized scale allows the clinician to evaluate a particular topography with greater detail, it makes comparison between examinations difficult because the scale may have changed in range and dioptric interval. A customizable option is also available where the clinician can determine the scale of the dioptric steps.

Placido devices use axial (sagittal), tangential (local), or refractive power maps to calculate radius of curvature [2].

The axial map measures the perpendicular distance from the tangent at a point to the optical axis and therefore has a spherical bias. This gives a global description of shape and may be less accurate in the corneal periphery and with irregular surfaces. On the other hand, a tangential map displays the radius of curvature of a point with respect to its neighbouring points along a specific meridian. It has a less spherical bias than an axial map and therefore may be preferred to assess the corneal periphery or in irregular corneas. The refractive map uses Snell's law to measure the focal power of the cornea.

The software provides the clinician with three options for delineating the major and minor axes for a given cornea. The orthogonal axes mark the major and minor axes as measured at the central 3-mm zone.

The zonal axes mark the major and minor axes at the 3-mm as well as the 5-mm and 7-mm zones. This allows the clinician to quickly assess if there is a shift in the major and minor axes with progression towards the corneal periphery. The instantaneous axes option draws a continuous line from the center of the cornea to the periphery, showing the true major and minor axes at any given diameter.

Data can also be manipulated by software to gather desired information. Cross-sectional maps display the elevation and depression of the anterior corneal surface along any given meridian. Difference maps can compare pre- and post-treatment corneal topographies by subtracting the first map from the second. Statistical indices, which are often used in clinical studies, can also be obtained using software analysis.

Current devices in the market place that are based on placido disk technology include the following:

1. Atlas 9000 Corneal Topographer
2. Tomey TMS Corneal Topographer
3. Magellan Mapper
4. EyeSys 3000 and EyeSys Vista
5. Galilea Dual Scheimpflug Analyzer (includes Scheimpflug tomography)
6. Oculus Keratograph
7. WaveLight Topolyzer and Topolyzer Vario (the images used in this chapter that are placido based were all obtained from the Topolyzer and Topolyzer Vario). The Topolyzer Vario includes pupil data at varying illumination levels and provides data on the pupil centroid shift at different degrees of dilation. The WaveLight devices are manufactured by Oculus and licenced to WaveLight and are essentially the same diagnostic devices as the Oculus Keratograph. They are however class IIB devices that register their therapeutic capabilities as opposed to just diagnostic abilities as in class IIA.

B) Corneal tomography
   a) Corneal tomography can be based on
   b) Scanning slit technology
   c) Scheimpflug technology

Scanning slit topography (e.g., Orbscan) is a projection-based method that uses a series of slit-beam images to generate data regarding anterior surface curvature, posterior surface curvature, and pachymetry [2]. Therefore, the cornea is represented as a three-dimensional (3D) structure. A slit lamp projects a beam at 45 degrees onto the cornea. Twenty slits are projected sequentially on the eye from the left side, and 20 slits from the right, for a total of 40 slits that produce 240 data points per slit. This produces an image that is a height map of the cornea relative to a best-fit sphere. The elevations and depressions are recorded in 5 μm increments. Height maps have a coloured reference scale and display elevations in warm colours and depressions in cool colours. The elevation of the anterior and posterior surfaces is determined and the difference between these surfaces provides corneal thickness or pachymetry. The instrument averages pachymetry in nine circles of 2-mm diameter located in the central cornea. It also averages pachymetry of eight circles located 3 mm from the visual axis in the mid-periphery. The Orbscan can calculate corneal spherical power. Astigmatic power maps represent the local astigmatism over the corneal surface, calculating the arithmetic difference of the principal curvatures for each data point [8, 9]. In addition, axial, tangential, and power maps are available, based on the same principles as the Placido disk systems.

The Orbscan II was the first elevation system with the capability to measure both the anterior and posterior corneal surfaces using a scanning-slit technique of optical cross-sectioning combined with Placido disc-based technology [10]. Measuring both corneal surfaces potentially offered diagnostic advantages compared with Placido disc-based technology and allowed the computation of a pachymetric map (corneal thickness is the difference between the anterior and posterior surfaces). The limitations of this device have been highlighted by many, particularly its variable ability to locate the posterior corneal surface and underestimations of corneal thickness after refractive surgery [11]. When comparing post-PRK eyes using Scheimpflug imaging, scanning slit topography and ultrasound pachymetry, the corneas measured thicker with Scheimpflug imaging than with scanning slit topography or ultrasound. With application of a correction factor, the Scheimpflug measurements were closer to the values obtained with ultrasound pachymetry and had better agreement than scanning-slit topography [12].

Scheimpflug photography can achieve a wide depth of focus, providing images that can include information from the anterior corneal surface through to the posterior crystalline lens capsule when the pupil is widely dilated. The Pentacam by Oculus combines a rotating Scheimpflug camera with a static camera to acquire multiple photographs of the anterior segment. The Scheimpflug camera rotates with a monochromatic slit light source around the optical axis to obtain the slit images. This rotating system performs a corneal scan from 0° to 180°, and each of the photographs is an image of the cornea at a specific angle. The static camera is placed opposite the centre of the pupil to detect the pupil's contours and control fixation and captures and corrects the eye's movements. The photographs are used in the reconstruction of the anterior and posterior corneal topographies from height data. The Pentacam can also provide analyses of corneal pachymetry, corneal wavefront aberrations, densitometry, and the complete anterior chamber. Using the Pentacam HR (High Resolution), Ambrosio and colleagues found that relational thickness was better than single-point pachymetric parameters for distinguishing normal corneas from those with keratoconus [13].

The Galilea Dual Scheimpflug Analyzer integrates a Placido disc and a dual rotating Scheimpflug system for corneal topography and three-dimensional analysis of the anterior segment. Like the other two devices, the Galilea covers the cornea, anterior chamber, and lens of the eye. During the rotating scan, Placido disc and Scheimpflug images are simultaneously acquired to obtain the information on the curvature and elevation of the cornea, respectively. The dual camera configuration captures two Scheimpflug slit images from opposite sides of the slit beam and simultaneously tracks decentration due to the eye's movements. The height data obtained from two corresponding slit images are averaged to improve the measurements of corneal elevation and thickness. The use of this device can be delegated to non-medical personnel after a study demonstrated that the pachymetry and keratometry readings from this device matched the Orbscan keratometry and Sonogage ultrasound pachymetry very well and showed strong concordance and high reproducibility, which would allow the examinations to be delegated to nonmedical personnel [14]

Rasterphotogrammetry (e.g., PAR Corneal Topography System) is another projection-based system that produces an elevation map of the cornea [2]. Its advantages are that it measures the entire corneal surface, up to 12 mm, and can also measure irregular or de-epithelialized corneas. A projector places a grid onto a corneal surface coated with fluorescein. Fluorescein produces light emissions from the surface of the cornea. Two or more camera systems at a different angle to the cornea from the projector, image the grid. The rays intersect in 3D space, creating the elevation map.

Current devices that are providing tomography of the anterior segment include the following and more:

A) Orbscan II and IIz Anterior Segment Analysis System
B) Pentacam and Pentacam HR(Oculus)
C) Precisio Surgical Tomographer (iVis Technologies)
D) Galilea Dual Scheimpflug Analyzer (includes placido disk topography)
E) WaveLight Oculyzer and Oculyzer II (the Scheimpflug images used in this chapter were all derived from the Oculyzer and Oculyzer II (High Definition).) The WaveLight devices are manufactured by Oculus and licenced to WaveLight and are essentially the same diagnostic devices as the Pentacam and Pentacam HR. They are however class IIB devices that register their therapeutic capabilities as opposed to just diagnostic abilities as in Class IIA.

A) OCT based systems

These systems typically combine placido disk topography and OCT pachymetry and anterior segment details.

1. Optovue Anterior Segment OCT Tomography
2. Visante Omni (Zeiss)

B) Combined topography / tomography and wavefront analysis systems

These systems typically combine wavefront aberrometry, topography, refraction, pupillometry and keratometry.

1. iTrace Combination Topography and Wavefront System (Tracey Technologies)
2. Nidek OPD Scan II – based on optical path difference technology
3. Topcon KR-1W
4. Topo-Aberrometry (Keratron Onda, Optikon)

The trend in anterior diagnostics has been the addition of more tests into one device in order to obtain more information than was possible before from a single special investigation. Combining anterior segment imaging using topography (corneal data), OCT and Scheimpflug imaging of the anterior segment (anterior segment data), wavefront data (entire eye refractive data) and even interferometry (axial length data) is leading to more accurate data and data that was not available before. It's not unconceivable that IOL power calculations will improve further due to these more comprehensive diagnostics. Extracting crystalline lens data by simple subtraction techniques (entire wavefront data minus corneal topography data) allows imaging on the lens's contribution to visual acuity and quality in ways that were simply not possible before.

Diagnostic and therapeutic Uses of Corneal Topography

Some diagnostic uses have been described earlier in this chapter but for clarity include:

1. Screening for laser refractive surgery, mostly excluding forme fruste keratoconus or frank keratoconus cases from undergoing corneal refractive surgery [4, 15-17].

2. Screening for cataract surgery by excluding corneal irregularities that may impact the performance of premium IOL's.
3. Measuring the effect of a corneal laser refractive or other shape altering procedure with the use of "difference maps" from pre-operative to post-operative.
4. Measuring the effect of corneal incisions such as primary incisions for cataract surgery and arcuate keratotomies for treating astigmatism.
5. Diagnosing and grading ectatic corneal disease including keratoconus, pellucid marginal degeneration and post-LASIK ectasia.
6. Measuring the effect of corneal cross-linking for keratoconus by evaluating pre-operative and post-operative average-K readings and K-Max (single steepest K-reading over the entire cornea).

The therapeutic uses of corneal topography and tomography include the following:

1. Providing guidance on where to place an incision.
2. Providing guidance on how large the incision/s should be.
3. Directly providing data to drive a laser ablation procedure:
   a) To expand a small optical zone
   b) To recentre a decentred optical zone
   c) To treat corneal irregularities
   d) To treat keratoconic corneas
   e) To allow placement of the centre of the ablation on a specific pupil centre. The Topolyzer Vario device provides information on the corneal topography and the pupil centre for a given pupil size. As the pupil dilates and constricts, it may not maintain the same geometrical centre due to uneven dilation and constriction. If the pupil centre shifts, this is called "pupil centroid shift" and will impact visual outcomes of laser refractive surgery if a treatment is centred on the photopic (small) pupil but when the pupil dilates and there is a pupil centroid shift, the ablation is in effect decentred for the larger pupil size. This pupil centroid shift information can be used therapeutically with laser surgery where a decision can be made to apply the centre of the ablation to the pupil centre corresponding to scotopic conditions. All of the above (3a-d) are performed using topographic data obtained from either a placido disk device (e.g. Topolyzer) or Scheimpflug-based device (e.g. Oculyzer). In order to purposely decentre an ablation to a pupil centre of choice, data is required from the Topolyzer Vario. Studies performed by this author have demonstrated equal efficacy using both Placido disk and Scheimpflug devices as tools for generating the ablation profile for topographically-guided customized corneal laser surgery[18]. Intuitively however, if the Oculyzer (Scheimpflug) contains better central data than the Topolyzer (Placido disk), then one would tend to use these maps to generate an ablation profile. Likewise, if the data on a particular cornea was more reliable on the Topolyzer rather than the Oculyzer, one would use the former with the better, more consistent data instead.

Using Corneal Topography in Corneal Refractive Surgery

Basic guidelines to using corneal topography in corneal refractive surgery were provided by Randleman at the ISRS Symposium (International Society of Refractive Surgeons) at the ISRS-American Academy of Ophthalmology Meeting in Chicago in November 2012.

There are 5 basic patterns to be seen in a cornea representing the most powerful (steepest, central area) part of the cornea:

a) Round
b) Oval
c) Symmetric bow-tie
d) Asymmetric bow-tie
e) No readily describable irregular pattern

For keratoconus and ectasia screening: there are 6 steps to follow in order to decide if the cornea is normal or not.

Step 1: Rule out contact lens warpage and ocular surface dryness
Step 2: Calculate the I-S ratio [7]
Step 3: Look for skewed radial axes (SRA) [7]
Step 4: Determine the steepest K-reading
Step 5: Look for topographic changes over time
Step 6: Check advanced imaging methods

The Randleman criteria [19], albeit imperfect, is a valuable tool in helping detect cases that are unsuitable for laser refractive surgery. Points are scored according to a list of criteria and the extent to which they are present as shown in the table below:

Parameter	Points				
	4	3	2	1	0
Topography pattern	FFKC	Inferior Steep SRA	-	Asymmetric Bow-tie	Symmetric Bow-tie
Residual Stromal Bed	< 240μ	240-259μ	260-279μ	280-299μ	>300μ
Age	-	18-21 yrs	22-25 yrs	26-29yrs	>30 yrs
Pre-operative pachymetry	<450μ	451-480μ	481-510μ	-	>510μ
MR (SE)	> -14	> -12-to < -14	> -10 to < -12	> -8 to < -10	< -8.00D

A score of 5 points or more represents too high a risk of ectasia to justify going ahead with laser refractive surgery. The Randleman criteria was configured after analyzing data from LASIK cases performed with microkeratomes. It is feasible that femto-LASIK will see fewer cases of ectasia due to thinner and more predictable flaps.

It is vital to validate maps prior to reading the topography: The following steps apply:

a) Identify the colour step scale.
b) Evaluate the quality of the scan (diameter scanned, centration and data loss).

c) Identify patterns:
   1) Normal / Symmetrical
   2) Suspicious:
      Asymmetry (mild)
      Focal steep / skewed radial axes (high)
   3) Abnormal:
      Keratoconus (early suspect FFKC)
      Pellucid Marginal Degeneration (PMD)

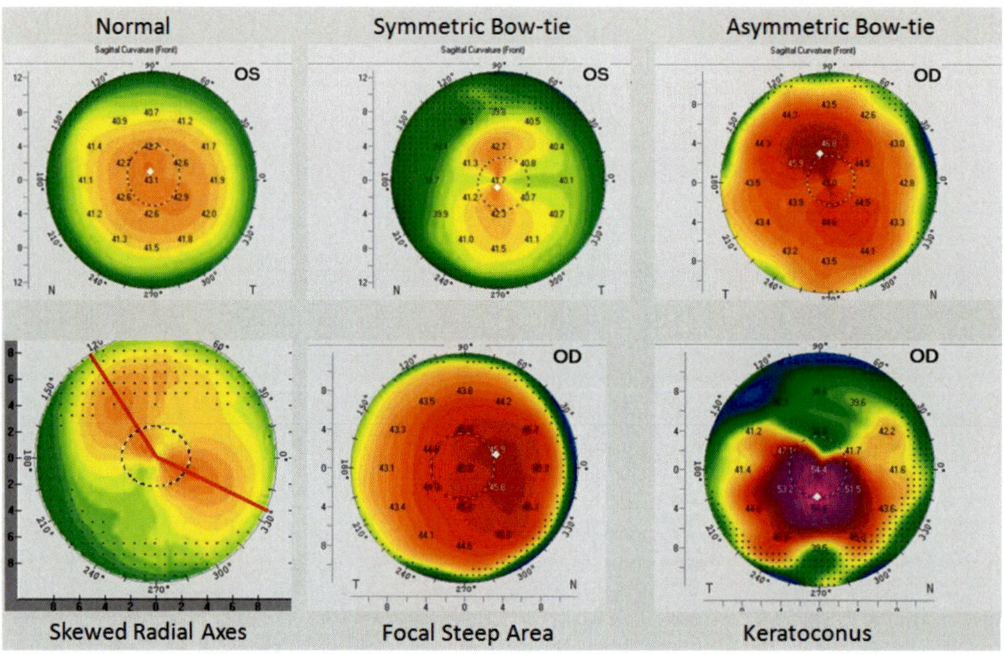

Additional data to analyse on tomography maps:

1. Location of the thinnest point.
2. Exact pachymetry measurement at this thinnest point.
3. Comparing the thinnest pachymetry to the pachymetry at pupil centre and corneal apex and the geometric distances between these 3 locations.
4. Peripheral / Central Corneal Thickness relationship.
5. Magnitude of anterior elevation / ectasia of anterior and posterior corneal surfaces.

A series of questions was asked of the 2012 ISRS / AAO audience before and after the didactic part of the lecture on corneal topography. Prior to the lecture, 43% of the audience perceived being able to recognize a specific abnormal pattern was the most important element to identify on any screening map while after the lecture 66% stated that the most important step was first identifying the image colour steps being utilised on the display. It is of vital importance to know the absolute keratometry values while reading a display. A "hot spot" in a cornea that has 40D K-readings and is 550 micron thick has different relevance to the same "hotspot" in a cornea of 460 micron and where the K-readings are 49D.

The most important screening metric is the subjective image evaluation according to the audience that was made up of experienced refractive surgeons as well as junior doctors and residents specializing in refractive surgery. It is important to note with elevation data what the reference sphere is in terms of diameter of radius and the reference shape (spherical versus toroid-elliptical).

Pearls from the Experts

Corneal topography and tomography are areas that are developing rapidly again with new devices and new combinations of functionality within devices. In an ever changing environment it is important to remember some basic considerations and the following tips from recognized experts within the field of cornea and corneal imaging are relevant in the author's opinion.

Yaron Rabinowitz

Corneal topography based on placido disk remains the most valuable device to detect forme fruste keratoconus. Adding OCT and wavefront to the diagnostics increases the yield of FFKC corneas detected during refractive surgery screening. Tangential maps provide better data for cone location and size than sagittal maps.

William Trattler

It is important to remember to refrain from wearing contact lenses for at least a week and preferably 2 weeks before doing the corneal topography. In the case of RGP contact lenses it is preferable to wait for 3 weeks and longer depending on findings. Dry eyes can negatively affect the scans. If scans are inadequate with the first measurements, treat the dry eyes first and then evaluate again once the tear film is better. Corneal topography has become a very important tool for the cataract surgeon for helping with the selection of premium IOL's and determining the suitability for corneal laser surgery "fine-tuning" post-cataract surgery if required.

Jack Holladay

The tangential map is different than an axial or refractive power map and displays the surface geometry of the cornea in more detail. It is the most sensitive map that can be created for the geometry of the anterior surface of the cornea. Previously, to look at the elevations of the anterior and posterior surfaces, a sphere was used as the reference shape; however, the cornea is normally a toric (astigmatic) prolate ellipsoid. Using a sphere as the reference, the central cornea is always above and the peripheral cornea always below. When astigmatism is present, the steep meridian is always above and the flatter meridian is always below the reference curve. Using a toric prolate ellipsoid, only the irregularities appear and make the normative data much tighter so that elevations on the posterior surface with forme fruste keratoconus are more sensitive. With the toric ellipsoid surface, the map easily detects abnormalities, such as keratoconus and pellucid marginal degeneration. Any central or paracentral elevation relative to the toric ellipsoid above 10 μm is considered pathologic. If the patient has a "hotspot" at the same point on the tangential, relative pachymetry and posterior elevation map, it is suggestive of keratoconus. Although there is often elevation on the anterior elevation map too, it is more variable due to the epithelial cell layer that can thin over the cone and thereby reduce or mask the increased anterior surface height.

Conclusion

Entire books and volumes have been dedicated to the topics of corneal topography and corneal tomography and it is not the intention of this chapter to attempt to cover the entire topic as it is simply too large for these few pages. The intention was to highlight the history and the way that corneal topography and tomography have and are developing to become key components of not just corneal surgery but also cataract surgery. Perusing the accompanying images will hopefully also refresh the memory of conditions to be aware of, details to look out for during interpretation of maps and appreciation for how the field has developed to make corneal refractive and cataract surgery safer and more effective than ever before.

References

[1] Klyce SD. Computer-Assisted Corneal Topography: High-Resolution Graphic Presentation and Analysis of Keratoscopy. *Investigative Ophthalmology & Visual Science.* 1984; 25(12): 1426-1435.

[2] Naidu S, Ocampo-Goldberg AC. Chapter 112 Corneal Topography. In Corbett MC, Rosen ES, O'Brart DPS in Corneal Topography: Principles and Applications. London, BMJ Books, 1999.

[3] Rabinowitz YS, Rasheed K. KISA% index: a quantitative videokeratography algorithm embodying minimal topographic criteria for diagnosing keratoconus. *Journal of Cataract & Refractive Surgery.* 1999; 25:1327-1335.

[4] Rabinowitz YS, McDonnell PJ. Computer-assisted corneal topography in keratoconus. *Refractive & Corneal Surgery.*1989; 5(6):400-408.

[5] Rabinowitz YS, Yang H, Brickman Y et al. Videokeratography database of normal human corneas. *British Journal of Ophthalmology.* 1996;80:610-616.

[6] Samalonis L. (2000). Innovator's lecture: Corneal topography in the 21st century. http://www.eyeworld.org/printarticle.php?id=1272.

[7] Wilson SE, Klyce SD. Quantitative descriptors of corneal topography. A clinical study. *Archives of Ophthalmology;* 1991, 109(3):349-353.

[8] Belin MW, Khachikian SS. An introduction to understanding elevation-based topography: how elevation data are displayed—a review. *Clinical and Experimental Ophthalmology*. 2009;37(1):14-29.

[9] Cairns G, McGhee CN. Orbscan computerized topography: attributes, applications, and limitations. *Journal of Cataract & Refractive Surgery*. 2005; 31(1):205-220.

[10] Barsam A. Technology for Keratoconus Screening. *Cataract & Refractive Surgery Today Europe;* 2012; 3:26-27.

[11] Hashemi H, Mehravaran S. Corneal changes after laser refractive surgery for myopia: comparison of Orbscan II and Pentacam findings *Journal of Cataract & Refractive Surgery*. 2007;33(5):841-847.

[12] Faramarzi A, Karimian F, Jafarinasab MR, et al. Central corneal thickness measurements after myopic photorefractive keratectomy using Scheimpflug imaging, scanning-slit topography, and ultrasonic pachymetry. *Journal of Cataract & Refractive Surgery*. 2010;36(9):1543-1549.

[13] Ambrósio R Jr, Caiado AL, Guerra FP, et al. Novel pachymetric parameters based on corneal tomography for diagnosing keratoconus. *Journal of Refractive Surgery*. 2011;27(10):753-758.

[14] Menassa N, Kaufmann C, Goggin M, et al. Comparison and reproducibility of corneal thickness and curvature readings obtained by the Galilei and the Orbscan II analysis systems. *Journal of Cataract & Refractive Surgery*. 2008;34(10):1742- 1747.

[15] Rabinowitz YS, Garbus J, McDonnell PJ. Computer-assisted corneal topography in family members of patients with keratoconus. *Archives of Ophthalmology*.1990; 108:365-37.

[16] Piccoli PM, Gomes AAC, Piccoli FVR. Corneal ectasia detected 32 months after LASIK for correction of myopia and asymmetric astigmatism. *Journal of Cataract and Refractive Surgery*. 2003; 29 (6); 1222–1225.

[17] Kymionis GD, Tsiklis N, Karp CL et al. Unilateral corneal ectasia after laser in situ keratomileusis in a patient with uncomplicated photorefractive keratectomy in the fellow eye. *Journal of Cataract and Refractive Surgery*. 2007; 33 (5); 859–861.

[18] Cummings AB, Mascharka N. Outcomes after topography-based LASIK and LASEK with the Wavelight Oculyzer and Topolyzer platforms. *Journal of Refractive Surgery*; 2010, 26(7):478-485.

[19] Randleman JB, Russell B, Ward MA. Risk factors and prognosis for corneal ectasia after LASIK. *Ophthalmology*. 2003;110(2): 267–275.

In: Current Understanding and New Techniques ...
Editor: Michael O'Keefe
ISBN: 978-1-62808-748-2

Chapter 12

Phakic Intraocular Lens Implants

Sarah Moran[*]
Mater Private Hospital, Dublin

Abstract

The success of corneal procedures in treating high refractive errors can be limited due to low predictability, regression, iatrogenic ectasia, optical aberrations, prolonged recovery and poor quality visual outcomes. In these cases, implantation of phakic intraocular lenses (pIOLs) offers many potential advantages.

The implantation of pIOLs has been shown to be an effective, safe, predictable and stable procedure to correct moderate and high refractive errors. Advantages include predictability, reversibility, high visual quality and quick visual rehabilitation, as well as preservation of accommodation. Phakic IOLs can also be used in children with bilateral significant ametropia or anisometropia, who are spectacle or contact lens noncompliant

Phakic IOLs can be classified according to the site of implantation in the eye. There are three main types of pIOLS; Angle-supported anterior chamber, iris-fixated anterior chamber, and posterior chamber pIOLs, each with distinct features, selection criteria, surgical technique, results, and complications. Complications are rare and generally related to the site of implantation. They include corneal endothelial cell loss, glaucoma, pigment deposits, chronic inflammation, glare/haloes, and lens dislocation. This chapter discusses in further detail the pre-operative evaluation, surgical technique and complications associated with each pIOL type.

Anterior segment optical coherence tomography (OCT) can now be used to precisely measure the shape, size and position of structures within the anterior segment, and determine pIOL position in the eye relative to the crystalline lens. The development of anterior segment imaging has many important clinical applications, allowing for increased safety profile and more accurate follow-up of pIOLs. Safety and functional outcomes continue to improve with developments in design and technology.

[*] sarmoran@gmail.com.

Introduction

Refractive surgery is continuing to evolve and expand as new technology and techniques become available. Laser corneal refractive surgery remains the most popular type of refractive procedure performed today. Despite ongoing advances in laser technology, the success of corneal procedures in treating high refractive errors can be limited due to low predictability, regression, iatrogenic ectasia, optical aberrations, prolonged recovery and poor quality visual outcomes. In these cases, implantation of phakic intraocular lenses (pIOLs) offers many potential advantages – a broader range of treatable refractive errors, quick vision recovery, stable refraction, and excellent quality vision. [1, 2]

Indications

Where patients are not suitable for keratorefractive procedures, intraocular procedures including pIOL implantation or refractive lens exchange (RLE) may be considered. RLE however is generally not considered in myopic pre-presbyopic patients as they can still accommodate, and the increased risk of retinal detachment is also a concern. [3] Therefore in young patients with high refractive errors who are unsuitable for keratorefractive procedures, pIOL implantation is an important option to consider.

Advantages of Phakic IOLs

Table 1. Advantages of phakic IOLs

• Reversibility
• Predictability
• Good visual quality
• Quick visual rehabilitation
• Preservation of accommodation [4]
• Preservation of corneal surface – option of bioptics
• Can be performed by non-refractive surgeons
• Retinal magnification in myopic eyes - potential gain of vision

Pre-Operative Evaluation

The preoperative workup for pIOL implantation should include manifest and cycloplegic refraction, uncorrected and best corrected visual acuity, pupillometry, anterior chamber depth measurement, corneal topography and pachymetry, endothelial cell count, anterior segment examination, intraocular pressure measurement, and dilated fundus examination.

Table 2. Anterior Chamber Depth Requirements

• Acrysof Phakic: >2.7mm
• Artisan/Artiflex: >2.7mm
• ICL: > 2.8mm for myopia, >3.0 mm for hyperopia
• PRL: >2.5mm

Table 3. Inclusion and Exclusion Criteria for pIOL Implantation

• **INCLUSION**
• Age > 21years
• Stable refraction for 1 year
• Ammetropia not amenable to laser refractive surgery
• Unsatisfactory vision +/- intolerance of contact lens/spectacles
• ECC > 2300cells/mm2
• Normal iris and pupil function
• Mesopic pupil size < 5.0 - 6.0mm
• **EXCLUSION**
• Active anterior segment disease
• Recurrent/chronic uveitis
• Cataract
• Macular/Retinal pathology

Types of Phakic Intraocular Lenses

Table 4. Phakic Intraocular Lens

1. Anterior Chamber iris-fixated
2. Angle-Supported anterior chamber
3. Posterior Chamber

Phakic IOLs can be classified according to the site of implantation in the eye. There are 3 main types; Angle-supported anterior chamber, iris-fixated anterior chamber, and posterior chamber, each with distinct features, selection criteria, surgical technique, results, and complications.

1. Angle-Supported Anterior Chamber Piols

The first minus-power anterior chamber pIOL to correct myopia in phakic eyes was implanted in 1953 by Strampelli. [5] Subsequently in 1959, Barraquer published the first series of myopic patients with angle-fixated pIOLs. [6] While initially promising, these lenses were abandoned due to high incidence of complications such as endothelial cell loss, iris atrophy, pupil ovalization, and chronic anterior uveitis. [7] It was nearly 30 years before pIOL design was re-visited and began to become more widely accepted. In 1986, Dvali and Baikoff designed a number of more advanced pIOLs with thinner, more flexible and highly polished haptics. The Vivarte/GBR (Ioltech) and the I-Care (Corneal Laboratories, Inc) pIOLs, which initially showed promising results, were withdrawn from the market due to concerns over endothelial cell loss.

Currently Available Angle-Supported PIOLs

As newer foldable pIOL models have been developed, the rigid PMMA angle-supported models are no longer widely in use. Few longterm studies exist, however angle supported anterior chamber IOLs generally appear to demonstrate good predictability, efficacy and safety.

1.1. Kelman-Duet

The Kelman Duet (Tekia, Inc.Irvine, CA) is an angle-supported pIOL with rigid PMMA haptic, and 6.3mm silicone optic, available in a dioptric range of -6.0D to -20.0D. It has a 2-piece design; the haptic is inserted into the AC through a 2.5mm incision, then the optic is inserted using an injector system. The IOL is then assembled in the AC. There are varying haptic sizes (12.0, 12.5, and 13.0mm), which are chosen based on the white-to-white measurement. The optics and haptics can be exchanged independently if necessary. One year follow-up results reported a mean endothelial cell loss of 5.43%, pupil ovalization of 10.1%, and haptic exchange or repositioning in 7.76%. [8] Longer-term results are not yet available.

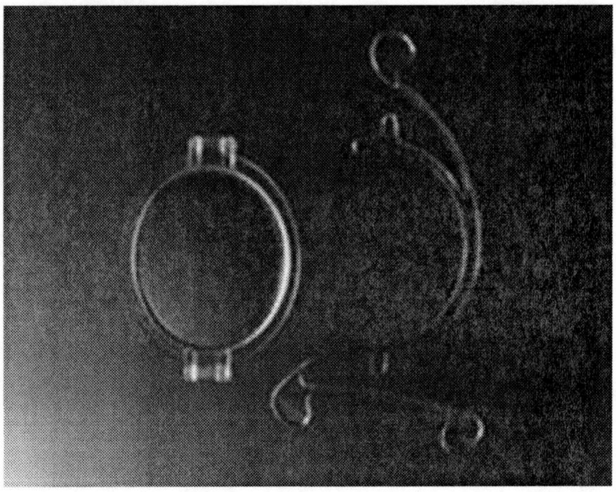

Image 1. Kelman-Duet IOL.

1.2. Acrysof

The Acrysof pIOL (Alcon, Inc.Fort Worth, Tx) is a single-piece hydrophobic acrylic angle-supported pIOL with a 6.0mm optic and overall length of 12.5 - 14.0mm, with a dioptric range of -6.0 to -16.5D. The pIOL is introduced into the anterior chamber with a Monarch (Alcon, Inc.). IOL delivery system through a 2.6mm or 3.2mm incision. Intraoperative gonioscopy can be used to confirm placement of the haptic footplates. A peripheral iridectomy is not required.

One-year results from a multicenter study [9] show excellent refractive correction and predictability, with acceptable safety in subjects with moderate-to-high myopia. The mean percentage change in central endothelial cell density at 1 year was -4.77 +/-8.04%. No pupil ovalization, pupillary block, or retinal detachment events were observed. One year results from a smaller study show endothelial cell loss of 4.04%. [10]

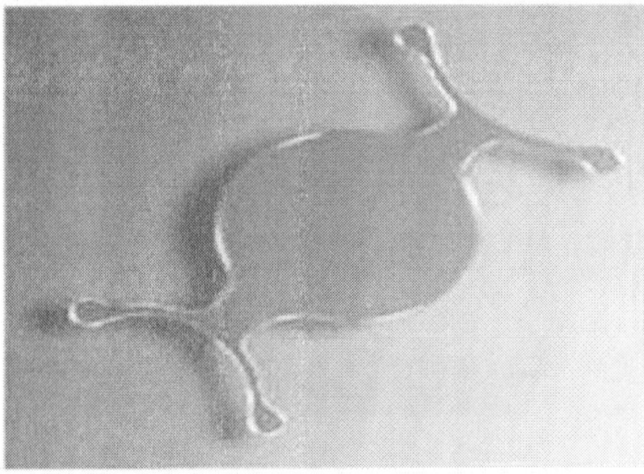

Image 2. Acrysof pIOL (Alcon Laboratories, Inc., Fort Worth, TX).

2. Iris-Fixated Anterior Chamber pIOLs

The iris-claw pIOL, designed by Jan Worst, was first implanted in 1978 to correct aphakia following cataract surgery. In 1986 this design was altered to a biconcave PMMA optic with an overall length of 8.5mm, and the pIOL was implanted in the first sighted myopic eye. [11] The design was further modified in 1991 to a convex-concave IOL, and in 1998 the name of the lens was changed to Artisan lens (Ophtec, Groningen, Netherlands) and Verisyse (Abbott Medical Optics, Santa Ana, CA.) in the US.

The iris-fixated pIOLs consist of an optic and 2 haptics, which are in the form of a lobster claw to enclavate iris tissue. The overall size of the lenses is 8.5mm for all eyes, except for a smaller and rarely used paediatric model. The haptics of the iris-fixated pIOL attach to the immobile, mid-peripheral iris stroma. The posterior face of the pIOL is vaulted to ensure optimal space in front of the natural lens, and also accounts for the forward displacement of the natural lens during accommodation. The distance from the edge of the optic to the corneal endothelium is approximately >1.0 mm, depending on the anterior chamber depth and the dioptric power. A toric version of the IOL for the correction of astigmatism has been available since 2001. To reduce surgically induced astigmatism a foldable version with silicon optic and PMMA haptics (Artiflex, Groningen, Ophthec) has more recently been developed. Iris-fixated pIOLs have the advantage of the longest clinical history and experience relative to other pIOLs. They are versatile, and various models are available which can be used in myopia, hyperopia, astigmatism, and aphakia, several studies have demonstrated long follow-up and all models, including toric models have shown good predictability, efficacy, and safety.

Table 5.

• IOL	• Optic size	• Overall length	• Dioptric Power
• Artisan Myopia	• 6.0mm	• 8.5mm	• -1.0 to -15.5D
• Artisan Myopia	• 5.0mm	• 8.5mm	• -1.0 to -23.5D
• Artisan Hyperopia	• 5.0mm	• 8.5mm	• +1.0 to +12.0D
• Artisan Toric	• 5.0mm	• 8.5mm	• 1 to 7.5D
• Artiflex Myopia	• 6.0mm	• 8.5mm	• -2.0 to -14.5D
• Artiflex Toric	• 6.0mm	• 8.5mm	• Sphere -1.0 to -13.5mm • Cylinder -1.0 to -5.0mm

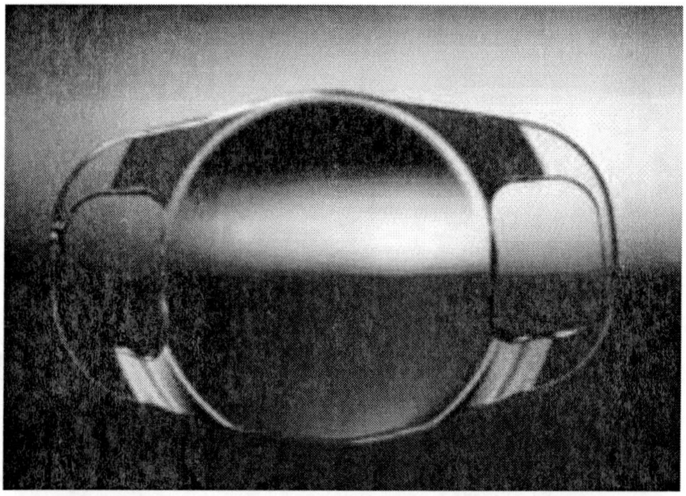

Image 3.Artisan Myopia IOL (Image courtesy of Ophtec, Groningen, The Netherlands).

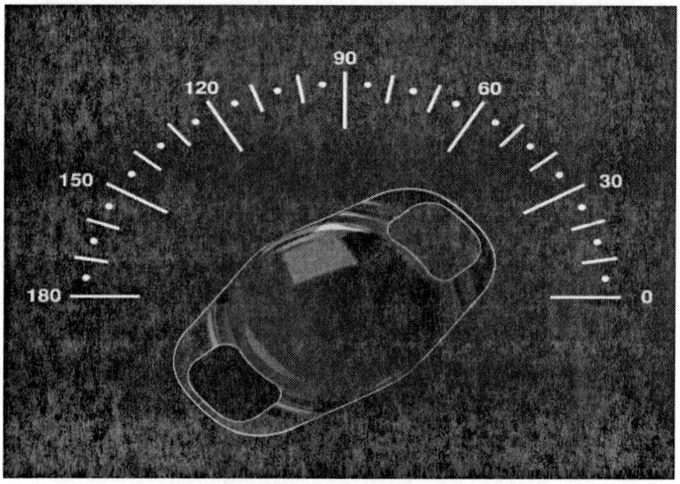

Image 4. Artisan Toric IOL (Image courtesy of Ophtec, Groningen, The Netherlands).

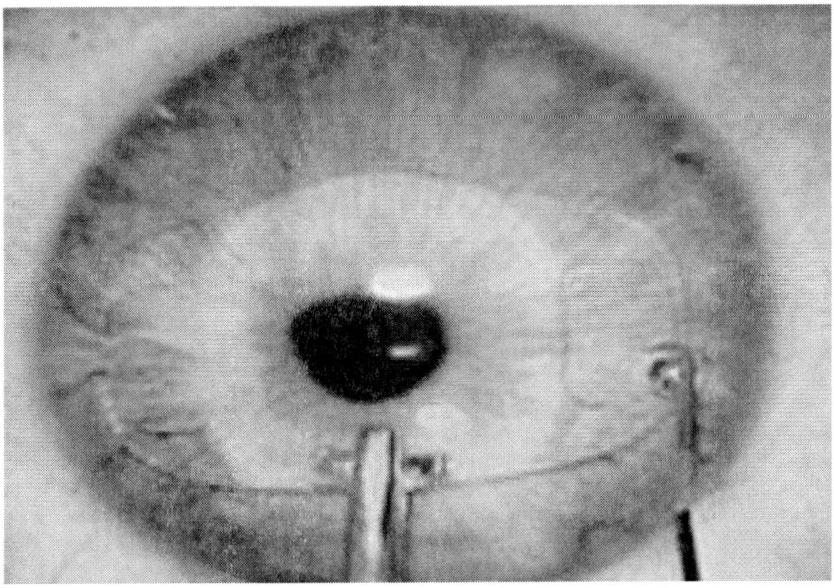

Image 5. Artisan IOL undergoing enclavation.

2.1. Surgical Technique: Artisan Iris-Fixated pIOL

The pIOL power is calculated using the van der Heijde and Fechner et al. formulas, based on subjective refraction, keratometry readings and anterior chamber depth. The procedure can be carried out under general, local or topical anaesthesia depending on the surgeon's preference. The pupil is constricted with pilocarpine 2% pre-operatively. A 6mm shelved clear corneal incision is made superiorly, and 2 paracenteses are made at 10 and 2 o'clock. Intra-operative pupillary constriction is maintained with an intracameral injection of acetylcholine chloride (Miochol E, Bausch & Lomb, Rochester, NY). The anterior chamber is filled with viscoelastic device. The pIOL is inserted into the anterior chamber using specialized implantation forceps, and rotated into a horizontal position. The pIOL is stabilized with holding forceps while the enclavation needle is introduced through the paracenteses, and used to push the iris tissue through the iris claw haptics. The same manouever is performed at the other enclavation site. A peripheral iridectomy is performed to prevent pupillary block. The corneal wounds are sutured with 10-0 nylon. Sutures are removed from 4 weeks post-operatively.

2.2. Artiflex Foldable Silicone pIOL

Insertion of the Artiflex foldable pIOL follows a similar surgical procedure however a smaller 3.0 - 3.2mm corneal incision is used. The incision is usually watertight but may require a single 10-0 nylon suture, which can be removed 2 weeks post-operatively.

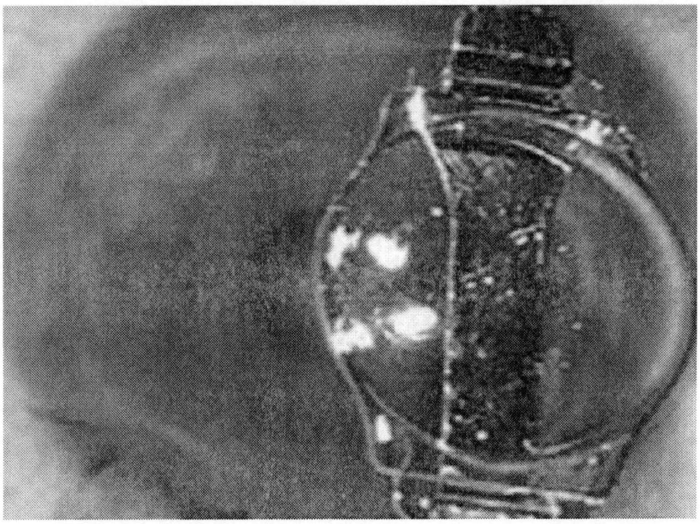

Image 6. Artiflex IOL placing instrument.

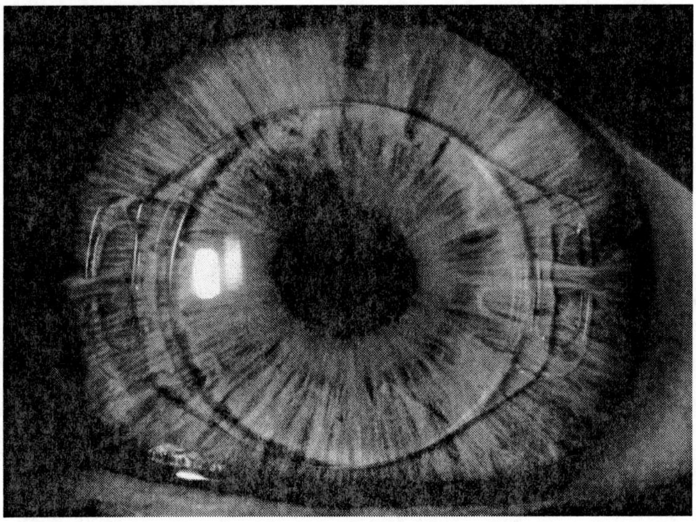

Image 7. Artiflex IOL in situ (Image courtesy of Ophtec BV, Groningen, The Netherlands).

3. Posterior Chamber Piols

Problems with anterior chamber pIOLs led towards development of posterior chamber pIOLs. In 1986, Fyodorov [12] developed a one-piece silicone "collar-button" pIOL with a concave anterior surface, which projected anteriorly through the pupil. The pIOL was fixated behind the iris plane by 2 haptics and had a total length of 8mm. Although initial results were encouraging, complications such as cataract formation, uveitis, glaucoma, and decentration occurred, which led to changes in IOL design. Several improved models have emerged since the Fyodorov pIOL. The following models are the most commonly used, and have shown good safety and efficacy in studies.

Current Posterior Chamber pIOL Models

3.1. Implantable Collamer Lens (STAAR Surgical)

The Implantable Collamer Lens (ICL) (Visian ICL. STAAR Surgical) is the most widely used posterior chamber pIOL. The pIOL is manufactured with collamer material, which consists of a copolymer (of hydroxyethylmethacrylate and benzophenone monomers),purified collagen, and water. The polymer material is soft, elastic, and hydrophilic. The ICL is available in powers ranging from -3.0 to -23.0D for myopic IOLs, +3.0 to +22.0D for hyperopic ICLs, and an added positive cylinder of +1.0 to +6.0 D for toric ICLS correcting myopia. The optic and overall diameters of the Visian ICL vary with refractive power, ranging from 4.9 mm (optic) / 12.1 mm (overall) to 5.8 mm (optic) / 13.7 mm (overall).

The current model is the Visian ICL V4, a rectangular single-piece IOL, 7.5-8.0m wide. In order to reduce contact of the pIOL with the anterior capsule of the crystalline lens, a forward vault is integrated into its plate-haptic design with a central convex/concave optical zone. The Visian ICLs are foldable, allowing for posterior chamber injection through a microscopic incision of 3.5 mm or smaller. The Visian ICL is positioned completely within the posterior chamber between the iris and crystalline lens. Numerous studies have shown that ICL pIOLs are predictable, safe, and stable. [13-18] However, there is a risk of cataract formation, pigment dispersion, and glaucoma. [19]

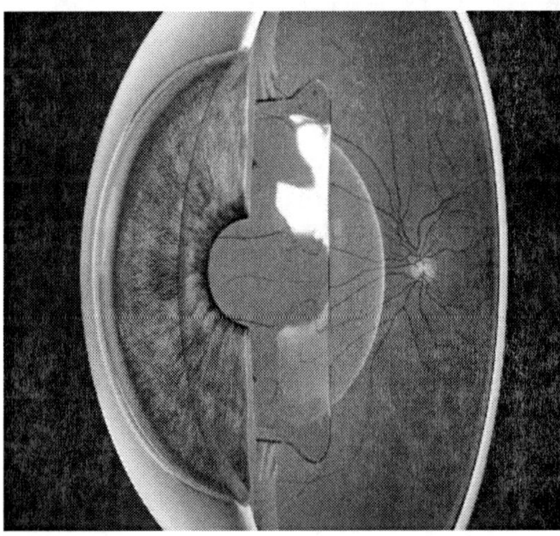

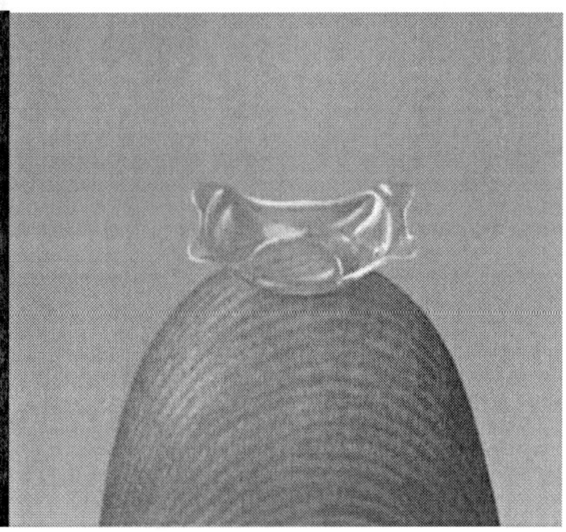

Image 8 & 9. Implantable Collamer Lens (Image courtesy of STAAR Surgical).

Surgical Technique

The pupil is dilated pre-operatively. Correct loading of the ICL in the cartridge and the injector is essential. The ICL is inserted through a sub-3.5mm incision. One or two side port paracenteses are created. The anterior chamber is filled with viscoelastic device. The cartridge is inserted bevel down and the ICL is carefully injected. As the IOL is unfolding, the bevel is twisted left or right to ensure correct orientation of the lens. The haptics are gently pushed under the iris using a blunt spatula and the IOL position and centration are checked. The pupil is constricted using intracameral acetylcholine chloride (MioChol E, Bausch & Lomb,

Rochester, NY). The viscoelastic device is removed and a peripheral iridectomy is performed. Alternatively peripheral iridotomies can be created pre-operatively with Nd:YAG laser.

3.2. Phakic Refractive Lens

The Phakic Refractive Lens (PRL:Zeiss Meditec) for the correction of myopia and hyperopia is a single-piece, convex-concave IOL made of ultra-thin, optically clear silicone. The PRL 100/101 is a single-piece, biconcave silicone IOL, with an optic diameter of 4.5-5.0mm and a total diameter of 10.8-11.3mm, and available in powers from -3 to -20D. The PRL 200 for high hyperopia has an optic diameter of 4.5mm and a total length of 10.6mm, and corrects from +3 to +15D.

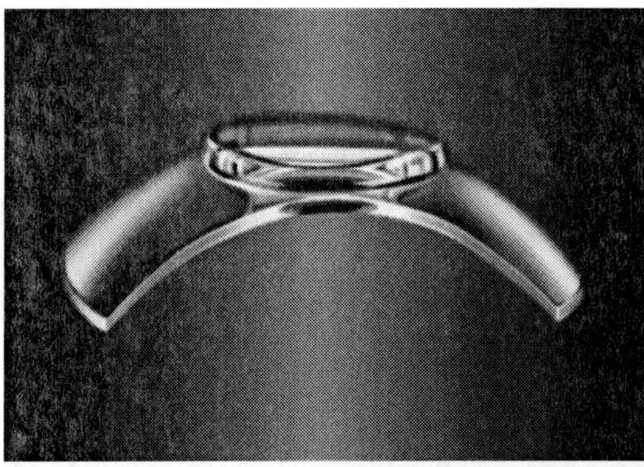
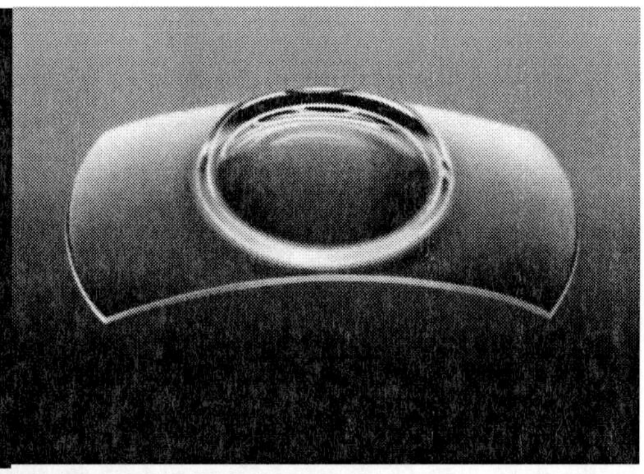

A B

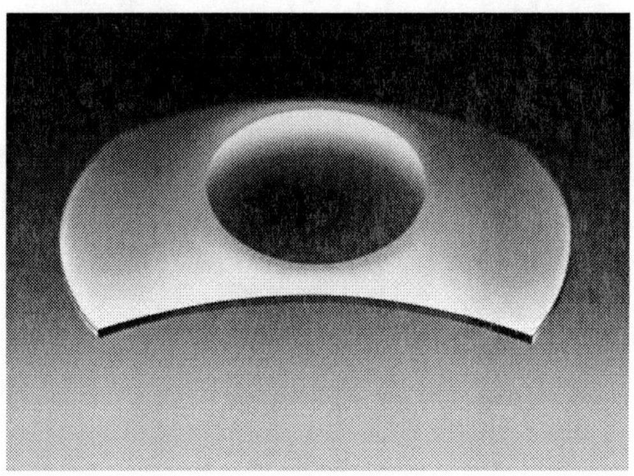

C

Image 10. A & B Myopic Lens, C. Hyperopic Lens.

This is a foldable pIOL, which can be inserted through a 3.2mm incision and floats on a layer of aqueous humour inside the posterior chamber. Lack of fixation is potentially problematic in terms of stability of centration, and rotation. For this reason, the PRL is not suitable for correction of astigmatism.

Table 6.

	• **PRL 100/101**	• **PRL 200**
• **Pathology**	• Myopia	• Hyperopia
• **Optic Diameter**	• 4.5/5mm	• 4.5mm
• **Total Diameter**	• 10.8/11.3mm	• 10.6mm
• **Material**	• Silicone	• Silicone
• **Lens design**	• Biconcave	• Convex-concave
• **Dioptre Range**	• -3 to -20D	• +3 to +15D
• **Anatomic Location**	• Posterior chamber	• Posterior chamber

Surgical Technique

The surgical technique for PRL implantation is almost identical to that of the ICL. A 3.2 mm clear corneal incision is made and two opposing paracenteses created. The PRL can be inserted with a Dementiev forceps or an injector system. The PRL unfolds slowly in the anterior chamber, the haptic initially lying anterior to the dilated iris. A long spatula or hook is used to gently place the haptics behind the iris. A miotic agent is inserted when the correct horizontal orientation has been verified. Two peripheral iridotomies, 90 degrees apart are mandatory to prevent pupil block as spontaneous rotation of the PRL can easily occur.

Complications of Phakic IOLs

Angle-Supported pIOL Complications:

1. Endothelial cell loss
   The main concern with anterior chamber pIOLs is loss of corneal endothelial cell loss. Preoperative examination should exclude patients with pre-existing low endothelial cell counts, or shallow anterior chambers as the risk to the corneal endothelium increases with decreasing distance between the pIOL and the endothelium. Endothelial cell losses appear to be greatest in the first post-operative year. A long-term follow-up study by Javaloy et al. found an endothelial cell loss of 10.6% in the first year, followed by a mean decrease of 1.8% per year thereafter. [20]
2. Pupil ovalization
   The position of the haptics in the sclerocorneal angle can lead to deformation of the iridosclerocorneal architecture, causing iris retraction or pupil ovalization. If severe this can result in glare and may be cosmetically unacceptable. Minor pupil ovalisation may be observed but if progressive may indicate entrapment of the iris root and is an indication for pIOL explantation.
3. Glare/Haloes
   The incidence of glare is dependent on the size and position of the optic, which varies with IOL design. The position of the pIOL in front of the pupil can lead to edge effects and optical aberration. The size of the scotopic pupil should be

considered pre-operatively; if significantly larger than the optic of the pIOL this will increase the chance of glare and discomfort and one should be cautious about implantation

4. Pigment deposits
   This condition is often seen in clinical practice although not frequently reported as it does not usually affect visual acuity
5. Pupil block Glaucoma
   To prevent pupil block glaucoma, either a preoperative laser iridotomy or intraoperative surgical iridectomy is recommended, as well as complete removal of viscoelastic devices from the anterior chamber at the end of surgery.
6. Cataract formation with anterior chamber pIOLs is much less frequent than in those with posterior chamber pIOLS, given the position of the pIOL away from the lens. A metaanalysis of cataract formation after pIOL implantation reported a total incidence of 1 .3% for anterior chamber pIOLs. [21]
7. Surgically induced astigmatism
8. Rotation of pIOL

Iris-Fixated pIOL Complications

1. Corneal Endothelial cell loss
   Endothelial cell loss may be secondary to surgical trauma, direct contact between the pIOL and the endothelium intraoperatively, or due to postoperative changes in pIOL position. Reports on the rate of endothelial cell loss vary. In our experience with Artisan pIOLs, endothelial cell loss 1.45% at 1 year, and neglible cell loss at 5 years. [22]
2. Pigment dispersion/Lens Deposits
   Pigmented precipitates may be noted on the pIOL commonly, however the effect on visual acuity is generally not of significance. Precipitates reduce with use of topical non-steroidal anti-inflammatories. Aetiology is unclear but may be secondary to iris disruption due to intraocular manipulation or pressure on the iris between the IOL and lens.

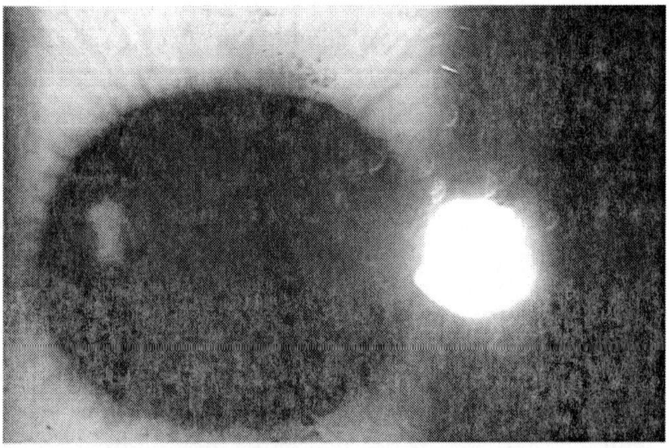

Image 11. Pigment precipitates on Artiflex IOL.

3. Surgically Induced Astigmatism (SIA)
   The non-foldable Artisan pIOL requires a 5-6mm incision, which may cause SIA, however according to the literature this is not as prevalent as one might expect. The foldable version further reduces SIA.
4. Glare/Haloes
   If the pupil diameter is larger than the optic, glare and haloes can result.
5. Chronic Inflammation/Uveitis
   This is a potential concern as the pIOL is directly fixated to the iris tissue and may cause pressure or shearing forces when the eye is moving or when patients rub their eye. This may lead to increased permeability of iris vessels, breakdown of the blood-aqueous barrier and release of inflammatory mediators.
6. Lens Dislocation
   Dislocation of one or both haptics may occur either spontaneously or secondary to trauma. Spontaneous dislocation of a haptic is thought to occur due to iris atrophy at the site of enclavation. In our experience the rate of dislocation is 2% in patients followed for up to 12 years postoperatively. Reenclavation of the pIOL is successful with no adverse effects on clinical outcomes.

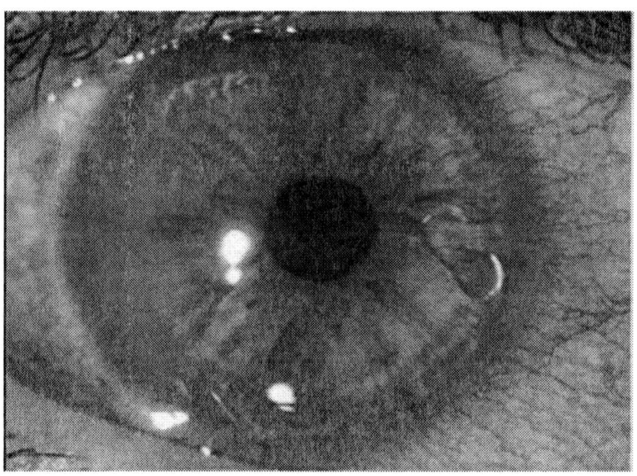

Image 12. Dislocation of Artisan IOL haptic.

7. Cataract Formation
   This is less with iris-fixated pIOLs as it is inserted over a miotic pupil and there is no contact with the crystalline lens.
8. Pupil ovalization
   This can occur if the pIOL is fixated assymmetrically, however it is usually not progressive.

Complication of posterior chamber pIOLs

1. Cataract Formation
   The overall incidence of cataract formation is much greater in posterior chamber pIOLs compared to anterior chamber pIOLs. A metaanalysis of 1210 eyes found an

incidence of 9.6%.[21] The most common form of cataract seen is anterior subcapsular. Possible causes are operative trauma, contact between the pIOL and the crystalline lens, and chronic subclinical inflammation.

2. Glare/Haloes
   This can result from a small optic diameter, particularly if there is decentration of the pIOL.
3. Endothelial cell loss
   Endothelial cell loss with pc-pIOLs is seen to be greatest in the first year after surgery, and then stabilize with time. It is thought to be caused mainly by surgical trauma.
4. Pupil block Glaucoma
   Due to the position of the pIOL the iris may be pushed forward and cause acute pupil block glaucoma, especially in hyperopic eyes. Preoperative or intraoperative iridotomies should be performed to prevent this.
5. Pigment dispersion
   Ultrasound biomicroscopy has shown contact between the posterior surface of the iris and the pIOL. A possible consequence of this is pigment dispersion and accumulation in the angle. However development of secondary glaucoma has not been observed.
6. IOL rotation/decentration
   Incorrect sizing may lead to IOL rotation or decentration.
7. Posterior dislocation
8. There have been rare reports of this serious complication, which may be attributed to pre-existing zonular defects, or pIOL rotation.

Table 7. Summary of Phakic IOL Complications

• **Angle-Supported**	• **Iris-Fixated**	• **Posterior Chamber**
• Pupil Ovalization	• Endothelial cell loss	• Cataract
• Endothelial cell loss	• Traumatic or spontaneous dislocation	• Endothelial cell loss
• Glare/Haloes	• Pupil-block glaucoma	• Posterior dislocation
• IOL rotation	• Pigment deposits on IOL	• Pupil block glaucoma
• Iris Atrophy	• Iris Atrophy	• Pigment dispersion
• Pigment deposits	• Glare/Haloes	• IOL rotation/ • decentration
• Pupil block glaucoma	• Pupil ovalization	• Glare/Haloes

Bioptics

The concept of bioptics was introduced over a decade ago, by Roberto Zaldivar of Buenos Aires. Bioptics refers to the use of laser refractive surgery following pIOL implantation to achieve maximal uncorrected distance visual acuity. This is a useful concept, which allows fine-tuning of refractive results, especially in patients with high refractive errors and astigmatism.

Anterior Segment Imaging and pIOLs

Anterior segment optical coherence tomography (OCT) can now be used to precisely measure the shape, size and position of structures within the anterior segment, and determine pIOL position in the eye relative to the crystalline lens. Baikoff et al. performed biometric studies of the anterior segment during accommodation using anterior segment OCT, and confirmed the Helmholtz theory of accommodation. [23] The anterior pole of the crystalline lens is shown to move forward by 30 μm with every diopter of accommodation, decreasing the distance between the anterior surface of the crystalline lens and the posterior surface of the ICL, thus increasing the risk of cataract formation. For iris-fixated pIOLs the distance between the pIOL and crystalline lens remains stable during accommodation. [4]

However the distance between the anterior pIOL surface and the corneal endothelium is seen to reduce during the accommodation process. This is of particular importance in anterior chamber pIOLs as it may be a factor in endothelial cell loss. Ageing changes of the crystalline lens also affects its position relative to pIOLs. The crystalline lens thickens with age, causing forward movement of the lens even while at rest, underlining the importance of long-term monitoring of patient with pIOLS. The development of anterior segment imaging therefore has many important clinical applications, allowing for increased safety profile and more accurate follow-up.

Use of Phakic IOLs in Children

Most children with refractive errors can be treated adequately and safely with spectacles or contact lenses, along with conventional therapy for amblyopia. However in certain subsets of children, traditional treatment is ineffective and further intervention is necessary. Currently, refractive surgery in children is performed only when conventional treatments have failed. In children with high refractive errors, spectacle tolerance can be reduced secondary to prismatic induced aberrations, limited field of view, as well as cosmetic appearance. Contact lenses can also be problematic in children due to difficulty with insertion and removal, infection, intolerance and expense. The particular pediatric subpopulations who may require refractive surgery include those with bilateral significant ametropia or anisometropia who are spectacle or contact lens noncompliant, as well as those with secondary high-refractive amblyopia in children with neurobehavioral disorders.

Table 8. Indications for phakic intraocular lens implantation in children

1.	High anisometropia, myopia, or hyperopia noncompliant with conventional treatment
2.	Bilateral high ametropia noncompliant with conventional treatment
3.	Secondary high-refractive amblyopia associated with neurobehavioral disorders

The pIOL implant of choice in the pediatric population is the anterior chamber Artisan iris-fixated pIOL, (Image 1 & 2) although the foldable Artiflex model which requires a smaller incision and less corneal sutures has been shown to be safe and effective also. Safe insertion and lower long-term risk for endothelial cell loss requires an anterior chamber depth of 3.2mm or greater. This may preclude the use of iris-fixated pIOLs in children younger than 3 years, and children with shallow anterior chambers, as can occur in children with high myopia following retinopathy of prematurity.

Reports of adverse events in the pediatric population are rare due to the limited number of surgeries performed; however it can be assumed that children would have a similar complication profile to the adult population; including cataract formation, uveitis, IOL dislocation, pigment dispersion, and endothelial cell loss. The most significant concern in the pediatric population is long-term corneal endothelial cell loss. This is particularly important given the long life expectancy of the child, as well as the potential for eye-rubbing. However experience in the pediatric population to date is limited, and this is compounded by difficulties in obtaining accurate endothelial cell counts in children. Data on endothelial cell loss in children with pIOLS is limited but available studies have shown an endothelial cell loss rate varying over the course of 3 to 5 years between 6.5% and 15.2%.

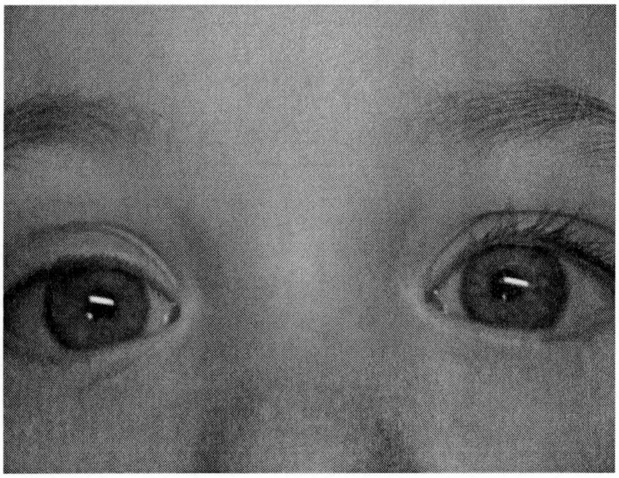

Image 13. Infant with bilateral iris-fixated phakic IOLs in situ.

Conclusion

The implantation of phakic IOLs has been shown to be an effective, safe, predictable and stable procedure to correct moderate and high refractive errors. Advantages include predictability, reversibility, high visual quality and quick visual recovery, as well as preservation of accommodation. There are 3 types of pIOL; angle-supported anterior chamber, iris-fixated anterior chamber, and posterior chamber. Complications are rare and generally related to the site of implantation. Safety and functional outcomes continue to improve with developments in design and technology.

References

[1] El Danasoury MA, El Maghraby A, Gamali TO. Comparision of iris-fixated Artisan lens implantation with excimer laser in situ keratomileusis in correcting myopia between -9.00 and -19.50 diopters: a randomized study. *Ophthalmology* 2002;109:955-64

[2] Sanders DR. Matched population comparison of the Visian implantable collamer lens and standard LASIK for myopia of -3.0 to -7.88 diopters. *J Refract Surg* 2007;23:537-53

[3] Colin J, Robinet A, Cochener B. Retinal detachment after clear lens extraction for high myopia:seven-year follow-up. *Ophthalmology* 1999;106:2281-4

[4] Guell JL, Morral M, Gris O, Gaytan J, Sisquella M, Manero F. Evaluation of Verisyse and Artiflex phakic intraocular lenses during accommodation using Visante optical coherence tomography. *J Cataract Refract Surg* 2007;33:1398-1404

[5] Strampelli B, Sopportabilita' di lenti acriliche in camera anteriore nella afachia e nei vizi di refrazione [Tolerance of acrylic lenses in the anterior chamber in aphakia and refraction disorders] *Ann Ottalmol Clin Oculist* 1954;80:75-82

[6] Barraquer J. Anterior chamber plastic lenses. Results of and conclusions from five years experience. *Trans Ophthalmol Soc UK* 1959;79:393-424

[7] Apple DJ, Brems RN, Park RB, Kavka-Van Norman D, Hansen SO, Tetz MR, Richards SC, Letchinger SD. Anterior chamber lenses. Part 1:complications and pathology and a review of designs. *J Cataract Refract Surg* 1987;13:157-174

[8] Alio JL, Pinero D, Bernabeu G, Galal A, Vargas JM, Ismail MM. The Kelman Duet phakic intraocular lens: 1-year results *.J Refract Surg*. 2007 Nov;23(9):868-79.

[9] Kohnen T, Knorz MC, Cochener B, Gerl RH, Arne J-L, Colin J, Alio JL, Belluci R, Marinho A. Acrysof phakic angle-supported intraocular lens for the correction of moderate to high myopia:one-year results of a multicenter European Study. *Ophthalmology* 2009;116:1314-1321

[10] Mastropasqua L, Toto L, Vecchiarino L, Doronzo E, Mastropasqua R, Di Nicola M. AcrySof cachet phakic intraocular lens in myopic patients: visual performance, wavefront error, and lens position. *J Refract Surg*. 2012 Apr;28(4):267-74. doi: 10.3928/1081597X-20120222-01. Epub 2012 Mar 1.

[11] Fechner PU, Worst JGF. A new concave intraocular lens for the correction of myopia. *Eur J Implant Refract Surg* 1989;1:41-43

[12] Fyodorov SN, Zuev VK, Aznabayev BM. Intraocular correction of high myopia with negative posterior chamber lens. *Ophthalmosurgery* (Moscow) 1991;3:57-58

[13] Lackner B, Pieh S, Schmidinger G, Simader C, Franz C, Deja-co-Ruhswurm I, Skorpik C. Long-term results of implantation of phakic posterior chamber intraocular lenses. *J Cataract Refract Surg* 2004; 30:2269-2276

[14] Implantable Contact Lens in the Treatment of Myopia (ITM) Study Group. U.S. Food and Drug Administration clinical trial of the Implantable Contact Lens for moderate to high myopia. *Ophthalmology* 2003;110:255-266

[15] Gonvers M, Othenin-Girard P, Bornet C, Sickenberg M. Implantable contact lens for moderate to high myopia;short-term follow-up f two models. *J Cataract Refract Surg* 2001;27:380-388

[16] Davidorf JM, Zaldivar R, Oscherow S. Posterior chamber phakic intraocular lens for hyperopia of +4 to +11D. *J Refract Surg* 1998;14:3-6-311
[17] Zalidivar R, Ricur G, Oscherow S. The phakic intraocular lens implant:in-depth focus on posterior chamber phakic IOLs. *Curr Opin Ophthalmol* 2000; 11:22-34
[18] Zaldivar R, Oscherow S, Ricur G. The STAAR posterior chamber phakic intraocular lens. *Int Ophthalmol Clin* 2000;40(3):237-244
[19] Jimenez-Alfaro I, Benitez del Castillo JM, Garcia-Feijoo J, Gil de Bernabe JG, Serrano de la Iglesia JM. Safety of posterior chamber phakic intraocular lenses for the correction of high myopia: anterior segment changes after posterior chamber phakic intraocular lens implantation. *Ophthalmology* 2001;108:90-99
[20] Javaloy J, Alio JL, Iradier MT, Abdelrahman AM, Javaloy T, Borras F. Outcomes of ZB5M angle-supported anterior chamber phakic intraocular lenses at 12 years. *J Refract Surg* 2007;23:147-158
[21] Chen L-J, Chang Y-J, Kuo JC, Rajagopal R, Azar DT. Metanalysis of cataract development after phakic intraocular lens surgery. *J Cataract Refract Surg* 2008;34:1181-1200
[22] Qasem Q, Kirwan C, O Keefe M. 5-year prospective follow-up of Artisan phakic intraocular lenses for the correction of myopia, hyperopia and astigmatism. *Ophthalmologica* 2010;224:283-290
[23] Baikoff G, Lutun E, Ferraz C. Anterior chamber optical coherence tomography study of human natural accommodation in a 19 year old albino. *J Cat Refract Surg* 2004;30:696-701

In: Current Understanding and New Techniques … ISBN: 978-1-62808-748-2
Editor: Michael O'Keefe

Chapter 13

Supracor

Andrea Ryan[1,*] ***and Michael O'Keefe***[2,†]
[1]Cork University Hospital, Cork, Ireland
[2]Mater Private Hospital, Dublin

Abstract

SUPRACOR® is a multifocal corneal excimer laser in situ keratomileusis (LASIK) - based procedure for ametropic presbyopia correction developed by Technolas Perfect Vision (Munich, Germany). The single step multifocal ablation profile is currently unique among pseudoaccommodative corneal procedures. There are no studies evaluating the SUPRACOR procedure in the peer-reviewed literature to date. The CE approval study supported by Technolas Perfect Vision and the authors' personal experience with the procedure (all surgery by M. O'Keefe) suggest a high level of spectacle independence can be achieved for distance and near vision. A degree of compromise is involved as with all presbyopia procedures. Refinements to the nomogram have the potential to reduce the enhancement rate. Careful patient selection is the key to successful outcomes.

Introduction

The correction of presbyopia remains a significant challenge for refractive surgeons and is considered by many to be the 'final frontier' of refractive surgery. A dynamic physiological process, accommodation is difficult to mimic or restore surgically. Numerous approaches have been developed, both accommodative and pseudoaccommodative, each with their own limitations and all involving some degree of compromise between the distance and near visual acuity outcomes.

Accommodative approaches to presbyopia correction have included insertion of accommodating intraocular lenses (IOLs)[1] and scleral expansion procedures [2] while

* andrearyan11@gmail.com.
† mokeefe@materprivate.ie.

pseudoaccommodative techniques have involved multifocal IOLs[3], corneal inlays[4], excimer laser-based multifocal ablations[5] and intrastromal femtosecond laser procedures[6].

A corneal approach is attractive to many surgeons as it is probably the least invasive, avoiding the potential risks of an intraocular procedure. Using a LASIK-based approach has the advantage of being a well-established and familiar technique with the possibility of easy enhancement if needed.

A variety of presbyopic LASIK ('presbyLASIK') procedures exist.[7-10] These are bifocal procedures that create a central hyperpositive corneal zone for near vision and peripheral corneal zone for distance vision (central presbyLASIK) or a central corneal zone for distance and midperipheral zone for near vision (peripheral presbyLASIK). Such multistep ablations can create transition zones within the optical zone and result in unwanted aberrations that can reduce vision.

SUPRACOR® (Technolas Perfect Vision GmbH, Munich, Germany) is a new-generation excimer laser pseudoaccommodative corneal treatment which can simultaneously treat a patient's distance and near correction. The SUPRACOR® treatment uses a progressive ablation profile to provide a smooth transition from distance to near correction in one step. In contrast to traditional 'presbyLASIK' treatments, the single step progressive ablation is multifocal and avoids a transition zone within the optical zone, therefore theoretically allowing for vision at all intermediate distances and reducing undesirable aberrations. This type of ablation is currently unique on the market.

The treatment is 'aberration-optimised' or designed to compensate for unwanted aberrations that may occur while harnessing beneficial higher order aberrations (HOAs) to improve depth of focus. Ordinarily, HOAs are felt to reduce the visual performance and wavefront-guided ablations aim to reduce or eliminate HOAs in standard myopic LASIK procedures. However, while HOAs will normally degrade vision, in certain circumstances, such as in presbyopia, the induction of specific HOAs can have a beneficial effect by improving the depth of focus.[11] It has been shown that the spherical aberration of the human eye shifts in a negative direction during normal accommodation.[12-14] Induction of negative spherical aberration on the cornea by excimer laser ablation can improve the depth of focus in presbyopic patients. SUPRACOR® induces a shift in spherical aberration in a negative direction to improve the depth of focus and provide additional pseudoaccommodation.

The SUPRACOR® procedure is designed to treat the full refractive range but is currently licensed in Europe for the treatment of hyperopic presbyopia. Trials are on-going in myopic, emmetropic and post-LASIK patients. The procedure aims for a target spherical equivalent (SE) refraction of -0.50D in both eyes.

The SUPRACOR® Procedure

The treatment is designed to be a bilateral LASIK procedure for use with the Technolas Excimer 217P workstation (Technolas Perfect Vision GmbH, Munich, Germany). A standard LASIK flap of ≥ 9mm and 110-120μm thickness is created with the use of a microkeratome or a femtosecond laser. The stromal bed is ablated in a unique profile in a 6mm optical zone centred on the pupil centre. The ablation profile applied by the laser in the treatment of hyperopic and myopic presbyopic eyes is shown in Figure 1. The central ‘bump’ is created by an extra 2000 pulses fired by the laser to give the near addition.

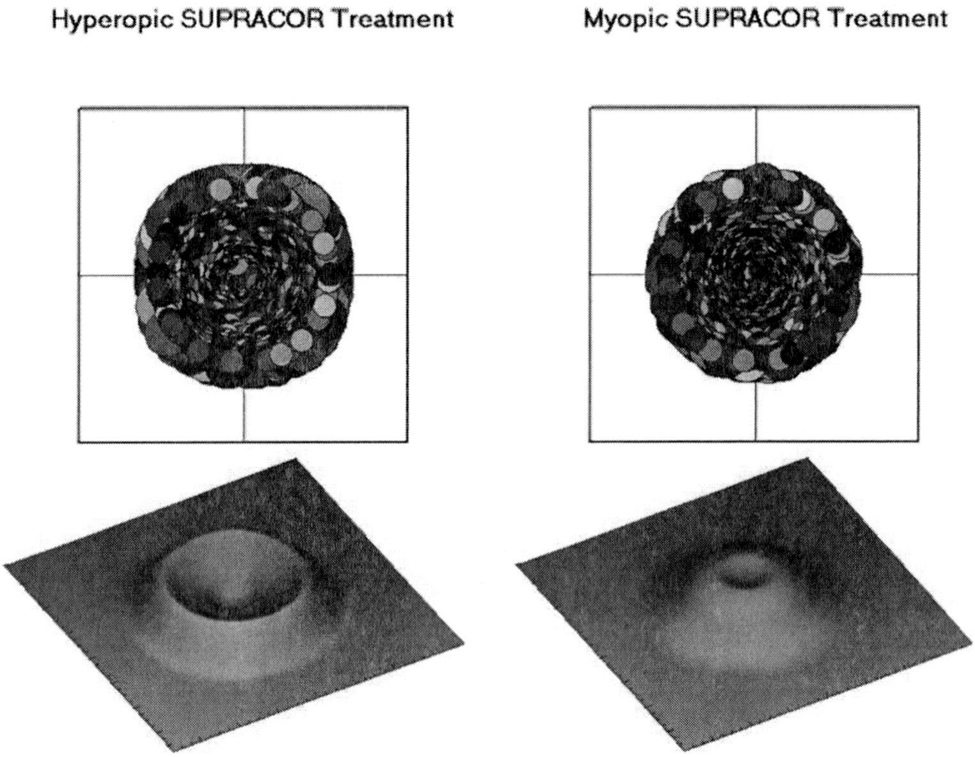

Figure 1. Ablation profile of SUPRACOR® in Hyperopic and Myopic Eyes (Courtesy of Technolas Perfect Vision).

Postoperatively, standard post-LASIK care is given. Artificial tear supplements are frequently required, especially in older patients.

Suitability Criteria for SUPRACOR® Treatment and Preoperative Assessment

The recommended inclusion criteria for SUPRACOR® for hyperopic presbyopic patients are provided in Table 1. Due to the multifocal nature of the procedure and the slightly myopic target SE refraction of -0.50D, a slight decrease in uncorrected distance visual acuity (UDVA) can be expected following SUPRACOR®. For this reason, patients should pass a ‘simulated test of decreased distance vision’ at the preoperative assessment to determine their suitability for the procedure. A trial frame with the best distance correction is placed before both eyes. An additional +0.50D is then placed in front of the distance correction to simulate the potential blur of multifocality. If the patient is unhappy with this level of UDVA, then they are not suitable for SUPRACOR® treatment.

Preoperative tests therefore should include measurement of UDVA and corrected distance visual acuity (CVDA) at near and distance, near addition, subjective refraction, cycloplegic refraction, corneal topography, assessment of tear film and simulated test of decreased distance vision.

Table 1.

Recommended Initial Inclusion Criteria for SUPRACOR® for Hyperopic Presbyopic Patients
❖ Age ≥ 47 years
❖ MRSE +0.75 to +3.0D
❖ Astigmatism ≤ 2D
❖ Maximum 0.75D difference between cycloplegic and manifest refraction
❖ Mean K reading 41-45D
❖ Angle kappa < 10 degrees
❖ Able to tolerate a near addition of +1.75D
❖ CDVA in both eyes ≥ 6/7.5 Snellen (0.8 Decimal)
❖ Usual LASIK restrictions
CCT >500μm
No evidence of keratoconus on corneal topography
Absence of significant dry eyes/ocular surface disease

Clinical Results Of SUPRACOR®

To date, there are no peer-reviewed reports on the outcome of SUPRACOR® treatment in the published literature. A European multicentre clinical study (referred to herein as the CE Study) has been carried out by Technolas Perfect Vision for the CE marking of SUPRACOR® (a mandatory conformity marking for products placed on the market in the European Economic Area). The authors of this chapter will also present their personal experience in treating hyperopic presbyopia by SUPRACOR® in an initial consecutive series of patients at the Mater Private Hospital (MPH), Dublin, Ireland and refer to this as the MPH study (all procedures by Professor Michael O'Keefe).

Patients

Table 2.

Baseline Characteristics of Patients Treated by SUPRACOR®		
	CE Study	MPH Study
Number of eyes	46	56
Mean Age in years (range)	55.5 (50-62)	57 (48-64)
Male/Female	49%/52%	25%/75%
Mean +/-SD Preoperative MRSE (D)	+1.67 +/-0.77	+1.90 +/-0.56
Follow-up	6 months	6 months
SD=standard deviation, MRSE=manifest refraction spherical equivalent, D=dioptres		

The baseline characteristics of the patients treated in the CE Study and MPH Study are shown in Table 2. Both studies evaluated the outcome of SUPRACOR® at 6 months postoperatively.

Efficacy

Distance Vision

The efficacy of SUPRACOR® in UDVA correction is shown in Table 3. Due to the 0.50D myopic SE target and the multifocal cornea, a UDVA of 6/6 or better is not the primary aim. Binocular UDVA of 6/6 or better is achieved in approximately 60% of patients, 6/9.5 or better in 92-96% and 6/12 or better in 96-100%. Binocular vision is considerably better than monocular vision. In the MPH Study, mean monocular UDVA at 6 months was 0.18 +/- 0.17 logMAR (Snellen equivalent 6/9 +/-1.7 lines) and mean binocular UDVA was 0.06 +/-0.12 (Snellen equivalent 6/7 +/-1.2 lines).

Table 3.

Cumulative Uncorrected Distance Visual Acuity	CE Study	MPH Study
Monocular		
6/6 or better	41%	21%
6/7.5 or better	78.5%	36%
6/9.5 or better	87%	70%
6/12 or better	93.5%	86%
Binocular		
6/6 or better	61%	57%
6/7.5 or better	96%	82%
6/9.5 or better	96%	92%
6/12 or better	100%	96%

Near Vision

Table 4.

Cumulative Uncorrected Near Snellen Visual Acuity	CE Study	Cumulative Uncorrected Near Ability on Vocational Reading Test	MPH Study
Monocular		Monocular	
6/6 or better	56.5%	N5 or better	53.5%
6/7.5 or better	85%	N6 or better	75%
6/9.5 or better	93.5%	N8 or better	79%
6/12 or better	96%	N10 or better	89%
Binocular		Binocular	
6/6 or better	83%	N5 or better	68%
6/7.5 or better	91%	N6 or better	82%
6/9.5 or better	96%	N8 or better	89%
6/12 or better	100%	N10 or better	96%

Near vision was assessed in the CE Study by near Snellen acuity. In the MPH Study, we measured near vision using the Vocational Reading test (N notation) and recorded the smallest print size (N5 being the smallest) that the patient could read comfortably at 40cm under photopic conditions. The results of near vision following SUPRACOR® are presented in Table 4.

The CE Study found that 87% of patients could read J2 or better on a Jaeger Reading test (approximately equivalent to N5) and the MPH Study found that 68% could read N5 or better and 89% N8 or better (approximately newspaper size print).

Predictability

Table 5 shows the mean manifest refraction spherical equivalent (MRSE) over time. The target was -0.50D SE at 6 months. The CE Study did not provide further data on predictability.

Table 5.

Manifest Refraction Spherical Equivalent Refraction (MRSE) over Time		
Mean +/-SD MRSE (D)	CE Study	MPH Study
Preoperative	+1.67 +/-0.77	+1.90 +/-0.56
1 month postoperative	-0.60 +/-0.56	...
3 month postoperative	-0.49 +/-0.42	-0.57 +/-0.64
6 month postoperative	-0.41 +/-0.39	-0.61 +/-0.72

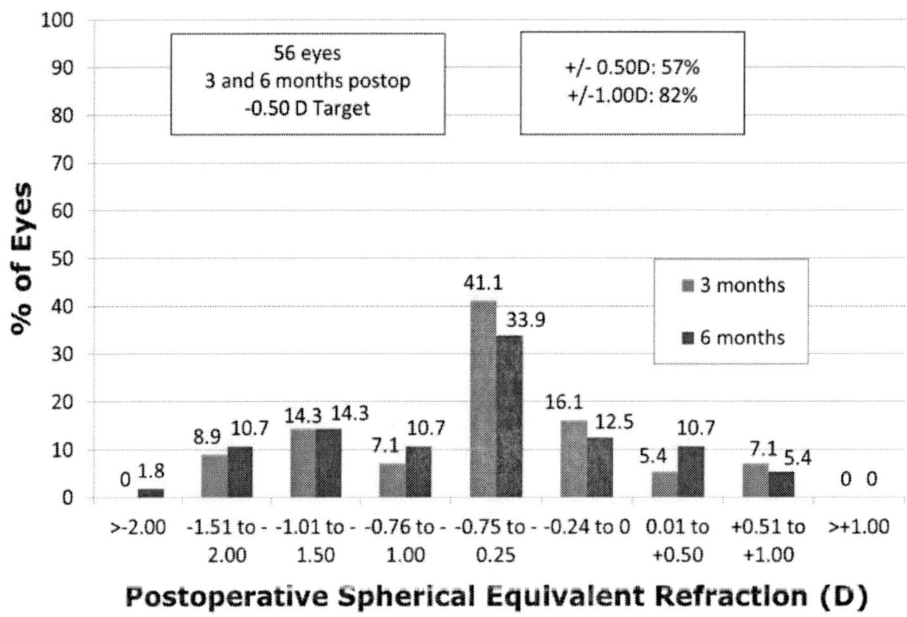

Figure 2. Accuracy of the Postoperative Spherical Equivalent Refraction following SUPRACOR®.

The MPH Study found 57% of eyes within 0.50D and 82% within 1D of the intended target at 6 months. The accuracy of the SE refraction in the MPH study is shown in Figure 2. The intended versus achieved SE refraction is shown in Figure 3 showing a relatively high degree of both under and overcorrections.

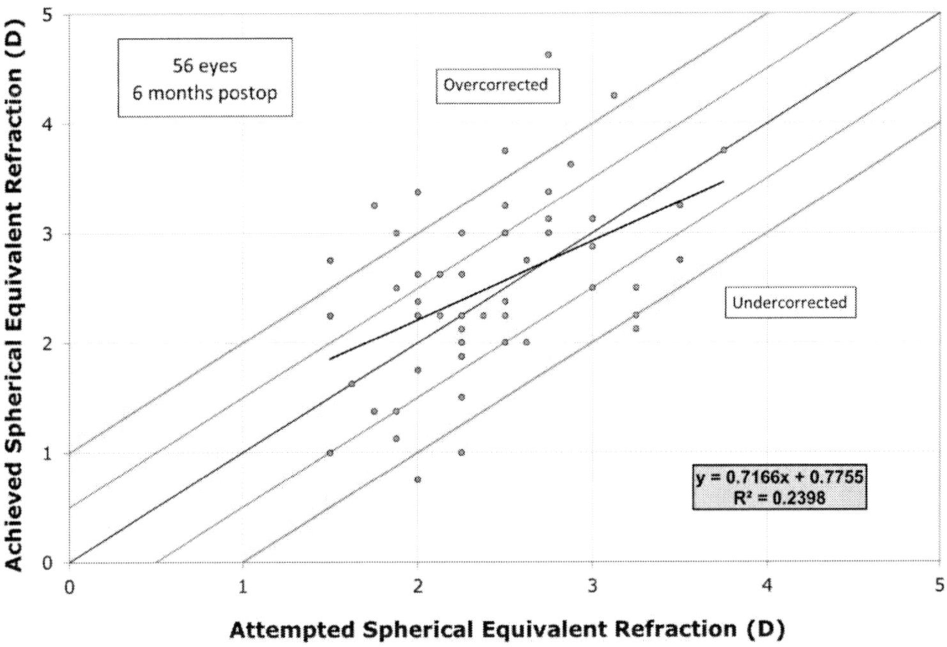

Figure 3. Attempted versus Achieved Spherical Equivalent Refraction for SUPRACOR®.

Stability

The CE Study reported that SE refraction remained stable after 1 month postoperatively. The MPH Study found that a mean myopic overcorrection continued to 6 months with 24% of patients experiencing a change in SE refraction of >0.50D between 3 and 6 months.

Safety

Change in lines of CDVA following SUPRACOR® is shown in Table 6. Substantially more lines of CDVA were lost in the MPH Study due to a much higher proportion of eyes having a preoperative CDVA of 6/4.8 or better in this study compared to the CE Study (38% in MPH Study versus 4% in CE Study). Even though monocular loss of ≥1 line was common in the MPH Study (14%), all eyes maintained CDVA of 6/9.5 or better. Monocular gain of ≥1 line of CDVA was achieved in 11% of eyes and binocular gain of ≥1 line in 17% of eyes in the CE Study and in 27% and 32% of eyes in the MPH Study, respectively.

Table 6.

Change in Lines of Corrected Distance Visual Acuity (CDVA) post SUPRACOR®		
	CE Study	MPH Study
Monocular		
Loss of 1 line of CDVA	4%	14%
Loss of ≥2 lines of CDVA	0	5%
Binocular		
Loss of 1 line of CDVA	4%	…
Loss of ≥2 lines of CDVA	0	3.6%

Complications

The CE Study did not report any complications. There were no serious intraoperative or postoperative complications in our MPH Study. Eighteen percent of our patients had symptoms or signs of dry eye at 3 months and 11% at 6 months. Fourteen percent reported sensitivity to light.

Re-Treatments

The CE Study did not report any re-treatments. During our 6 month follow-up study, no re-treatments were performed as the refraction did not appear to be fully stabilised. Five of our patients (18%) had a re-treatment on their dominant eye to enhance the UDVA after 6 months. The mean re-treated SE was -0.98 +/- 0.60 D. One of these 5 subjects also had a re-treatment on the non-dominant eye of +1.00D to improve the uncorrected reading ability. The mean logMAR UDVA prior to re-treatment was 0.32 +/-0.09 (Snellen equivalent 6/13 +/-0.9 lines) and improved to 0 logMAR (6/6 Snellen equivalent) postoperatively. Correction of the distance myopic refraction did not reduce the near vision. Post re-treatment, all patients could read N5 binocularly. Monocular reading ability in the re-treated eyes was N5 in 60%, N8 in 20% and N12 in 20%.

Patient Functioning and Satisfaction

The CE Study reported that 100% of patients felt that they 'lived a life without glasses' at 6 months postoperatively and all would recommend the procedure to their friends. 96% could read newspaper print, mobile phone messages and menus and 78% could read package inserts of prescription medication. In the MPH Study, 93% reported that they were totally independent of reading glasses, 4% partly independent and 4% (1 subject) wholly dependent on reading glasses for near work at 6 months. This latter subject subsequently had successful enhancement. Good light is needed with 25% reporting difficulty reading in dim lighting conditions. Eighty two per cent of patients were satisfied with their distance vision and the dis-satisfied 18% underwent retreatment to successfully enhance the UDVA.

Discussion

The results of our first consecutive series of patients treated by SUPRACOR® presented in this chapter are promising. The SUPRACOR procedure certainly provides satisfactory near vision in phototopic reading conditions. Patients should be advised of the light dependency of the near vision. The main limitation of the procedure is a reduction in distance vision. A degree of compromise in distance vision is to be expected in all multifocal and presbyopia procedures. However, it is our opinion that the predictability of the procedure in terms of the refractive accuracy is not sufficient at present. The mean postoperative MRSE was close to the target of -0.50D in both our own study and in the CE Study. However, our patients were slightly more myopic and demonstrated a wider standard deviation than in the CE Study. Our patients continued to show a slight myopic shift from 3 to 6 months postoperatively and it is our impression that the refraction takes at least 6 months to stabilise.

We observed an overcorrection towards greater degrees of myopia than intended quite frequently with 27% of eyes more myopic than -1.0D at 6 months postoperatively. We found that enhancement could be readily performed, however, and successfully improved the distance vision without compromising the near vision, at least binocularly. A nomogram adjustment is required to improve the predictability of the primary procedure and reduce the enhancement rate. Following the results in our initial cohort of patients, we have adjusted our nomogram and now employ an asymmetrical approach targeting emmetropia in the dominant eye and -0.50D myopia in the non-dominant eye. Preliminary results would suggest that this is a better approach.

It could be argued that induced myopia was largely responsible for the reading ability seen in our patients. However, similar near vision was observed in eyes that were myopic and eyes that were emmetropic or hyperopic at 6 months - 78% of eyes with myopia of 0.50D or more and 77% of emmetropic/hyperopic eyes (MRSE $\geq$0) could read N8 or better. This indicates that the SUPRACOR® procedure does create a true multifocal effect on the cornea. All of our patients showed induction of negative spherical aberration on wavefront aberrometry analysis as intended by the treatment procedure thus aiding in the provision of pseudoaccommodation.

As regards safety, we did observe a relatively high rate of monocular loss of lines of CDVA. Binocular loss was much less. All patients did maintain monocular CDVA of at least 6/9.5. Preoperative CDVA of at least 6/7.5 in each eye is recommended. A substantially greater proportion of patients gained lines of CDVA in our study. The loss of lines of CDVA is a potential limitation of many presbyopia procedures. Similar and greater losses in CDVA have been reported in other corneal pseudoaccommodative techniques. Using a bi-aspheric ablation profile PresbyMAX® (SCHWIND eye-tech-solutions GmbH and Co. KG, Kleinostheim, Germany), Uthoff et al. found 15% monocular loss of $\geq$2 lines of CDVA and 13% binocular loss of $\geq$2 lines of CDVA at 6 months in the treatment of presbyopic hyperopes, emmetropes and myopes. [15] No hyperope gained a line of CDVA in that study. In a study of central presbyLASIK in presbyopic hyperopes, Alio et al. reported a loss of maximum 2 lines of CDVA in 28%. [9]

Some of the possible reasons proposed for reduced CDVA in pseudoaccommodative corneas include the reduced light striking the retina from any focal length reducing the contrast sensitivity, the pupil size reduction that occurs in the phototopic conditions used to test CDVA causing the hyperpositive central cornea to be utilised for distance vision and the need for adaptation to the multifocal cornea. In addition, we found that ocular surface dryness occurred commonly and may play a role in reducing CDVA. The routine placement of immediate postoperative punctal plugs for 3 to 6 months is now our preferred practice and has reduced the incidence of dry eye and improved CDVA in our patients. Centration of the treatment is also very important as decentred ablations causing unwanted aberrations could reduce CDVA.

Conclusion

SUPRACOR® can provide a high level of spectacle independence for distance and near vision. Careful patient selection for the procedure is vital. Managing patient expectation preoperatively is of paramount importance. Patients should be made aware that a degree of compromise in distance vision is to be expected and enhancement may be required. While a rapid improvement in near vision can be expected, distance vision improves more gradually and may take 6 months to stabilise. Occupational visual demands should be taken into consideration in preoperative assessment as patients with a high demand for excellent distance or near vision such HGV drivers, jewellers etc should be avoided. Further nomogram adjustment has the potential to improve the primary outcome.

Disclosure

The authors of this chapter have no financial or proprietary interest in any of the materials or methods mentioned.

References

[1] Sheppard, AL; Bashir, A; Wolffsohn, JS; Davies, LN. Accommodating intraocular lenses: a review of design concepts, usage and assessment methods. *Clin Exp Optom* 2010; 93: 441-52.

[2] Malecaze, FJ; Gazagne, CS; Tarroux, MC; Gorrand, JM. Scleral expansion bands for presbyopia. *Ophthalmology* 2001; 108: 2165-71.

[3] Cillino, S; Casuccio, A; Di Pace, F; Morreale, R; Pillitteri, F; Cillino, G , et al. One-year outcomes with new-generation multifocal intraocular lenses. *Ophthalmology* 2008; 115: 1508-16.

[4] Yilmaz, OF; Alagoz, N; Pekel, G; Azman, E; Aksoy, EF; Cakir, H , et al. Intracorneal inlay to correct presbyopia: Long-term results. *J Cataract Refract Surg* 2011; 37: 1275-81.

[5] Alio, JL; Amparo, F; Ortiz, D; Moreno, L. Corneal multifocality with excimer laser for presbyopia correction. *Curr Opin Ophthalmol* 2009; 20: 264-71.

[6] Menassa, N; Fitting, A; Auffarth, GU; Holzer, MP. Visual outcomes and corneal changes after intrastromal femtosecond laser correction of presbyopia. *J Cataract Refract Surg* 2012; 38: 765-73.

[7] Telandro, A. Pseudo-accommodative cornea: a new concept for correction of presbyopia. *J Refract Surg* 2004; 20: S714-7.

[8] Pinelli, R; Ortiz, D; Simonetto, A; Bacchi, C; Sala, E; Alio, JL. Correction of presbyopia in hyperopia with a center-distance, paracentral-near technique using the Technolas 217z platform. *J Refract Surg* 2008; 24: 494-500.

[9] Alio, JL; Chaubard, JJ; Caliz, A; Sala, E; Patel, S. Correction of presbyopia by technovision central multifocal LASIK (presbyLASIK). *J Refract Surg* 2006; 22: 453-60.

[10] El Danasoury, AM; Gamaly, TO; Hantera, M. Multizone LASIK with peripheral near zone for correction of presbyopia in myopic and hyperopic eyes: 1-year results. *J Refract Surg* 2009; 25: 296-305.

[11] Rocha, KM; Vabre, L; Chateau, N; Krueger, RR. Expanding depth of focus by modifying higher-order aberrations induced by an adaptive optics visual simulator. *J Cataract Refract Surg* 2009; 35: 1885-92.

[12] Lopez-Gil, N; Fernandez-Sanchez, V; Legras, R; Montes-Mico, R; Lara, F; Nguyen-Khoa, JL. Accommodation-related changes in monochromatic aberrations of the human eye as a function of age. *Invest Ophthalmol Vis Sci* 2008; 49: 1736-43.

[13] Ivanoff, A. On the influence of accommodation on spherical aberration in the human eye, an attempt to interpret night myopia. *J Opt Soc Am* 1947; 37: 730.

[14] Koomen, M; Tousey, R; Scolnik, R. The spherical aberration of the eye. *J Opt Soc Am* 1949; 39: 370-6.

[15] Uthoff, D; Polzl, M; Hepper, D; Holland, D. A new method of cornea modulation with excimer laser for simultaneous correction of presbyopia and ametropia. *Graefes Arch Clin Exp Ophthalmol* 2012;

In: Current Understanding and New Techniques … ISBN: 978-1-62808-748-2
Editor: Michael O'Keefe

Chapter 14

Corneal Inlays

Caroline Baily * ***and Michael O'Keefe*** ǂ
Mater Private Hospital, Dublin, Ireland

Abstract

There have been numerous surgical procedures performed for the treatment of presbyopia over the past decade. Many of these procedures have demonstrated unpredictable visual outcomes, regression and irreversibility, and hence have not gained general acceptance. In recent times, due to advances in femtosecond laser and availability of more biocompatible materials, we have seen a resurgence of interest in corneal inlays. The earliest stromal inlays, made of flint glass and plexiglass, were introduced in the 1940's but caused significant problems with stromal necrosis. Twenty years later, corneal inlays were manufactured using hydrogels, however, problems with biocompatibility and surgical difficulties still remained. These surgical issues have been solved in recent years with the introduction of newer more biocompatible hydrogels. There are currently three main categories of corneal inlays commercially available. This includes small-aperture inlays, space-occupying inlays and refractive-add inlays. Each category has a distinctly unique mode of action and hence, unique advantages and disadvantages.

Introduction

In recent times the focus of interest in refractive surgery has shifted towards the treatment of presbyopia. Many surgical methods have been proposed [1-7], however, no one procedure has emerged as having widespread acceptance due to the various disadvantages associated with presbyopic procedures including regression, limited effectiveness, irreversibility, expense and complications. Corneal implants or inlays have been available for decades, however, the earlier studies have reported numerous complications with corneal necrosis, vascularisation and nutrition. [8-16] Due to recent advances in laser technology and inlay

* Carolinebaily@yahoo.com
ǂ mokeefe@materprivate.ie

biomechanics, coupled with the growing demand for presbyopic procedures, we have seen a resurgence of interest in the use of corneal inlays.

The Evolution of Corneal Inlays

The concept of the corneal inlay has been around for decades. The continued drive to find a satisfactory presbyopic procedure coupled with advantages such as potential reversibility, ease of insertion, removal and repositioning, the ability to combine with other refractive procedures and the absence of complications from 'removing' tissue in conventional laser has kept the concept of keratophakia alive. Keratophakia involves the 'addition' of material which changes the shape of the cornea and may or may not include a refractive-add within the lens substance. There were significant challenges with early intrastromal inlays, [11, 16] however, the introduction of more advanced biocompatible materials and increasingly sophisticated laser systems have allowed significant development and maturation of the existing technology. [17-20]

Dr. José Ignacio Barraquer of Bogota, Colombia was the first to pioneer corneal inlays in 1949. [21] His early experiments tried two different approaches. The first approach involved the implantation of donor corneal tissue by shaping frozen tissue with a cryolathe. His later approach involved the use of synthetic corneal inlays made of flint glass and plexiglass. These inlays caused significant problems with oedema, vascularisation, anterior stromal necrosis, ulceration and extrusion. He concluded that corneal implants had to be chemically inactive and should not compromise the corneal circulation or apply excessive tension on the corneal tissue.

About 20 years later, in 1961, Knowles [8] pioneering the concept that a water-impermeable intrastromal implant interfered with the maintenance of normal corneal physiology by blocking the movement of water molecules, glucose and lactate and therefore contributing to the corneal thinning and ulceration that occurred in the tissue overlying a water-impermeable inlay. Thus, an inlay that would be sufficiently permeable to water, glucose and lactate molecules was deemed superior. The advent of hydrogels offered solutions to many of the concerns relating to transport within the cornea. Hydrogel is a network of polymer chains that are hydrophilic and highly absorbent, containing up to 99.9 % water. They also possess a degree of flexibility very similar to natural tissue due to the high water content.

Claes H. Dohlman [16] of Boston, USA, first described the use of a glyceryl methacrylate (GMA) hydrogel (88% water) within the stroma of rabbit and cat in 1967. Several problems existed with these initial inlays including stromal necrosis and deposition of opaque proteins on the lens surface. Mester et al. [22] investigated intrastromal implants made of hydroxyethylmethacrylate (HEMA), which are composed of 38 % water. There were no extrusions in rabbit corneas during the 18 month follow-up period. This led to interest surrounding corneal inlay thickness and shape. McCarey et al. [9] implanted the Permalens (Perfilcon-A) in rabbit eyes and concluded that the implant depth, the rigidity of the material, the hydrogel hydration in situ and the diameter of the implant needed to be better defined. Following on from this numerous studies carried out by Werblin et al. [14, 15] and McDonald et al. [10] continued to validate the use of hydrogels in corneal tissue.

Early inlays used in humans included the Kerato-Gel [12] (Allergan Medical Optics, Irvine, CA, USA) made from lidofilcon A, a hydrogel with an equilibrium water content of 68 % used for correction of aphakia. Reported limitations of the procedure included irregular microkeratome resections, loss of best-corrected visual acuity, and induced astigmatism. The Chiron inlay (Bausch and Lomb, Rochester, NY, USA) was a hydrogel meniscus lens with a power ranging from + 1.50 to + 3.50 diopters (D) used for treatment of presbyopia. The PermaVision intracorneal lens (Anamed, Lake Forest, CA, USA) was composed of a hydrogel, Nutrapore, with a water content of 78 %. This 5.0-5.5 mm diameter lens (30-60 μm thickness) was used to alter corneal curvature in the treatment of hyperopia. However, the reported refractive and surgical outcomes for this device were less than satisfactory. [23] This was followed by the IntraLens (ReVision Optics, Inc., Lake Forest, CA, USA) which similarly altered the corneal curvature. The technologies and principles applied in the PermaVision and IntraLens served as the precursor model for the Vue+ corneal inlay (formerly the PresbyLens, ReVision Optics, Inc.). The Microlens (BioVision AG, Brüggs, Switzerland) was the first annular-add inlay to be used. It had a diameter of 3 mm with a central thickness of 20 μm and a central opening to facilitate nutrient flow. This lens was renamed the InVue, the precursor to the ICOLENS (Neoptics AG, Hünenberg, Switzerland). The ICOLENS is similar to its precursor lens regarding the bifocal design; however it has the addition of several key advancements, including the specific pocket-cutting algorithm with the femtosecond laser (Femto LDV, Ziemer Ophthalmic Systems, Port, Switzerland), the unique preloaded deployment device and the development of the custom-designed surgical instruments; the “Opener” and “Repositioner”. The Flexivue (Presbia, Amsterdam, Netherlands) is also an annular-add corneal inlay with similar properties to the ICOLENS.

Corneal Physiology and Inlays

In order to ensure the integrity of the cornea is maintained following inlay implantation it is important to respect the unique and complex physiology of corneal tissue. The first aim is to facilitate the transfer of nutrients via diffusion across an avascular structure. Larreau et al[24] found that when the lens was placed at 3/4 of the corneal thickness, the influence of the inlay diffusivity was smaller than at more anterior or posterior placements. The diffusivity of the inlay affects the way nutrients will be transported through the cornea. Glucose transport is affected to a greater degree than oxygen as the latter can diffuse through the anterior and posterior surfaces of the cornea. The second aim of inlay implantation is to ensure that oxygen from the tear film and glucose from the aqueous humour can pass via the inlay to the keratocytes. Thus, the inlay must be semi-permeable. The third aim is to ensure that the organisation of the corneal structure is not disrupted as this is a major factor in corneal transparency. Keratocytes are specialised fibroblasts that play a key role in stromal remodeling, healing and transparency by producing and maintaining the extracellular matrix of the corneal stroma. It is possibly that an intrastromal implant might potentially affect the precisely orchestrated functioning of the keratocytes resulting in changes that could alter corneal transparency. [13, 25-27]

Categories of Corneal Inlays

The three main categories of corneal inlay currently available are outlined in Table 1.

Table 1. Categories of corneal inlays

Category	Inlay	Mechanism of action	Manufacturer
Refractive-add inlay	ICOLENS	Bifocal lens	Neoptics AG
	Invue Lens	Bifocal lens	Biovision AG (acquired by Neoptics AG)
	Flexivue Micro-Lens	Bifocal lens	Presbia Coöperatief U.A.
Small-aperture inlay	KAMRA (Acufocus)	Pinhole effect	AcuFocus Inc.
Space-occupying inlay	Vue+	Central corneal steepening	ReVision Optics Inc.

1. KAMRA Inlay (AcuFocus)

Mechanism of Action

This corneal inlay was designed to increase the depth of field based on the principle of small-aperture optics with the goal of improving uncorrected near and intermediate vision without markedly affecting distance vision.

Physical Properties

The sixth generation KAMRA inlay (ACI-7000 PDT) is a microperforated artificial aperture with a 3.8 mm outer diameter and 1.6 mm inner diameter and a thickness of 5 μm (Figure 1 and 2). The inlay is composed of polyvinylidene fluoride (PVDF) and carbon. Carbon black is incorporated to make it opaque. It has 8400 laser-drilled holes (diameter 5 to 11μm) which are arranged in a pseudorandomised pattern to allow sufficient nutritional flow through the inlay. The holes allow unwanted additional light to pass through the inlay such that the average light transmission through the annulus of the lens is 5 %.[18] The prior generation KAMRA inlay (ACI-7000) had 1600 mircroperforations and was 10 μm thick.

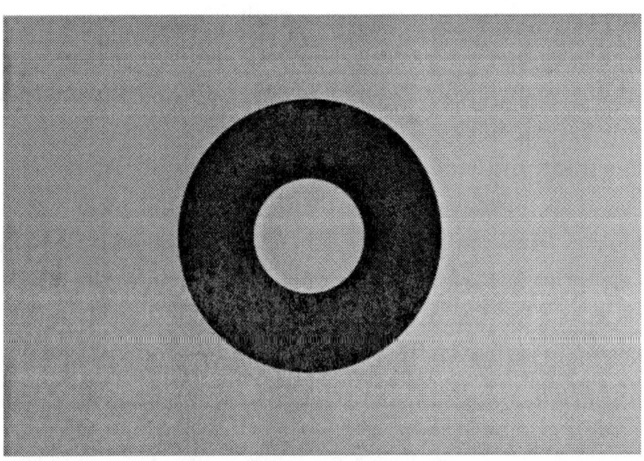

Figure 1. The KAMRA inlay.

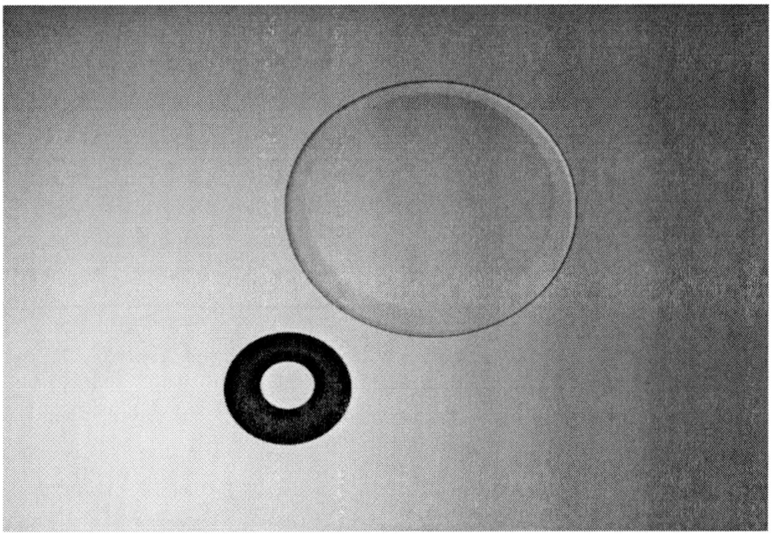

Figure 2. The KAMRA inlay compared for size against a regular soft contact lens.

Patient Selection

Those suitable include emmetropic, ammetropic, or post-LASIK presbyopes aged between 45 to 60 years old. They should have an uncorrected near visual acuity (UNVA) of 20/40 or worse and a best corrected distance acuity (CDVA) of at least 20/20 in both eyes. Additional criteria include a minimum central corneal thickness (CCT) of 500 μm, and a minimum endothelial cell count (ECC) of 2000 cells/mm^2 with a corneal power between 41.00 and 47.00 D in all meridians. Exclusion criteria include latent hyperopia (defined as a difference of $\geq$ 1.00 D between the manifest and cycloplegic refraction), previous ocular surgery (other than PRK or LASIK), anterior or posterior segment pathology, patients taking systemic medications with significant ocular side-effects and immunosuppressive disorders. [18]

Surgical Technique

The KAMRA corneal inlay is centered on the line of sight in the non-dominant eye following creation of a corneal flap or pocket using a femtosecond laser. The line of sight is identified by marking the centre of the cornea with a marker using the first Purkinje reflex with the patient fixating on the microscope or excimer laser fixation light. In patients with a large angle kappa, the inlay will be positioned between the pupil centre and first Purkinje reflex. Seyeddain et al. [28] described implantation of the ACI-7000 through a superior-hinged flap in the non-dominant eye created using a 60 kHz femtosecond laser (Intralase, Abbott Medical Optics, Inc.) while Yilmaz et al. [20] reported implantation of the ACI-7000 through a superior-hinged lamellar flap using a Schwind-Carriazo pendular mechanical microkeratome with a 170 mm cutting head. Dexl et al. [18] reported implantation of the KAMRA (ACI-7000 PDT) through a temporal pocket using both Intralase (60 kHz and 150 kHz laser systems) and Femto LDV (Ziemer Ophthalmic Systems AG) femtosecond laser systems. The inlay is positioned either in the lamellar pocket or on the stromal bed using specific forceps. Centration is rechecked at the end of the procedure with the patient fixating on the microscope light.

Refractive Outcomes

Dexl et al. [18] reported implantation of the current generation KAMRA corneal inlay (ACI 7000 PDT) in 24 eyes. At 12 months, they found 92% of patients to be reading Jaeger (J) 3 or better with a mean uncorrected near visual acuity (UNVA) of J2 in their inlay eye. Mean uncorrected intermediate visual acuity (UIVA) in the inlay eye was 20/25 at 12 months, a statistically significant improvement from pre-op. Mean distance visual acuity (UDVA) was 20/20 in the surgical eye and 20/16 binocularly. All patients maintained binocular CDVA of 20/16 or better throughout the follow-up period. Patients also reported statistically significant improvements in near and intermediate task performance and no reduction in ability to perform distance related tasks, including driving at night. No inlay was removed or recentered. Seyeddain et al. [27] described implantation of the prior generation inlay (ACI-7000) in 32 patients. In this report, they described mean UNVA improved from J7/8 at pre-op to J2 at 1 month and reached J1 at 3 years with 97% of eyes having UNVA of J3 or better. Mean UDVA was 20/20 with all eyes achieving 20/32 or better at three years. Nine eyes (28.3%) lost one line of CDVA in the inlay eye, however no patients lost a line of binocular CDVA. No inlay was removed. Yilmaz et al. [20] published four year results of the prior generation inlay (ACI-7000) in 39 patients. All patients (n = 22) had two or more lines of improvement in UNVA with no compromise in distance acuity. The mean final UNVA was 20/20 with 96% reading J1or better with an UDVA of 20/40 or better in all eyes. Four inlays were removed during the study (one due to a button-hole flap, two due to refractive shift and one due to a thin flap of 58 μm). The published data suggests that this small-aperture inlay demonstrates excellent UNVA results with little compromise in UDVA or CDVA.

2. ICOLENS

Mechanism of Action

The ICOLENS is a bifocal design with a central zone for distance and peripheral positive refractive zone for near. There are three options of near add; + 1.25 D, + 1.75 D, + 2.25 D and three options of distance correction; SE 0.0 D, SE 0.5 D, SE 1.0 D, therefore, the pairing of near add and distance will give you nine different lens types.

Physical Properties

The ICOLENS has a diameter of 3 mm with an edge thickness of 15 μm with a central hole measuring 150μm to facilitate nutrient flow (Figure 3). It is a copolymer of HEMA (2-hydroxyethyl methacrylate) and MMA (methyl methacrylate) which have hydrogel properties.

Patient Selection

Those suitable for inlay implantation include subjects aged between 45 to 65 years of age with an uncorrected near visual acuity UNVA of ≤ 20/50 and UDVA ≥ 20/30. They should have a corrected near visual acuity (CNVA) and CDVA ≥ 20/20 with a SE refraction for distance ranging between -0.25 and + 1.00 D with no more than ± 1.00 D of astigmatism. All subjects should be wearing full-time reading glasses for near visual tasks for a minimum of one year and have clearly determined ocular dominance (Dolman and Porta method). Pupils should be round and central with a diameter of ≤ 4.5 mm measured at "mesopic high" on the Procyon pupillometer (Procyon Instruments Ltd, London, UK) in the non-dominant eye. All subjects should have a CCT of > 500 µm and ECC density of > 2000 cells/mm^{2}. Exclusion criteria includes dry eye syndrome, any previous corneal surgery that may interfere with pocket creation, any acute or chronic ocular disease, any medication that could interfere with ordinary healing process or any inability to comply with the follow-up regime. (Baily et al., ongoing pilot study at Mater Private Hospital Dublin Ireland, unpublished data)

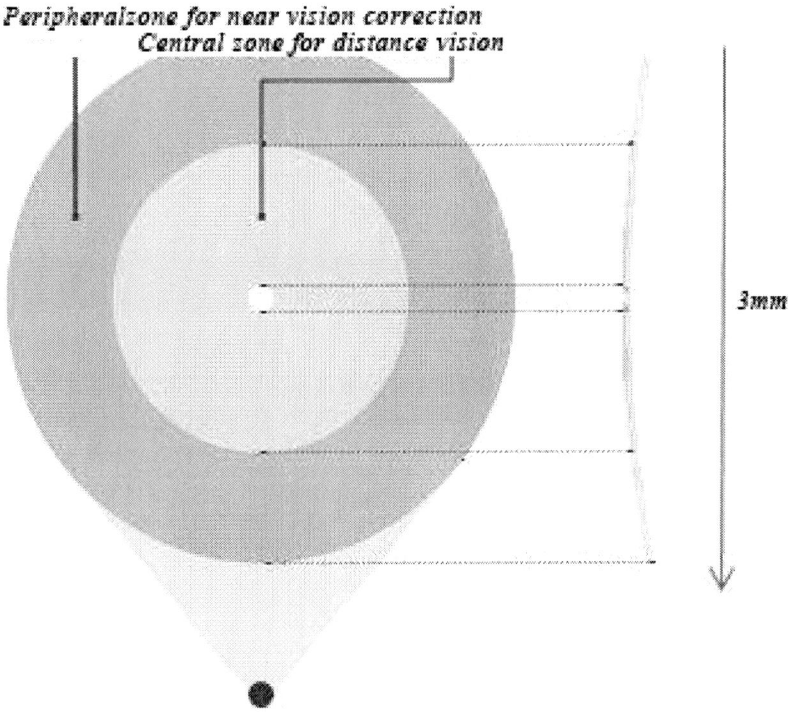

Figure 3. The ICOLENS corneal inlay.

Surgical Technique

The preparation and draping regimens are similar to those used for any patient undergoing a laser refractive procedure. The ICOLENS is inserted through either a temporal or superior corneal pocket (Figure 4) created using the Femto LDV laser system (Ziemer Ophthalmic Systems, Port, Switzerland). The inlay is positioned over the line of sight which is identified by placing the patient under a surgical microscope and asking the patient to fixate on the fixation light. A surgical marker is then used to highlight the center of the entrance pupil. The pocket is then created with the Femto LDV following selection of the appropriate suction ring size and corneal pocket depth. The choice of pocket depth is determined by the central corneal thickness. The preloaded device (Figure 5 and 6) is then inserted smoothly into the corneal pocket until the hole located on the leaves is centric to the mark on the cornea. Once correctly positioned the leaves of the preloaded unit are pulled back releasing the ICOLENS and the preloaded unit is then gently removed from the pocket by pulling the handle backwards. If the lens is slightly off position the repositioning instrument

"Repositioner" can be inserted into the pocket and used to move the lens by applying gentle pressure to the inferior lens surface. Positioning is checked at the end of the procedure (Figure 7).

(Baily et al., ongoing pilot study at Mater Private Hospital Dublin Ireland, unpublished data).

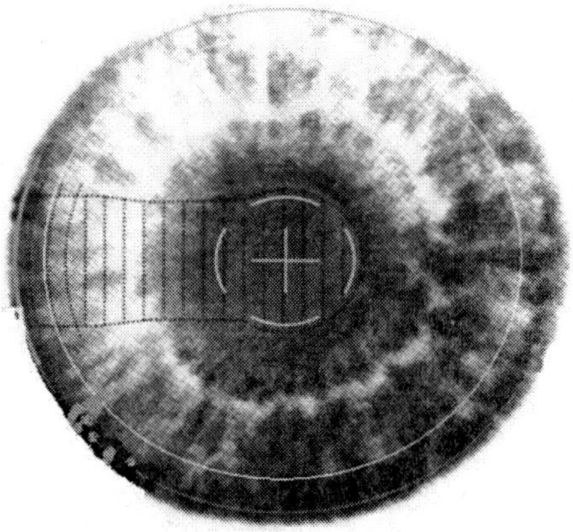

Figure 4. The ICOLENS pocket created using femtosecond laser with an estimated diameter of 3.4mm and depth of 300μm.

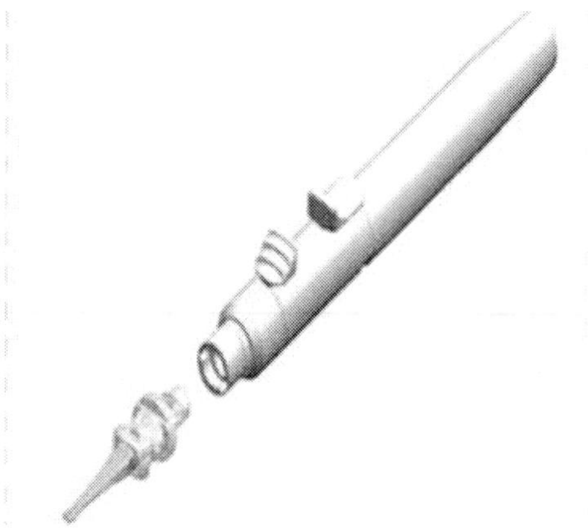

Figure 5. The reusable deployment handle of the ICOLENS system attaches to the sterile preloaded tip containing the inlay.

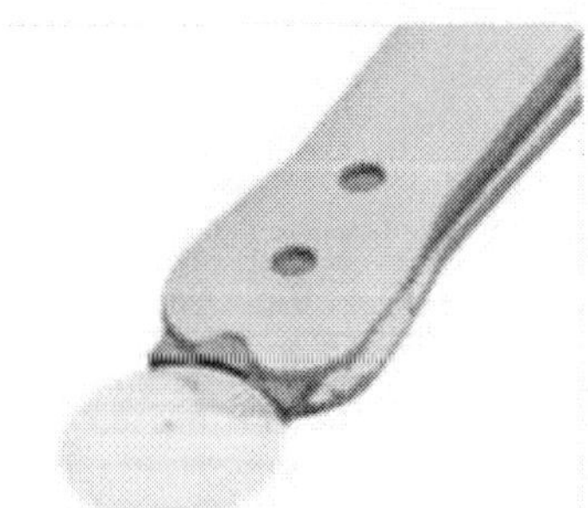

Figure 6. The sterile preloaded device containing the ICOLENS inlay.

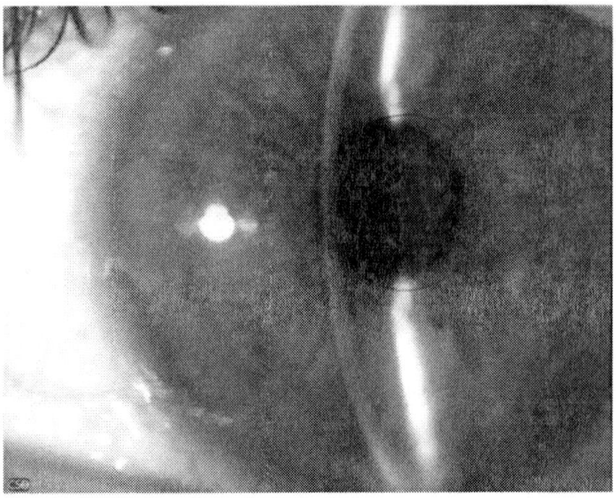

Figure 7. The ICOLENS positioned centrally within the corneal pocket.

Refractive Outcomes

In a series of 52 patients performed as a part of a pilot study in the Mater Private Hospital Dublin (Baily et al., unpublished data), the mean UNVA in the surgical eye improved preoperatively from N18/N24 to N8 postoperatively ($p = 0.000$). There was a mean ± SD loss of 1.69 ± 2.04 lines of UDVA ($p = 0.000$) in the surgical eye and a mean ± SD gain of 0.56 ± 1.01 lines of vision binocularly ($p = 0.000$). There were 11 implants explanted due to minimal or no improvement in UNVA. There were no significant adverse events reported during the study.

3. Flexivue Micro-Lens

Mechanism of Action

The Flexivue lens has similar mechanism of action and physical properties to the ICOLENS.

Surgical Technique

Limnopoulou et al. [19] describe implantation of this inlay, centered on the line of sight, inside a corneal pocket created in the patient's nondominant eye, using a femtosecond laser.

Refractive Outcomes

At 12 months follow-up they reported UNVA of 20/32 or better in 75% of operated eyes with mean UDVA statistically significantly decreased from 20/20 preoperatively to 20/50 postoperatively. Mean binocular UDVA was not significantly altered. A total of 17 patients lost one line of CDVA and no patients lost 2 lines of CDVA in the operated eye. No intra- or postoperative complications occurred throughout the study. [19]

4. Invue Lens

Mechanism of Action

The Invue Lens is the precursor lens to the ICOLENS and therefore has similar mechanism of action and physical properties. [17]

Patient Selection

Those suitable for inlay implantation include those aged between 45 and 60 years of age with and UNVA of ≤ 20/50 and UDVA of ≥ 20/30. They should have a CNVA and CDVA ≥ 20/20 with a SE refraction for distance ranging between - 0.75 and + 0.75 D with no more than ± 1.00 D of astigmatism. They should be in reading glasses for a minimum of one year and have a CCT of > 500 μm and ECC density of > 2000 cells/mm^2. [17]

Surgical Technique

The Invue Lens is inserted through a temperonasal pocket using a mechanical microkeratome (Visitome 20-10 Microkeratome, Biovision AG, Brüggs, Switzerland). The line of sight is identified and marked using the excimer laser centration device (Allegretto 400 Hz laser; WaveLight Laser Technologie AG, Erlangen, Germany). The peripheral cornea is marked using a radial peripheral marker using the marked line of sight as the center point. The suction ring in then applied on the cornea aligned with the radial marks. Following vacuum build-up the 1.2 mm blade creates a pocket with a 3.5 mm diameter set at approximately 3/5 of the corneal depth. The inlay is then inserted using an inserting device. [17]

Refractive Outcomes

Bouzoukis et al. [17] at 12 months post-implantation reported UNVA of 20/32 or better in 98 % of surgical eyes and UDVA of 20/40 or better in 93% of surgical eyes. They described an UDVA of 20/25 or better in all patients binocularly. Three patients lost one line of CDVA in the surgical eye but the inlay was not removed as they were satisfied with their binocular near and distance vision. There were no complications reported during the 12 month follow-up period.

5. Vue+

Mechanism of Action

The inlay adds a microscopic change in curvature in the range of 2 to 3 mm to the centre of the cornea, creating a multifocal cornea and therefore facilitating near and intermediate focusing ability.

Physical Properties

The lens has a diameter of 2 mm and a thickness of about 150 μm. It is made of a soft malleable micro-porous hydrogel material (Figure 8).

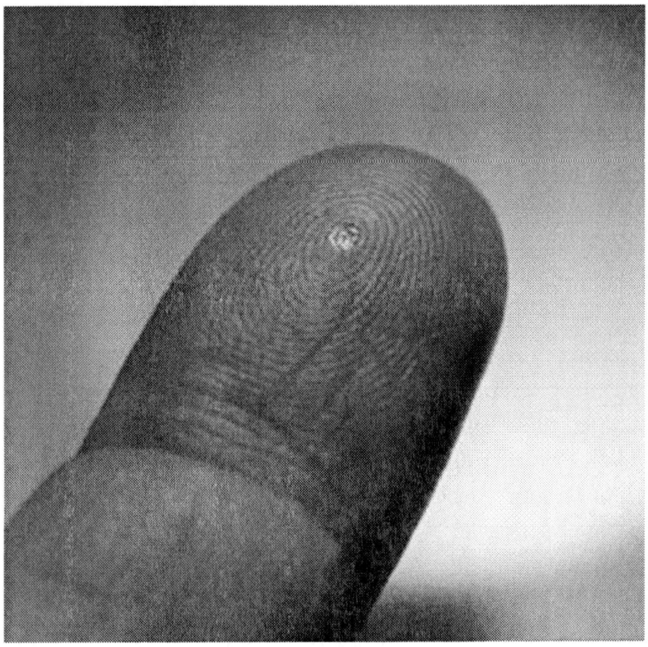

Figure 8. The relative size of the Vue+ Inlay.

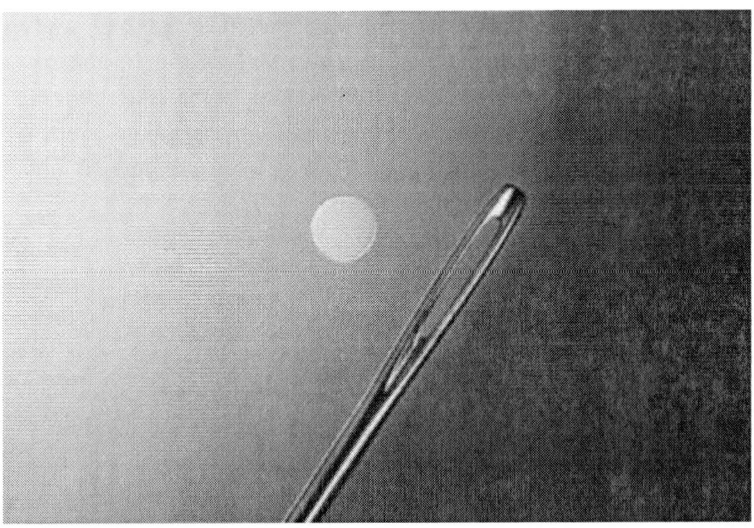

Figure 9. The Vue+ inserting device.

Surgical Technique

The Vue+ in placed on the cornea through an open LASIK flap with care taken during placement using to avoid wrinkling (Figure 9).

Refractive Outcomes

There is no published data available on the Vue +.

The Downside to Inlay Technology

Even the most advanced technology has its negatives and intrastomal corneal inlays are no exception. The insertion of a corneal inlay does not offer the perfect solution to presbyopia as only one eye is corrected. It is essential to ensure patient expectations are managed appropriately pre-operatively. Reading vision may still be problematic in dim light, when reading for a prolonged period of time or if the print is very small. The majority of patients will become independent but not completely free of glasses for near vision. Therefore inlays may be unsuitable for poorly motivated individuals or those with unrealistic expectations.

Additionally, certain patients may take longer to adapt to their post-inlay vision due to an element of presumed 'neuroadaption'. It is also possible that they may never 'adapt', and they will have an unexplained unsatisfactory outcome. This may be due to ambiguous dominance at the outset and, hence, ensuring clear ocular dominance is a key inclusion criteria.

Another important factor is centration. This is critical to the effective functioning of the inlay and is essential in ensuring an optimum outcome. The KAMRA has recently introduced an electronic alignment system, the AcuTarget System (AcuFocus Inc.) which effectively deals with this issue.

There have been some concerns with the KAMRA inlay regarding the cosmesis of this implant in pale irides and fundal examination in those requiring regular retinal assessments. However, Seyeddain et al. [28] found that the thin aperture did not prevent fundal examination with a wide-field lens and despite the fact that the ring was visible during Goldmann fundoscopy they explained that small movements of the 3-mirror contact glass the shadow of the inlay moved enough for sufficient inspection of the entire retina.

Going forward it will be important to determine if corneal inlays are truly 'reversible' with no alteration to the pre-operative refraction or if they are just 'removable'. Further studies will need to determine this key point.

Future

Corneal inlays will continue to evolve as to does the technology. More sophisticated laser systems will ensure smoother wound planes and more rapid healing. Electronic alignment systems will improve centration and more advanced intraoperative inlay delivery systems will aim to simplify the surgical procedure and reduce the surgical learning curve. It is also possible that preoperative contact lenses may be introduced to assist in identifying those patients who may experience neuroadaptation issues post-implantation.

Conclusion

Corneal inlays are emerging as an effective option for the successful treatment of presbyopia in emmetropic and ammetropic patients. They offer the unique advantage of removability and exchangeability and only require a monocular refractive procedure. It is important, however, to highlight the paucity of long-term follow-up data surrounding these devices which is essential in ultimately appraising their safety and value to the aging population.

References

[1] Alio Jl, Chaubard Jj, Caliz A, Sala E, Patel S. Correction Of Presbyopia By Technovision Central Multifocal Lasik (Presbylasik). *J Refract Surg* 2006;22:453-460.

[2] Iida Y, Shimizu K, Ito M. Pseudophakic Monovision Using Monofocal And Multifocal Intraocular Lenses: Hybrid Monovision. *J Cataract Refract Surg* 2011;37:2001-2005.

[3] Klaproth Ok, Titke C, Baumeister M, Kohnen T. [Accommodative Intraocular Lenses--Principles Of Clinical Evaluation And Current Results]. *Klin Monbl Augenheilkd* 2011;228:666-675.

[4] Menassa N, Fitting A, Auffarth Gu, Holzer Mp. Visual Outcomes And Corneal Changes After Intrastromal Femtosecond Laser Correction Of Presbyopia. *J Cataract Refract Surg* 2012;38:765-773.

[5] Qazi Ma, Pepose Js, Shuster Jj. Implantation Of Scleral Expansion Band Segments For The Treatment Of Presbyopia. *Am J Ophthalmol* 2002;134:808-815.

[6] Reilly Cd, Lee Wb, Alvarenga L, Caspar J, Garcia-Ferrer F, Mannis Mj. Surgical Monovision And Monovision Reversal In Lasik. *Cornea* 2006;25:136-138.

[7] Tomita M, Watabe M, Ito M, Tsuru T. Conductive Keratoplasty For The Treatment Of Presbyopia: Comparative Study Between Post- And Non-Lasik Eyes. *Clin Ophthalmol* 2011;5:231-237.

[8] Knowles Wf. Effect Of Intralamellar Plastic Membranes On Corneal Physiology. *Am J Ophthalmol* 1961;51:1146-1156.

[9] Mccarey Be, Andrews Dm. Refractive Keratoplasty With Intrastromal Hydrogel Lenticular Implants. *Invest Ophthalmol Vis Sci* 1981;21:107-115.

[10] Mcdonald Mb, Mccarey Be, Storie B Et Al. Assessment Of The Long-Term Corneal Response To Hydrogel Intrastromal Lenses Implanted In Monkey Eyes For Up To Five Years. *J Cataract Refract Surg* 1993;19:213-222.

[11] Mester U, Roth K, Dardenne U. [Trial With 2-Hydroxy-Ethyl-Methacrylate Lenses As Keratophakia Material]. *Ber Zusammenkunft Dtsch Ophthalmol Ges* 1974;72:326-329.

[12] Steinert Rf, Storie B, Smith P Et Al. Hydrogel Intracorneal Lenses In Aphakic Eyes. *Arch Ophthalmol* 1996;114:135-141.

[13] Sweeney Df, Vannas A, Hughes Tc Et Al. Synthetic Corneal Inlays. *Clin Exp Optom* 2008;91:56-66.

[14] Werblin Tp, Patel As, Barraquer Ji. Initial Human Experience With Permalens Myopic Hydrogel Intracorneal Lens Implants. *Refract Corneal Surg* 1992;8:23-26.

[15] Werblin Tp, Peiffer Rl, Binder Ps, Mccarey Be, Patel As. Eight Years Experience With Permalens Intracorneal Lenses In Nonhuman Primates. *Refract Corneal Surg* 1992;8:12-22.

[16] Dohlman Ch, Refojo Mf, Rose J. Synthetic Polymers In Corneal Surgery. I. Glyceryl Methacrylate. *Arch Ophthalmol* 1967;77:252-257.

[17] Bouzoukis Di, Kymionis Gd, Panagopoulou Si Et Al. Visual Outcomes And Safety Of A Small Diameter Intrastromal Refractive Inlay For The Corneal Compensation Of Presbyopia. *J Refract Surg* 2012;28:168-173.

[18] Dexl Ak, Seyeddain O, Riha W Et Al. One-Year Visual Outcomes And Patient Satisfaction After Surgical Correction Of Presbyopia With An Intracorneal Inlay Of A New Design. *J Cataract Refract Surg* 2012;38:262-269.

[19] Limnopoulou An, Bouzoukis Di, Kymionis Gd Et Al. Visual Outcomes And Safety Of A Refractive Corneal Inlay For Presbyopia Using Femtosecond Laser. *J Refract Surg* 2013;29:12-19.

[20] Yilmaz Of, Alagoz N, Pekel G Et Al. Intracorneal Inlay To Correct Presbyopia: Long-Term Results. *J Cataract Refract Surg* 2011;37:1275-1281.

[21] Barraquer Ji. Queratoplatica Refractiva. *Estudies E Informaciones Oftalmoloqiaces* 1949;2:10.

[22] Mester U, Roth K, Dardenne Mu. Versvche Mit 2-Hydroxyaethylmethcrylatlinsen Als Kerotophakiematerial. *Ber Ophthalmol Ger* 1972;72:326.

[23] Verity Sm, Mcculley Jp, Bowman Rw, Cavanagh Hd, Petroll Wm. Outcomes Of Permavision Intracorneal Implants For The Correction Of Hyperopia. *Am J Ophthalmol* 2009;147:973-977.

[24] Larrea X, De Court, Feingold V, Burger J, Buchler P. Oxygen And Glucose Distribution After Intracorneal Lens Implantation. *Optom Vis Sci* 2007;84:1074-1081.

[25] Boote C, Dennis S, Newton Rh, Puri H, Meek Km. Collagen Fibrils Appear More Closely Packed In The Prepupillary Cornea: Optical And Biomechanical Implications. *Invest Ophthalmol Vis Sci* 2003;44:2941-2948.

[26] Conrad Gw, Funderburgh Jl. Eye Development And The Appearance And Maintenance Of Corneal Transparency. *Trans Kans Acad Sci* 1992;95:34-38.

[27] Maurice Dm. The Transparency Of The Corneal Stroma. *Vision Res* 1970;10:107-108.

[28] Seyeddain O, Hohensinn M, Riha W Et Al. Small-Aperture Corneal Inlay For The Correction Of Presbyopia: 3-Year Follow-Up. *J Cataract Refract Surg* 2012;38:35-45.

In: Current Understanding and New Techniques ... ISBN: 978-1-62808-748-2
Editor: Michael O'Keefe

Chapter 15

Management of Keratoconus

Edward Loane*[*] and William J. Power
Royal Victoria Eye and Ear Hospital, Dublin, Ireland

Abstract

Keratoconus is a non-inflammatory corneal ectasia that causes progressive corneal thinning and steepening, resulting in variable progressive visual impairment and reduced visual quality, due to progressive myopia and irregular astigmatism. It is usually bilateral and affects about 1 in 2000 younger individuals of both sexes and all ethnicities. The precise aetiology of keratoconus is unknown. Classification of keratoconus may be based on morphologic findings, topographic or index-based findings, and the Amsler-Krumeich classification. Classifying the severity of the disease guides appropriate, individualised management strategies for each patient. Management is centred around: (1) treating any associated atopic disease, (2) establishing whether or not the disease is progressing and treating this with corneal collagen cross-linking, if appropriate, and (3) visual rehabilitation, with any combination of spectacle or contact lens correction, implantation of intra-corneal ring segments, implantation of phakic intraocular lenses, refractive laser surgery, keratoplasty (penetrating or deep anterior lamellar).

Introduction

Keratoconus is a non-inflammatory corneal ectasia that results in progressive corneal thinning and steepening, with the cornea typically assuming a conical shape. This results in progressive myopia and irregular astigmatism, with variable progressive visual impairment and reduced visual quality. [1] It is usually a bilateral condition, although it may be asymmetrical, [2; 3] and if acute corneal hydrops occurs, it may result in corneal scarring.

Keratoconus affects approximately 1 in 2000 individuals in the general population. [4] It affects males and females equally and usually presents in the mid to late teens and early

[*] edwardloane@yahoo.com

twenties. Keratoconus tends to be progressive until the early thirties, when it often stabilises, but it may progress at any age. [2] It occurs in all ethnic groups. [1; 4; 5]

The precise aetiology of this condition is unknown, but it is believed to be related to genetic, biochemical and environmental influences, in particular eye rubbing.[6-8] Increased proteinase enzyme activity coupled with reduced activity of proteinase inhibitors results in stromal protein digestion and biomechanical instability of the cornea.[9; 10] Keratoconus is more common in individuals with underlying atopic disease (allergic eye disease, hay fever, eczema, asthma) and it is certainly more common in people with Down syndrome (the incidence may be as high as 1 in 20 in this group), who tend to rub their eyes vigorously. [5; 11] It is also associated with connective tissue disorders such as Ehlers-Danlos syndrome, osteogenesis imperfecta and joint hypermobility. [12-14]

Classification of Keratoconus

Classifying keratoconus is important because the severity of the disease at the time of diagnosis will affect the individual management approach and the results achievable for each patient. There are several classification systems for keratoconus based on morphologic findings, topographic or index-based findings, and the Amsler-Krumeich classification. [15; 16]

Morphologic Classification

There are three cone patterns in keratoconus:

1. *Nipple cone*: diameter of the cone is ≤ 5mm, it is round in shape and is usually inferonasally located.
2. *Oval cone*: diameter of the cone is > 5mm, it is ellipsoid in shape and is usually inferotemporally located.
3. *Globus cone*: the cone is generalized, located throughout 75% of the cornea.

Topographic Classification

Keratoconus can be classified topographically according to the elevation maps, the corneal thickness map or the curvature maps. Corneal topography enables detection of different patterns of keratoconus. Keratoconus is diagnosed or at least suspected, based on the detection of typical patterns characterizing irregularity, in combination with more than one of a number of topographic criteria. [15]

Topographic patterns characterizing irregularity on the anterior curvature map:

1. Central or paracentral round steepening
2. Central oval steepening
3. Superior steepening

4. Inferior steepening
5. Generalized irregular curvature
6. Symmetric bow tie
7. Symmetric bow tie with a skewed steepest radial axis
8. Asymmetric bow tie with inferior steepening
9. Asymmetric bow tie with superior steepening
10. Asymmetric bow tie with a skewed steepest radial axis
11. Butterfly pattern
12. Claw pattern
13. Junctional pattern

Topographic criteria for diagnosing keratoconus:
Features on the saggital curvature map:

1. Steep K reading > 48 dioptres (D)
2. Maximum K > steep K by > 1D
3. Skewed steepest radial axis > 22°
4. Superior-inferior difference on the 5mm circle > 2.5D
5. Inferior-superior difference on the 5mm circle > 1.5D
6. Corneal astigmatism on either surface > 6D
7. Against the rule astigmatism is suspicious for keratoconus

Features on the thickness map:

1. Cone or bell shape
2. Superior-inferior difference at the 5mm circle > 30μm
3. Thinnest location < 470μm
4. Thickness at pachymetry apex minus the thickness at the thinnest location > 10μm
5. Y-coordinate value at the thinnest location > 500μm
6. Difference in thickness between both eyes at the thinnest location > 30μm

Features on the elevation maps:

1. Isolated island or tongue-like extension on either surface on the best-fit sphere mode
2. Values > 12μm within the central 5mm zone on the anterior elevation map on the best-fit toric ellipsoid mode
3. Values > 17μm within the central 5mm zone on the posterior elevation map on the best-fit toric ellipsoid mode

A further refinement of the Amsler-Krumeich classification of keratoconus has been suggested by Alió et al. that would take account of the root mean square of coma-like aberrations. [17]

Amsler-Krumeich Classification

Stage	Mean central K	Minimum corneal thickness	Myopia and/or astigmatism	Central corneal clarity
I	< 48D	> 500μm	< 5D	No scarring
II	48-53D	400-500μm	5-8D	No scarring
III	53-55D	300-400μm	8-10D	No scarring
IV	> 55D	< 300μm	Not measurable	Scarring

Patient Assessment

Once the diagnosis of keratoconus has been made, the patient must be evaluated according to certain parameters so that they can be appropriately managed. The parameters that must be considered include the following: patient's age, sex, progression, contact lens tolerance, refractive error and visual acuity, corneal transparency, corneal thickness, K max. [15]

Age

Younger patients have a much greater probability of having progressive disease. Younger patients exhibit a greater response to treatment by virtue of the fact that their corneas are more elastic than older patients. There is a greater risk of complications with corneal collagen cross linking (CXL) in patients older than 35 years of age. [18]

Sex

Oestrogen is a stimulus for progression of keratoconus, which may be seen in pregnancy. [19] As a result, CXL may need to be repeated following pregnancy.

Progression

Progression of keratoconus usually occurs before the age of 30 years old, and is less common thereafter, although it may progress at any age. [1; 4] Progression is defined as an increase in K max of > 1D, or corneal thinning by > 30μm at the thinnest location, or an increase in corneal astigmatism by > 1D within a six month interval. [15] Therefore, patients younger than 30 years of age should be monitored at six-monthly intervals to screen for progression. If progression is detected, CXL should be performed, if appropriate.

Contact Lens Tolerance

It is important to establish contact lens (CL) tolerance, as this is traditionally a mainstay of management of non-progressive keratoconus. It must be borne in mind that rigid gas permeable (RGP) CL wear should be stopped for a minimum of two weeks prior to evaluation of keratoconus in order to correctly assess corneal topography.

Refractive Error and Visual Acuity

The refractive error and the discrepancy between the uncorrected visual acuity (UCVA) and the best spectacle corrected visual acuity (BSCVA) should be assessed and may guide management. The higher the refractive error, the more likely it is that keratoplasty will be required for visual rehabilitation.

Corneal Transparency

Central corneal scarring will generally result from previous acute hydrops and in such cases is an indication for keratoplasty. A clear cornea with significant Vogt's striae is suggestive of advanced disease and in such cases keratoplasty may well be the best management option.

Corneal Thickness

The thinner the cornea, the more advanced the disease is. Furthermore, CXL should only be performed in corneas with a preoperative thickness of at least 400μm at the thinnest location. Implantation of intra-corneal ring segments (ICRS) also requires at least 400μm of corneal tissue at the site of implantation of the ICRS. [20]

K Max

The K max is a key variable in diagnosing and determining the stage of keratoconus, as well as the likelihood of progression. Furthermore, K readings > 58D are associated with a higher risk of complications following CXL, and poorer outcomes with ICRS implantation. [18; 21]

Management

Management of keratoconus varies according to the severity of the disease and whether or not it is progressive. In assessing the patient with keratoconus, it is essential to determine both of these issues. Since keratoconus may be associated with atopy, it is important to actively discourage eye rubbing and to treat any underlying allergic eye disease in the first instance. [6] Management may then consist of non-surgical and surgical interventions, which should be aimed at firstly stabilising the progression of keratoconus if it is progressive and, secondly, visual rehabilitation. Management strategies may include any combination of the following: spectacle correction, CLs, CXL, ICRS, phakic intra-ocular lens (pIOL) implantation, refractive laser surgery, and keratoplasty (lamellar or penetrating) [Figure 1]. Each of these treatment modalities will be discussed in turn.

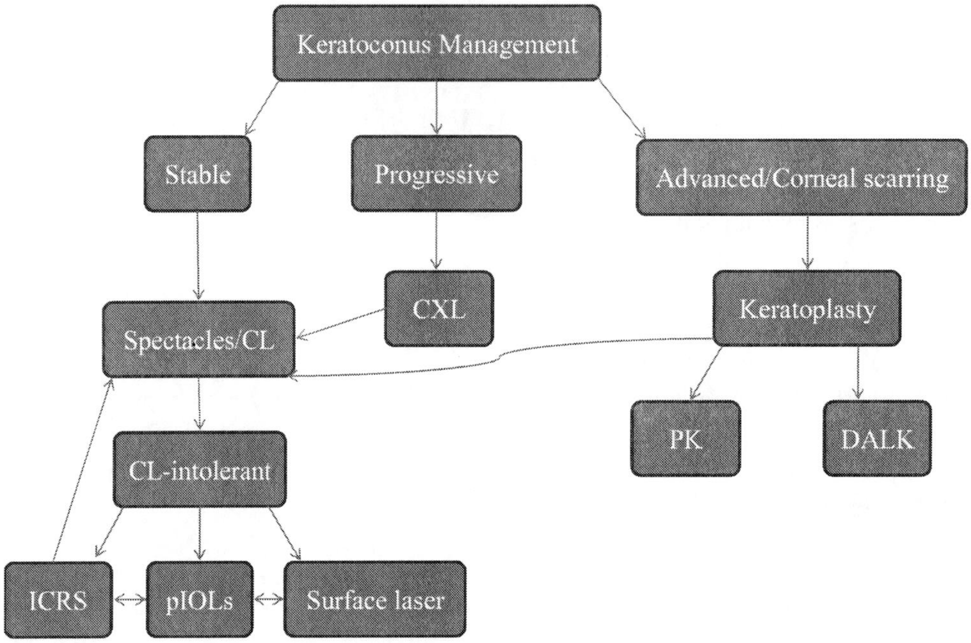

Figure 1. Summary management of keratoconus.

Spectacle Correction

Early to moderate keratoconus, which is non-progressive, can be sufficiently managed with spectacle correction alone. [4] However, once a significant degree of irregular astigmatism develops, adequate visual correction with spectacles is not possible.

Contact Lenses

When spectacle correction is insufficient, CLs should be considered. CLs provide a regular refracting surface, as the space between the irregular corneal surface and the posterior surface of the CL becomes filled with tear fluid. CLs for keratoconus may be either soft, RGP, hybrid (rigid centrally with a soft surrounding edge), or 'piggyback' (RGP lens worn over a soft lens, with the soft lens mainly providing comfort, but each providing a degree of visual correction). However, RGP lenses are the most commonly used type, as others cannot correct the higher levels of irregular astigmatism that result from more advanced keratoconus. [22; 23] In advanced cases where the cornea is very irregular, it may not be possible to achieve an adequate lens fit with any corneal CL, and gas permeable scleral CLs may be an option in such patients. [24]

CL fitting involves one of three strategies for CL support: apical clearance, apical touch or three-point touch. Three-point touch is probably the best fitting technique, with light apical contact and greater paracentral corneal contact, as this provides good visual correction, some control of disease progression, good wearing comfort, and it may be associated with lesser progression of central corneal scarring. [16; 25-27]

If there is no significant difference between the UCVA and the BSCVA, the patient may either be amblyopic or may have significant higher order aberrations (HOAs). If amblyopia is the cause, there will be no significant improvement in BCVA when measured over a fitted RGP lens; thus, CLs can also have a diagnostic role in keratoconus. [15]

Corneal Collagen Cross Linking

CXL with Riboflavin (Vitamin B_2) and ultraviolet A (UVA at 370nm) is the first treatment that appears to stabilise keratoconus. This procedure was developed in Germany towards the end of the twentieth century and was first reported to halt the progression of keratoconus in 2003. [28-30] The aim of the procedure is to stabilise the condition by increasing the biomechanical stability of the cornea by increasing its resistance to enzymatic digestion. [31] This increase in the biomechanical strength of the cornea has been demonstrated by stress-strain experiments on cross-linked and non-cross-linked human and porcine corneal tissue. [32] It is believed that this stability is achieved by the formation of cross-links between adjacent collagen molecules and proteoglycans in the extracellular matrix, although there is no direct evidence as yet for such formation, as these cross-links cannot be seen microscopically. [29] Riboflavin acts as a photosensitizer, producing free radicals that activate the lysyl oxidase pathway, and the absorption of riboflavin by the corneal stroma also prevents damage to deeper ocular structures including the corneal endothelium, lens and retina, provided the cornea is of normal thickness. [29] More recently, it has been shown that singlet oxygen and free carbonyl groups in corneal tissue are essential for the photochemical generation of collagen cross-links. Furthermore, other mechanisms for the photochemical generation of cross-links in corneal collagen have been postulated, including: imidazolone production which can form new covalent bonds with molecules such as histidine; and/or a self-activation product of riboflavin itself (2,3-butanedione) could be formed that would react with endogenous carbonyl groups of the corneal stroma. [33]

Since the initial report by Wollensak et al. in 2003, in which they showed stabilisation of keratoconus in patients with up to four years of follow-up, clinical studies have demonstrated the efficacy of CXL in stabilising keratoconus in 98-100% of treated eyes with up to six years of follow-up. Indeed, many studies, including the initial one, have demonstrated improvements in vision and reduced corneal power measurements with no adverse effects on the corneal endothelium, which theoretically may be damaged by the procedure. [30; 34-38] These positive findings have also been replicated in a paediatric population, in whom it is well recognised that rapid and dramatic disease progression may occur. This study by Vinciguerra *et al.,* with two years of follow up, showed continued improvements in visual acuity (both UCVA and BSCVA), refractive measurements, topography and aberrometry (HOAs), with no demonstrable endothelial toxicity recorded over the follow-up period. [39] However, it is important to explicitly counsel patients that the aim of the procedure is to halt the progression of keratoconus and not to improve vision, as improvements are not seen in all patients. [30; 38]

CXL is performed with topical anaesthesia under sterile conditions. Topical pilocarpine should also be instilled preoperatively to reduce the potential exposure of the lens and retina to UVA irradiation. To minimise the risk of corneal endothelial cell damage from UVA exposure, it must be ensured that the minimum preoperative corneal thickness is > 400μm. This is because cell culture studies have shown a cytotoxic threshold level of 0.35 mW/cm^2, which is twice the irradiance incident on the endothelium in eyes with a minimum preoperative corneal thickness of > 400μm, confirmed by *in vivo* preclinical studies. [40-42] Riboflavin is a hydrophilic compound that cannot easily be absorbed through the intact corneal epithelium and, therefore, initial studies and most practitioners advocate epithelial debridement as part of the CXL procedure, to facilitate riboflavin absorption into the corneal stroma. [29; 35; 43] Reported techniques of CXL involve debridement of the central 6-9mm of the corneal epithelium, followed by the application of either isotonic (in cases with minimum preoperative corneal thickness > 450μm) or hypotonic (in cases with corneal thickness between 400-450μm) riboflavin 0.1% drops to the de-epithelialised cornea every 2-5 minutes for an initial 5-30 minutes and then every 3-5 minutes for a further 30 minutes with UVA exposure at 3 mW/cm^2 during the latter 30 minutes of the procedure.[34-39; 43] Recent debate has centred around methods of reduced epithelial disturbance to facilitate stromal riboflavin absorption, trans-epithelial CXL using different formulations of riboflavin or iontophoretic delivery, and methods of accelerated CXL using higher UVA fluence over a shorter duration of time (as short as one minute, versus the previously standard 30 minutes) to deliver the same total dose of UVA to the cornea. [44-53]

Overall, CXL is a safe procedure, but the eye may be quite painful for the first few days while it is re-epithelialising, although perceived pain decreases significantly on each consecutive day, and has also been shown to correlate with age (younger patients tend to experience greater pain following CXL). [54] Post-operative pain management is with systemically administered analgesics and a bandage soft CL. During the re-epithelialisation phase there is a risk of infectious keratitis, which may be severe resulting in irreversible corneal scarring and visual loss. [55-59] This risk is minimised by the use of topical antibiotics during the first post-operative week and instructions to the patient not to remove or replace the bandage CL themselves. Mid-stromal haze occurs in almost all patients but typically disappears by 6-12 months, and may be facilitated by the use of topical steroids post-operatively, although it is generally self-limiting. [60-62]

Despite treatment, some patients will continue to progress. [34] Patients older than 35 years and patients with maximum keratometric values of > 58 D are at the greatest risk of complications and/or progression following primary CXL. [18] If further progression occurs following primary CXL, it is reasonable to repeat the CXL procedure provided the cornea is sufficiently thick, although the results of repeated CXL are unclear to date. [34] Longer term follow-up studies are required to determine the long term stability and safety of this very promising procedure which has not yet received FDA approval in the USA, although it is the subject of intense international clinical research. [63]

Intra-Corneal Ring Segments

Intra-corneal ring segments (ICRS) were initially proposed as a potential treatment for myopia or hyperopia over 20 years ago. [64; 65] Indeed, the first generation was a complete

360° ring called the intrastromal corneal ring or KeraVision ring. It was more than 10 years later before their use was proposed in the management of keratoconus. [66] ICRS are poly(methyl methacrylate) (PMMA) segments, of which there are three main types that differ in terms of their size, shape and number: (1) Intacs® corneal implants (paired), which are the largest and most commonly used (Addition Technology Inc., California, USA); (2) Ferrara Ring segments (paired), which are intermediate in size (Mediphacos Inc, Belo Horizonte, Brazil); and (3) Bisantis segments (four segments), which are the smallest (Optikon 2000 SpA and Soleko SpA, Rome, Italy). Intacs® are hexagonal in cross-section, Ferrara Rings are triangular and Bisantis segments are oval. A newer Intacs® SK ICRS is now available, with a smaller inner diameter and an oval cross-section, for use in patients with steeper corneas and higher K max values. They all act to flatten the centre of the cornea based on the Barraquer thickness law, which states that when material is added to the corneal periphery or when tissue is removed from the centre of the cornea, a flattening effect occurs centrally. [67] Varying degrees of flattening can be achieved based on the number of segments implanted, their diameter and thickness, and their position relative to the corneal centre or the centre of the cone. Nomograms are available from each company guiding the choice of segment to implant. ICRS implantation does not affect the progression of keratoconus which, to date, can only be influenced by CXL, but it can temporarily improve the UCVA and facilitate fitment of CLs, delaying the need for keratoplasty, or possibly even obviating the need for keratoplasty if combined with CXL. [68] Furthermore, it is a minimally invasive and reversible procedure that is not associated with a high incidence of significant complications. [69]

Patients with keratoconus who have become CL intolerant due to poor fitment and who have clear corneas that are at least 400μm thick at the point of ICRS implantation are suitable for this treatment. [20] Colin et al. were the first to report on this treatment in the year 2000, following its initial use by them in 1997. [66] They published their one year follow-up results in 2001, showing that corneal steepening and astigmatism associated with keratoconus were reduced, and visual acuity was improved with treatment in almost all eyes of the 10 patients treated. [70] In 2003 Boxer Wachler et al. reported a retrospective series of 74 eyes of 50 keratoconus patients who underwent Intacs® implantation. [71] They found that 45% of eyes gained two lines in BSCVA and 72% of eyes had similar gains in UCVA with significantly reduced irregular astigmatism at postoperative follow-up. Their series included eyes with and without corneal scarring and, perhaps surprisingly, the greatest improvements in BSCVA were seen in the scarred eyes, but improvements in UCVA were greater in eyes with clear corneas. However, interestingly, significant improvements were seen in both groups. A prospective study by Colin in 2006 in 57 eyes with keratoconus and clear corneas showed significant improvements in objective visual outcomes, with BSCVA of 20/40 or better being achieved by 74% of patients following Intacs® implantation, compared to 53% preoperatively. [69] Also in 2006, Alió et al. reported a retrospective series of 25 keratoconic eyes implanted with Intacs® suggesting that better results, in terms of visual and topographic improvements, can be expected in patients with preoperative mean K values ≤ 53D and a relatively low spherical equivalent, whereas poorer outcomes can be expected in patients with mean K values ≥ 55D. [21] This finding was supported by more recent research in a larger cohort (219 keratoconic eyes) that showed more significant improvements in eyes with Stage I or II keratoconus compared to eyes with Amsler-Krumeich Stage III keratoconus, but all stages still showed improvements following ICRS implantation. [72] However, several other studies have suggested that Intacs® implantation can also be beneficial and safe in advanced keratoconus. [73; 74] Furthermore, implantation of the newer, smaller Intacs® SK ICRS has shown particularly promising results in moderate to advanced cases of keratoconus, possibly making it the implant of choice in such cases. [75-78]

The ICRS channels may be dissected mechanically or fashioned with a femtosecond laser. [79] The femtosecond laser presents obvious advantages in terms of speed and reproducibility, with a lower risk of complications, particularly anterior or posterior perforation, but there is a significant cost implication with this method. [80] Nonetheless, the advantages in terms of safety are significant. One series using the mechanical dissection technique reported complications in almost one third of their cases (6/20) regarding thinning and segment exposure. [81] By comparison, there is a low risk of corneal epithelial defects or corneal oedema with the femtosecond laser and it is not necessary to suture the keratotomy with this method. However, epithelial plugs at the incision site, granulomatous deposits around the ICRS, and keratitis can occur with either method of channel creation. [80; 82] In terms of refractive outcomes, there does not seem to be any significant difference between either method, although using the femtosecond laser may afford certain advantages. [83]

Phakic Intra-Ocular Lens Implantation

As outlined previously, implantation of ICRS in patients with clear corneas and CL intolerance is a very useful, safe and reversible method of improving both UCVA and BSCVA, often facilitating the re-fitting of CLs, and deferring the need for keratoplasty for visual rehabilitation in patients with keratoconus. However, some patients will remain CL intolerant or will have significant residual ametropia, such that additional surgical options should be considered. [20]

The implantation of pIOLs in patients with keratoconus was first reported by Leccisotti et al. in 2003, who implanted angle-supported anterior chamber pIOLs in a small number of eyes with early keratoconus. [84] Two years later Budo et al. reported a very small series of eyes (n=6) implanted with Artisan toric pIOLs (Ophtec BV, Groningen, The Netherlands), in which five had improvement in BSCVA and all of which had a significant reduction in spherical equivalent refraction. [85] Larger studies (largest, n=17) using both Artisan and Artiflex pIOLs have been published more recently, with positive outcomes in all reports and no significant reduction in endothelial cell counts recorded. [86-88] Both spherical and toric collamer posterior chamber pIOLs (e.g. the Visian ICL™, STAAR® Surgical, Nidau, Switzerland) have been implanted by several other groups, reporting good outcomes in terms of refractive results, stability and safety profiles. [89-93] However, one group did conclude that, although the refractive error was corrected by the implantation of the collamer pIOL, the associated aberrations meant that the final visual quality was sub-optimal. [94]

The assessment of a patient with keratoconus regarding their possible suitability for pIOL implantation, in order to improve the visual results that can be obtained, should include a complete ophthalmic clinical examination. Prospective patients should have an anterior chamber depth of > 2.8mm and an endothelial cell count > 2500 cells/mm^2. Their corneal irregularity should not be so severe as to make optical correction of their sphero-cylindrical error impossible with a spherical or toric IOL. This may be ascertained by evaluating their preoperative BSCVA and comparing it with RGP CL-corrected distance VA to determine how the patient feels about this type of lens-corrected VA. A suitable candidate for pIOL implantation should have a BSCVA of 20/40 or better. [89] Implantation of pIOLs should not be undertaken in patients with progressive disease, so it should either be performed when progression has stopped, or it should be following CXL. [86; 87; 95] Consideration must also be given to the potential risk posed for cataract progression and/or complications arising from changes in anterior segment morphology on implantation of a pIOL. [96; 97]

Larger, randomized controlled studies with longer follow-up are needed to decide which type of lens is best to use and to evaluate the safety, predictability, and stability of pIOL implantation in patients with keratoconus.

Refractive Laser Surgery

Photorefractive keratectomy (PRK) uses the excimer laser to ablate a small amount of tissue from the corneal stroma, permanently altering the shape of the anterior corneal surface and its refractive power. The first report on the use of this technique in patients with keratoconus was in 1994 by Mortensen and Ohrström, who treated five eyes with PRK to reduce the steepness of the cone, deferring penetrating keratoplasty. [98] In four of these eyes the astigmatism was reduced and the VA improved; no complications during 6-12 months of follow-up were noted. They concluded that the traditional contraindication to this treatment in patients with keratoconus may be exaggerated; however, their follow-up was very short and it is well known that refractive correction in patients with keratoconus, by whatever means, may be complicated by the unstable nature of the disease, leading to a progressive refractive error. For this reason, some authorities advocate avoiding irreversible, 'subtractive' therapies in keratoconus and suggest alternative means of refractive correction, such as CLs or ICRS, both of which may be considered reversible and 'additive'. [99-101] Nevertheless, further study by Mortensen et al. in a larger cohort, with longer follow-up (6-46 months, with a mean of 22 months), also reported good outcomes. [102]

More recently, wavefront-supported and topography-guided PRK has been performed in patients ranging from mild or forme fruste keratoconus to mild-moderate keratoconus (Amsler-Krumeich Stage II), and has been shown to be effective in treating the associated myopia and astigmatism and/or reducing the severity of several indices used to describe the degree of keratoconus. [103-106]

Photoastigmatic refractive keratectomy (PARK) is another approach that has been taken to the treatment of myopia and astigmatism in forme fruste and mild keratoconus. In 2007, Alpins and Stamatelatos reported a retrospective study of 45 eyes of 29 patients with stable, mild or forme fruste keratoconus that underwent PARK for myopic astigmatism, with a follow-up of between 1-10 years. [107] They used vector planning, a technique that takes account of the ocular residual astigmatism (ORA, or non-corneal astigmatism) in every case, to enable treatment parameters to combine topographic and refractive data in a systematic paradigm. This technique of vector planning facilitates a greater reduction in corneal astigmatism than treatment using only refractive parameters, resulting in fewer second- and third-order aberrations. Inclusion criteria for this study were: BCVA of $\geq$ 20/40; a non-progressive cone, with refractive and corneal stability for at least 2 years; age $\geq$ 25 years. Exclusion criteria were: patients with average K readings $\geq$ 50D; visible ectasia or scarring under slit-lamp examination; residual stromal bed less than 300μm (allowing for an epithelial thickness of 60μm). One year postoperatively, UCVA was ≥ 20/40 in all eyes, ≥ 20/30 in 89% of eyes, and ≥ 20/20 in 56% of eyes. The BCVA preoperatively and at one year was ≥ 20/20 in 89% of eyes and ≥ 20/30 in 100% of eyes. One eye lost two lines of Snellen acuity, six eyes lost one line, 22 eyes were unchanged, 13 eyes gained one line, and three eyes gained two lines of Snellen acuity. No cases progressed over the follow-up period. Thus, PARK was deemed to be safe and effective for the treatment of myopia and astigmatism in this carefully selected group of patients.

If considering PRK treatment in a patient with keratoconus, it is worth taking account of the following criteria developed by Gulani and Nordan: [108]

- Patient is symptomatic with reduced VA, double vision, or glare; patient cannot tolerate CLs; spectacle or CL correction is limited and/or unsuccessful
- Clinical examination and signs characteristic of keratoconus
- BCVA ≥ 20/30 (even with RGP CL trial). BCVA < 20/40 would favour ICRS implantation
- Refraction is stable on review of prior clinical examinations
- Astigmatism higher than myopia/hyperopia is preferred
- Corneal thickness > 400μm at the thinnest point; the treatment plan should not leave the thinnest point < 350μm post-operatively
- Corneal scarring, if present, should be less than the anterior one third in depth
- The patient must understand that using an excimer laser in patients with keratoconus is an off-label procedure and that if their ectasia deteriorates due to laser treatment or natural progression, they could be a candidate for other corrective procedures, such as ICRS implantation or keratoplasty

Keratoplasty

Penetrating Keratoplasty

For many years, penetrating keratoplasty (PK) has been the mainstay of treatment for advanced keratoconus, when the combination of significant visual loss, corneal scarring, and intolerance or failure of other treatment strategies exists. A recent report from the Michigan Corneal Transplantation Patient Registry on corneal graft survival in this patient group showed that allograft rejection was most likely to occur in the first two years (probability: 41%, standard error: 3%), graft failure had a 20-year probability of 12% (standard error: 3%), and there was a 20-year probability of 10% (standard error: 4%) for keratoconus recurrence in the graft. [109] Other long term reports on visual outcomes following PK for keratoconus have shown good results, with 73-91% of eyes achieving a BCVA of ≥ 20/40.[110-114] These results are testament to the long term efficacy and the role that PK continues to have in the management of advanced keratoconus, despite the slow visual rehabilitation that inevitably ensues after PK due to iatrogenic astigmatism and anisometropia, and the recent advances that have been made with alternative techniques, in particular deep anterior lamellar keratoplasty. [115]

Deep Anterior Lamellar Keratoplasty

Eyes with keratoconus generally retain a healthy endothelium, even following repeated episodes of corneal hydrops. Allograft rejection after PK is usually endothelial in origin, therefore, techniques that do not interfere with the host endothelium potentially offer advantages in this regard, along with the benefits afforded by not having to perform 'open sky' surgery. [116] Furthermore, the cornea is tectonically stronger postoperatively and earlier postoperative cessation of steroid treatment is also possible. [117] The concept of anterior lamellar keratoplasty has been around for many years, but it is only within the last 15 years that the technique of deep anterior lamellar keratoplasty (DALK) has been refined and more commonly used in patients with keratoconus. [118-121] Various different techniques for performing DALK have been described, including Melles' technique, intrastromal air- and/or saline-assisted dissection, the 'Big Bubble' technique, or variations of the 'Big Bubble' technique and, more recently, femtosecond laser-assisted techniques ('IntraBubble'). [121-130] Nonetheless, there is a significant learning curve with this technique and it remains technically more challenging and more time-consuming than PK, in spite of the potential advantages. [131; 132] No doubt this explains, at least in part, the findings of Jones et al. that, of the 2372 first time grafts for keratoconus performed in the UK between 1999 and 2005, 81% were PK and only 19% were DALK.[133]

The achievement of a smooth donor-host interface is central to good quality vision postoperatively following DALK. [120] This has been facilitated first by the microkeratome and, more recently, by the femtosecond laser, the use of which has been shown to result in superior outcomes, particularly when baring of Descemet's membrane is possible. [134-136]

Comparative studies between the outcomes following PK and DALK are still somewhat equivocal, with each surgical approach having advantages and disadvantages in certain respects, or else being shown to have very similar outcomes. [115; 116; 137; 138] Several recent large studies have shown that 78-83% of patients will achieve a BCVA $\geq$ 20/40 following DALK, which compares reasonably well with the visual outcomes following PK (see above). [117; 139; 140] However, it would still appear that patients who have a PK for keratoconus have a greater chance of attaining 20/20 VA postoperatively compared to those having a DALK. In 2009, Jones et al. reported from their very large series (PK n=1136; DALK n=234) that at two years postoperatively, 33% of patients who had a PK achieved a BCVA of $\geq$ 20/20, compared with 22% of patients who had a DALK (p=0.0007). [133] An older report by Watson et al. from 2004 found that, in patients with keratoconus, those in the PK group were twice as likely to achieve a BCVA of $\geq$ 20/20 compared with those in the DALK group (64% vs. 32%). [141] More recently, similar visual outcomes have been reported with both treatments, including those relating to visual quality, such as contrast sensitivity function and HOAs, evaluated in a prospective, randomised case series of 174 eyes of 140 patients.[142] Endothelial cell loss seems to be less following DALK than following PK. [117;143;144]

Further refinements in the techniques used to perform DALK are necessary in order for it to become more widely adopted as the popular choice for keratoplasty in patients with keratoconus.

Conclusion

The decision tree in keratoconus management has grown from one of riding out the wave of progression, to active measures to halt the progression of this ectatic disease. Indeed, the introduction of CXL has radically altered the management approach to keratoconus, which, a little over ten years ago, centred on RGP CL fitting when spectacle correction no longer sufficed, and keratoplasty where CL intolerance prevailed. Over the last decade, once keratoconus progression has been halted, either naturally or with CXL, new interventions for visual rehabilitation including ICRS, pIOL implantation, and refractive laser techniques have significantly added to the ophthalmic surgeon's armamentarium for managing keratoconus. Nowadays, the management approach can be summarised under two key headings: corneal shape stabilisation and visual rehabilitation.

Future management of keratoconus will undoubtedly centre on refinements of the above techniques and the strategic application of appropriate combination therapies in a systematic manner. These refinements are already underway, with investigators seeking to determine which combination strategies might be best. Kanellopoulos found that same day simultaneous CXL and topography-guided PRK are superior to sequential CXL and PRK in patients with progressive keratoconus. [145] Spadea and Paroli have recently reported that customized PRK and CXL provided safe and effective results in the management of corneal regularisation for refractive purposes after previous lamellar keratoplasty for keratoconus. [146] Further similar investigations, preferably in randomised controlled studies with longer follow-up are necessary to determine which strategies work best, their safety, predictability and stability, in an effort to ultimately defer or obviate the need for keratoplasty.

References

[1] Krachmer Jh, Feder Rs, Belin Mw. Keratoconus And Related Noninflammatory Corneal Thinning Disorders. *Surv Ophthalmol* 1984 Jan;28(4):293-322.

[2] Kennedy Rh, Bourne Wm, Dyer Ja. A 48-Year Clinical And Epidemiologic Study Of Keratoconus. *Am J Ophthalmol* 1986 Mar 15;101(3):267-73.

[3] Zadnik K, Steger-May K, Fink Ba, Joslin Ce, Nichols Jj, Rosenstiel Ce, Et Al. Between-Eye Asymmetry In Keratoconus. *Cornea* 2002 Oct;21(7):671-9.

[4] Rabinowitz Ys. Keratoconus. *Surv Ophthalmol* 1998 Jan;42(4):297-319.

[5] Weed Kh, Macewen Cj, Giles T, Low J, Mcghee Cn. The Dundee University Scottish Keratoconus Study: Demographics, Corneal Signs, Associated Diseases, And Eye Rubbing. *Eye* (Lond) 2008 Apr;22(4):534-41.

[6] Krachmer Jh. Eye Rubbing Can Cause Keratoconus. *Cornea* 2004 Aug;23(6):539-40.

[7] Jafri B, Lichter H, Stulting Rd. Asymmetric Keratoconus Attributed To Eye Rubbing. *Cornea* 2004 Aug;23(6):560-4.

[8] Jacobs Ds, Dohlman Ch. Is Keratoconus Genetic? *Int Ophthalmol Clin* 1993;33(2):249-60.

[9] Andreassen Tt, Simonsen Ah, Oxlund H. Biomechanical Properties Of Keratoconus And Normal Corneas. *Exp Eye Res* 1980 Oct;31(4):435-41.

[10] Zhou L, Sawaguchi S, Twining Ss, Sugar J, Feder Rs, Yue By. Expression Of Degradative Enzymes And Protease Inhibitors In Corneas With Keratoconus. *Invest Ophthalmol Vis Sci* 1998 Jun;39(7):1117-24.

[11] Cullen Jf, Butler Hg. Mongolism (Down's Syndrome) And Keratoconus. *Br J Ophthalmol* 1963 Jun;47:321-30.:321-30.

[12] Robertson I. Keratoconus And The Ehlers-Danlos Syndrome: A New Aspect Of Keratoconus. *Med J Aust* 1975 May 3;1(18):571-3.

[13] Beckh U, Schonherr U, Naumann Go. [Autosomal Dominant Keratoconus As The Chief Ocular Symptom In Lobstein Osteogenesis Imperfecta Tarda]. *Klin Monbl Augenheilkd* 1995 Apr;206(4):268-72.

[14] Woodward Eg, Morris Mt. Joint Hypermobility In Keratoconus. *Ophthalmic Physiol Opt* 1990 Oct;10(4):360-2.

[15] Sinjab Mm. *Keratoconus: When, Why And Why Not - A Step By Step Systematic Approach. First Ed.* New Delhi: Jaypee Brothers Medical Publishers Ltd; 2012.

[16] Romero-Jimenez M, Santodomingo-Rubido J, Wolffsohn Js. Keratoconus: A Review. *Cont Lens Anterior Eye* 2010 Aug;33(4):157-66.

[17] Alio Jl, Shabayek Mh. Corneal Higher Order Aberrations: A Method To Grade Keratoconus. *J Refract Surg* 2006 Jun;22(6):539-45.

[18] Koller T, Mrochen M, Seiler T. Complication And Failure Rates After Corneal Crosslinking. *J Cataract Refract Surg* 2009 Aug;35(8):1358-62.

[19] Bilgihan K, Hondur A, Sul S, Ozturk S. Pregnancy-Induced Progression Of Keratoconus. *Cornea* 2011 Sep;30(9):991-4.

[20] Ertan A, Colin J. Intracorneal Rings For Keratoconus And Keratectasia. *J Cataract Refract Surg* 2007 Jul;33(7):1303-14.

[21] Alio Jl, Shabayek Mh, Belda Ji, Correas P, Feijoo Ed. Analysis Of Results Related To Good And Bad Outcomes Of Intacs Implantation For Keratoconus Correction. *J Cataract Refract Surg* 2006 May;32(5):756-61.

[22] Zadnik K, Barr Jt, Edrington Tb, Everett Df, Jameson M, Mcmahon Tt, Et Al. Baseline Findings In The Collaborative Longitudinal Evaluation Of Keratoconus (Clek) Study. *Invest Ophthalmol Vis Sci* 1998 Dec;39(13):2537-46.

[23] Lim N, Vogt U. Characteristics And Functional Outcomes Of 130 Patients With Keratoconus Attending A Specialist Contact Lens Clinic. *Eye* (Lond) 2002 Jan;16(1):54-9.

[24] Segal O, Barkana Y, Hourovitz D, Behrman S, Kamun Y, Avni I, Et Al. Scleral Contact Lenses May Help Where Other Modalities Fail. *Cornea* 2003 May;22(4):308-10.

[25] Mcmonnies Cw. Keratoconus Fittings: Apical Clearance Or Apical Support? *Eye Contact Lens* 2004 Jul;30(3):147-55.

[26] Edrington Tb, Gundel Re, Libassi Dp, Wagner H, Pierce Ge, Walline Jj, Et Al. Variables Affecting Rigid Contact Lens Comfort In The Collaborative Longitudinal Evaluation Of Keratoconus (Clek) Study. *Optom Vis Sci* 2004 Mar;81(3):182-8.

[27] Zadnik K, Barr Jt, Steger-May K, Edrington Tb, Mcmahon Tt, Gordon Mo. Comparison Of Flat And Steep Rigid Contact Lens Fitting Methods In Keratoconus. *Optom Vis Sci* 2005 Dec;82(12):1014-21.

[28] Sporl E, Huhle M, Kasper M, Seiler T. [Increased Rigidity Of The Cornea Caused By Intrastromal Cross-Linking]. *Ophthalmologe* 1997 Dec;94(12):902-6.

[29] Spoerl E, Huhle M, Seiler T. Induction Of Cross-Links In Corneal Tissue. *Exp Eye Res* 1998 Jan;66(1):97-103.
[30] Wollensak G, Spoerl E, Seiler T. Riboflavin/Ultraviolet-A-Induced Collagen Crosslinking For The Treatment Of Keratoconus. *Am J Ophthalmol* 2003 May;135(5):620-7.
[31] Spoerl E, Wollensak G, Seiler T. Increased Resistance Of Crosslinked Cornea Against Enzymatic Digestion. *Curr Eye Res* 2004 Jul;29(1):35-40.
[32] Wollensak G, Spoerl E, Seiler T. Stress-Strain Measurements Of Human And Porcine Corneas After Riboflavin-Ultraviolet-A-Induced Cross-Linking. *J Cataract Refract Surg* 2003 Sep;29(9):1780-5.
[33] Mccall As, Kraft S, Edelhauser Hf, Kidder Gw, Lundquist Rr, Bradshaw He, Et Al. Mechanisms Of Corneal Tissue Cross-Linking In Response To Treatment With Topical Riboflavin And Long-Wavelength Ultraviolet Radiation (Uva). *Invest Ophthalmol Vis Sci* 2010 Jan;51(1):129-38.
[34] Raiskup-Wolf F, Hoyer A, Spoerl E, Pillunat Le. Collagen Crosslinking With Riboflavin And Ultraviolet-A Light In Keratoconus: Long-Term Results. *J Cataract Refract Surg* 2008 May;34(5):796-801.
[35] Caporossi A, Mazzotta C, Baiocchi S, Caporossi T. Long-Term Results Of Riboflavin Ultraviolet A Corneal Collagen Cross-Linking For Keratoconus In Italy: The Siena Eye Cross Study. *Am J Ophthalmol* 2010 Apr;149(4):585-93.
[36] Vinciguerra P, Albe E, Trazza S, Rosetta P, Vinciguerra R, Seiler T, Et Al. Refractive, Topographic, Tomographic, And Aberrometric Analysis Of Keratoconic Eyes Undergoing Corneal Cross-Linking. *Ophthalmology* 2009 Mar;116(3):369-78.
[37] Coskunseven E, Jankov Mr, Hafezi F. Contralateral Eye Study Of Corneal Collagen Cross-Linking With Riboflavin And Uva Irradiation In Patients With Keratoconus. *J Refract Surg* 2009 Apr;25(4):371-6.
[38] Asri D, Touboul D, Fournie P, Malet F, Garra C, Gallois A, Et Al. Corneal Collagen Crosslinking In Progressive Keratoconus: Multicenter Results From The French National Reference Center For Keratoconus. *J Cataract Refract Surg* 2011 Dec;37(12):2137-43.
[39] Vinciguerra P, Albe E, Frueh Be, Trazza S, Epstein D. Two-Year Corneal Cross-Linking Results In Patients Younger Than 18 Years With Documented Progressive Keratoconus. *Am J Ophthalmol* 2012 Sep;154(3):520-6.
[40] Wollensak G, Sporl E, Reber F, Pillunat L, Funk R. Corneal Endothelial Cytotoxicity Of Riboflavin/Uva Treatment In Vitro. *Ophthalmic Res* 2003 Nov;35(6):324-8.
[41] Wollensak G, Spoerl E, Wilsch M, Seiler T. Endothelial Cell Damage After Riboflavin-Ultraviolet-A Treatment In The Rabbit. *J Cataract Refract Surg* 2003 Sep;29(9):1786-90.
[42] Spoerl E, Mrochen M, Sliney D, Trokel S, Seiler T. Safety Of Uva-Riboflavin Cross-Linking Of The Cornea. *Cornea* 2007 May;26(4):385-9.
[43] O'brart Dp, Chan E, Samaras K, Patel P, Shah Sp. A Randomised, Prospective Study To Investigate The Efficacy Of Riboflavin/Ultraviolet A (370 Nm) Corneal Collagen Cross-Linkage To Halt The Progression Of Keratoconus. *Br J Ophthalmo*l 2011 Nov;95(11):1519-24.

[44] Alhamad Ta, O'brart Dp, O'brart Na, Meek Km. Evaluation Of Transepithelial Stromal Riboflavin Absorption With Enhanced Riboflavin Solution Using Spectrophotometry. *J Cataract Refract Surg* 2012 May;38(5):884-9.

[45] Raiskup F, Pinelli R, Spoerl E. Riboflavin Osmolar Modification For Transepithelial Corneal Cross-Linking. *Curr Eye Res* 2012 Mar;37(3):234-8.

[46] Kissner A, Spoerl E, Jung R, Spekl K, Pillunat Le, Raiskup F. Pharmacological Modification Of The Epithelial Permeability By Benzalkonium Chloride In Uva/Riboflavin Corneal Collagen Cross-Linking. *Curr Eye Res* 2010 Aug;35(8):715-21.

[47] Leccisotti A, Islam T. Transepithelial Corneal Collagen Cross-Linking In Keratoconus. *J Refract Surg* 2010 Dec;26(12):942-8.

[48] Filippello M, Stagni E, O'brart D. Transepithelial Corneal Collagen Crosslinking: Bilateral Study. *J Cataract Refract Surg* 2012 Feb;38(2):283-91.

[49] Koppen C, Wouters K, Mathysen D, Rozema J, Tassignon Mj. Refractive And Topographic Results Of Benzalkonium Chloride-Assisted Transepithelial Crosslinking. *J Cataract Refract Surg* 2012 Jun;38(6):1000-5.

[50] Kanellopoulos Aj. Long-Term Safety And Efficacy Follow-Up Of Prophylactic Higher Fluence Collagen Cross-Linking In High Myopic Laser-Assisted In Situ Keratomileusis. *Clin Ophthalmol* 2012;6:1125-30. Doi: 10.2147/Opth.S31256. Epub;2012 Jul 18.:1125-30.

[51] Celik Hu, Alagoz N, Yildirim Y, Agca A, Marshall J, Demirok A, Et Al. Accelerated Corneal Crosslinking Concurrent With Laser In Situ Keratomileusis. *J Cataract Refract Surg* 2012 Aug;38(8):1424-31.

[52] Hao J, Li Sk, Liu Cy, Kao Ww. Electrically Assisted Delivery Of Macromolecules Into The Corneal Epithelium. *Exp Eye Res* 2009 Dec;89(6):934-41.

[53] Stojanovic A, Chen X, Jin N, Zhang T, Stojanovic F, Raeder S, Et Al. Safety And Efficacy Of Epithelium-On Corneal Collagen Cross-Linking Using A Multifactorial Approach To Achieve Proper Stromal Riboflavin Saturation. *J Ophthalmol* 2012;2012:498435. Doi: 10.1155/2012/498435. Epub;2012 Jul 30.:498435.

[54] Ghanem Vc, Ghanem Rc, De Or. Postoperative Pain After Corneal Collagen Cross-Linking. *Cornea* 2013 Jan;32(1):20-4.

[55] Dhawan S, Rao K, Natrajan S. Complications Of Corneal Collagen Cross-Linking. *J Ophthalmol* 2011;2011:869015. Doi: 10.1155/2011/869015. Epub;2011 Dec 27.:869015.

[56] Koppen C, Vryghem Jc, Gobin L, Tassignon Mj. Keratitis And Corneal Scarring After Uva/Riboflavin Cross-Linking For Keratoconus. *J Refract Surg* 2009 Sep;25(9):S819-S823.

[57] Rama P, Di Mf, Matuska S, Paganoni G, Spinelli A. Acanthamoeba Keratitis With Perforation After Corneal Crosslinking And Bandage Contact Lens Use. *J Cataract Refract Surg* 2009 Apr;35(4):788-91.

[58] Pollhammer M, Cursiefen C. Bacterial Keratitis Early After Corneal Crosslinking With Riboflavin And Ultraviolet-A. *J Cataract Refract Surg* 2009 Mar;35(3):588-9.

[59] Perez-Santonja Jj, Artola A, Javaloy J, Alio Jl, Abad Jl. Microbial Keratitis After Corneal Collagen Crosslinking. *J Cataract Refract Surg* 2009 Jun;35(6):1138-40.

[60] Mazzotta C, Balestrazzi A, Baiocchi S, Traversi C, Caporossi A. Stromal Haze After Combined Riboflavin-Uva Corneal Collagen Cross-Linking In Keratoconus: In Vivo Confocal Microscopic Evaluation. *Clin Experiment Ophthalmol* 2007 Aug;35(6):580-2.

[61] Seiler T, Hafezi F. Corneal Cross-Linking-Induced Stromal Demarcation Line. *Cornea* 2006 Oct;25(9):1057-9.

[62] Raiskup F, Hoyer A, Spoerl E. Permanent Corneal Haze After Riboflavin-Uva-Induced Cross-Linking In Keratoconus. *J Refract Surg* 2009 Sep;25(9):S824-S828.

[63] Nih Clinical Trials *Http://Clinicaltrials.Gov/Ct2/Results?Term=Corneal+Collagen+Cross+Linking&Search=Search.* 2012. 30-12-2012. Ref Type: Internet Communication

[64] Fleming Jf, Wan Wl, Schanzlin Dj. The Theory Of Corneal Curvature Change With The Intrastromal Corneal Ring. *Clao J* 1989 Apr;15(2):146-50.

[65] Burris Te, Ayer Ct, Evensen Da, Davenport Jm. Effects Of Intrastromal Corneal Ring Size And Thickness On Corneal Flattening In Human Eyes. *Refract Corneal Surg* 1991 Jan;7(1):46-50.

[66] Colin J, Cochener B, Savary G, Malet F. Correcting Keratoconus With Intracorneal Rings. *J Cataract Refract Surg* 2000 Aug;26(8):1117-22.

[67] Barraquer Ji. Modification Of Refraction By Means Of Intracorneal Inclusions. *Int Ophthalmol Clin* 1966;6(1):53-78.

[68] Kymionis Gd, Grentzelos Ma, Diakonis Vf, Pallikaris Ai, Pallikaris Ig. Nine-Year Follow-Up Of Intacs Implantation For Keratoconus. *Open Ophthalmol J* 2009 Dec 8;3:77-81. Doi: 10.2174/1874364100903010077.:77-81.

[69] Colin J. European Clinical Evaluation: Use Of Intacs For The Treatment Of Keratoconus. *J Cataract Refract Surg* 2006 May;32(5):747-55.

[70] Colin J, Cochener B, Savary G, Malet F, Holmes-Higgin D. Intacs Inserts For Treating Keratoconus: One-Year Results. Ophthalmology 2001 Aug;108(8):1409-14.

[71] Boxer Wachler Bs, Christie Jp, Chandra Ns, Chou B, Korn T, Nepomuceno R. Intacs For Keratoconus. *Ophthalmology* 2003 May;110(5):1031-40.

[72] Alfonso Jf, Lisa C, Fernandez-Vega L, Madrid-Costa D, Montes-Mico R. Intrastromal Corneal Ring Segment Implantation In 219 Keratoconic Eyes At Different Stages. Graefes Arch Clin Exp Ophthalmol 2011 Nov;249(11):1705-12.

[73] Shetty R, Kurian M, Anand D, Mhaske P, Narayana Km, Shetty Bk. Intacs In Advanced Keratoconus. *Cornea* 2008 Oct;27(9):1022-9.

[74] Ertan A, Kamburoglu G. Intacs Implantation Using A Femtosecond Laser For Management Of Keratoconus: Comparison Of 306 Cases In Different Stages. *J Cataract Refract Surg* 2008 Sep;34(9):1521-6.

[75] Fahd Dc, Jabbur Ns, Awwad St. Intrastromal Corneal Ring Segment Sk For Moderate To Severe Keratoconus: A Case Series. *J Refract Surg* 2012 Oct;28(10):701-5.

[76] Niknam S, Shamshiri M, Shahrzad Ss, Alipour A, Rajabi Mb, Rajabi Mt. Treatment Of Moderate To Severe Keratoconus With 6-Mm Intacs Sk. *Int J Ophthalmol* 2012;5(4):513-6.

[77] Khan Mi, Injarie A, Muhtaseb M. Intrastromal Corneal Ring Segments For Advanced Keratoconus And Cases With High Keratometric Asymmetry. *J Cataract Refract Surg* 2012 Jan;38(1):129-36.

[78] Sansanayudh W, Bahar I, Kumar Nl, Shehadeh-Mashour R, Ritenour R, Singal N, Et Al. Intrastromal Corneal Ring Segment Sk Implantation For Moderate To Severe Keratoconus. *J Cataract Refract Surg* 2010 Jan;36(1):110-3.

[79] Rabinowitz Ys, Li X, Ignacio Ts, Maguen E. Intacs Inserts Using The Femtosecond Laser Compared To The Mechanical Spreader In The Treatment Of Keratoconus. *J Refract Surg* 2006 Oct;22(8):764-71.

[80] Ertan A, Kamburoglu G, Bahadir M. Intacs Insertion With The Femtosecond Laser For The Management Of Keratoconus: One-Year Results. *J Cataract Refract Surg* 2006 Dec;32(12):2039-42.

[81] Kanellopoulos Aj, Pe Lh, Perry Hd, Donnenfeld Ed. Modified Intracorneal Ring Segment Implantations (Intacs) For The Management Of Moderate To Advanced Keratoconus: Efficacy And Complications. *Cornea* 2006 Jan;25(1):29-33.

[82] Levy J, Lifshitz T. Keratitis After Implantation Of Intrastromal Corneal Ring Segments (Intacs) Aided By Femtosecond Laser For Keratoconus Correction: Case Report And Description Of The Literature. *Eur J Ophthalmol* 2010 Jul;20(4):780-4.

[83] Pinero Dp, Alio Jl, El Kb, Coskunseven E, Morbelli H, Uceda-Montanes A, Et Al. Refractive And Aberrometric Outcomes Of Intracorneal Ring Segments For Keratoconus: Mechanical Versus Femtosecond-Assisted Procedures. *Ophthalmology* 2009 Sep;116(9):1675-87.

[84] Leccisotti A, Fields Sv. Angle-Supported Phakic Intraocular Lenses In Eyes With Keratoconus And Myopia. *J Cataract Refract Surg* 2003 Aug;29(8):1530-6.

[85] Budo C, Bartels Mc, Van Rg. Implantation Of Artisan Toric Phakic Intraocular Lenses For The Correction Of Astigmatism And Spherical Errors In Patients With Keratoconus. *J Refract Surg* 2005 May;21(3):218-22.

[86] Izquierdo L, Jr., Henriquez Ma, Mccarthy M. Artiflex Phakic Intraocular Lens Implantation After Corneal Collagen Cross-Linking In Keratoconic Eyes. *J Refract Surg* 2011 Jul;27(7):482-7.

[87] Guell Jl, Morral M, Malecaze F, Gris O, Elies D, Manero F. Collagen Crosslinking And Toric Iris-Claw Phakic Intraocular Lens For Myopic Astigmatism In Progressive Mild To Moderate Keratoconus. *J Cataract Refract Surg* 2012 Mar;38(3):475-84.

[88] Sedaghat M, Nsari-Astaneh Mr, Zarei-Ghanavati M, Davis Sw, Sikder S. Artisan Iris-Supported Phakic Iol Implantation In Patients With Keratoconus: A Review Of 16 Eyes. *J Refract Surg* 2011 Jul;27(7):489-93.

[89] Navas A, Tapia-Herrera G, Jaimes M, Graue-Hernandez Eo, Gomez-Bastar A, Ramirez-Luquin T, Et Al. Implantable Collamer Lenses After Intracorneal Ring Segments For Keratoconus. *Int Ophthalmol* 2012 Oct;32(5):423-9.

[90] Alfonso Jf, Palacios A, Montes-Mico R. Myopic Phakic Staar Collamer Posterior Chamber Intraocular Lenses For Keratoconus. *J Refract Surg* 2008 Nov;24(9):867-74.

[91] Kamiya K, Shimizu K, Kobashi H, Komatsu M, Nakamura A, Nakamura T, Et Al. Clinical Outcomes Of Posterior Chamber Toric Phakic Intraocular Lens Implantation For The Correction Of High Myopic Astigmatism In Eyes With Keratoconus: 6-Month Follow-Up. *Graefes Arch Clin Exp Ophthalmol* 2011 Jul;249(7):1073-80.

[92] Alfonso Jf, Fernandez-Vega L, Lisa C, Fernandes P, Gonzalez-Meijome Jm, Montes-Mico R. Collagen Copolymer Toric Posterior Chamber Phakic Intraocular Lens In Eyes With Keratoconus. *J Cataract Refract Surg* 2010 Jun;36(6):906-16.

[93] Alfonso Jf, Lisa C, Fernandez-Vega L, Madrid-Costa D, Poo-Lopez A, Montes-Mico R. Intrastromal Corneal Ring Segments And Posterior Chamber Phakic Intraocular Lens Implantation For Keratoconus Correction. *J Cataract Refract Surg* 2011 Apr;37(4):706-13.
[94] Kurian M, Nagappa S, Bhagali R, Shetty R, Shetty Bk. Visual Quality After Posterior Chamber Phakic Intraocular Lens Implantation In Keratoconus. *J Cataract Refract Surg* 2012 Jun;38(6):1050-7.
[95] Kymionis Gd, Grentzelos Ma, Karavitaki Ae, Zotta P, Yoo Sh, Pallikaris Ig. Combined Corneal Collagen Cross-Linking And Posterior Chamber Toric Implantable Collamer Lens Implantation For Keratoconus. *Ophthalmic Surg Lasers Imaging* 2011 Feb 17;42 Online:E22-5. Doi: 10.3928/15428877-20110210-05.:E22-E25.
[96] Gonvers M, Bornet C, Othenin-Girard P. Implantable Contact Lens For Moderate To High Myopia: Relationship Of Vaulting To Cataract Formation. *J Cataract Refract Surg* 2003 May;29(5):918-24.
[97] Chung Ty, Park Sc, Lee Mo, Ahn K, Chung Es. Changes In Iridocorneal Angle Structure And Trabecular Pigmentation With Staar Implantable Collamer Lens During 2 Years. *J Refract Surg* 2009 Mar;25(3):251-8.
[98] Mortensen J, Ohrstrom A. Excimer Laser Photorefractive Keratectomy For Treatment Of Keratoconus. *J Refract Corneal Surg* 1994 May;10(3):368-72.
[99] Schmitt-Bernard Cf, Lesage C, Arnaud B. Keratectasia Induced By Laser In Situ Keratomileusis In Keratoconus. *J Refract Surg* 2000 May;16(3):368-70.
[100] Hori-Komai Y, Toda I, Sano-Kato N, Tsubota K. Reasons For Not Performing Refractive Surgery. *J Cataract Refract Surg* 2002 May;28(5):795-7.
[101] Reznik J, Salz Jj, Klimava A. Development Of Unilateral Corneal Ectasia After Prk With Ipsilateral Preoperative Forme Fruste Keratoconus. *J Refract Surg* 2008 Oct;24(8):843-7.
[102] Mortensen J, Carlsson K, Ohrstrom A. Excimer Laser Surgery For Keratoconus. *J Cataract Refract Surg* 1998 Jul;24(7):893-8.
[103] Koller T, Iseli Hp, Donitzky C, Ing D, Papadopoulos N, Seiler T. Topography-Guided Surface Ablation For Forme Fruste Keratoconus. *Ophthalmology* 2006 Dec;113(12):2198-202.
[104] Bahar I, Levinger S, Kremer I. Wavefront-Supported Photorefractive Keratectomy With The Bausch & Lomb Zyoptix In Patients With Myopic Astigmatism And Suspected Keratoconus. *J Refract Surg* 2006 Jun;22(6):533-8.
[105] Cennamo G, Intravaja A, Boccuzzi D, Marotta G, Cennamo G. Treatment Of Keratoconus By Topography-Guided Customized Photorefractive Keratectomy: Two-Year Follow-Up Study. *J Refract Surg* 2008 Feb;24(2):145-9.
[106] Guedj M, Saad A, Audureau E, Gatinel D. Photorefractive Keratectomy In Patients With Suspected Keratoconus: Five-Year Follow-Up. *J Cataract Refract Surg* 2013 Jan;39(1):66-73.
[107] Alpins N, Stamatelatos G. Customized Photoastigmatic Refractive Keratectomy Using Combined Topographic And Refractive Data For Myopia And Astigmatism In Eyes With Forme Fruste And Mild Keratoconus. *J Cataract Refract Surg* 2007 Apr;33(4):591-602.
[108] Gulani Ac, Nordan Lt, Alpins N, Stamatelatos G. Excimer Laser Photorefractive Keratectomy For Keratoconus. In: Wang M, Editor. *Keratoconus & Keratoectasia:*

Prevention, Diagnosis, And Treatment. First Ed. Thorofare: Slack Incorporated; 2009. P. 145-51.
[109] Niziol Lm, Musch Dc, Gillespie Bw, Marcotte Lm, Sugar A. Long-Term Outcomes In Patients Who Received A Corneal Graft For Keratoconus Between 1980 And 1986. *Am J Ophthalmol* 2012 Oct 27;(12):10.
[110] Basu S, Reddy Jc, Vaddavalli Pk, Vemuganti Gk, Sangwan Vs. Long-Term Outcomes Of Penetrating Keratoplasty For Keratoconus With Resolved Corneal Hydrops. *Cornea* 2012 Jun;31(6):615-20.
[111] Pramanik S, Musch Dc, Sutphin Je, Farjo Aa. Extended Long-Term Outcomes Of Penetrating Keratoplasty For Keratoconus. *Ophthalmology* 2006 Sep;113(9):1633-8.
[112] Paglen Pg, Fine M, Abbott Rl, Webster Rg, Jr. The Prognosis For Keratoplasty In Keratoconus. *Ophthalmology* 1982 Jun;89(6):651-4.
[113] Lim L, Pesudovs K, Coster Dj. Penetrating Keratoplasty For Keratoconus: Visual Outcome And Success. *Ophthalmology* 2000 Jun;107(6):1125-31.
[114] Zadok D, Schwarts S, Marcovich A, Barkana Y, Morad Y, Eting E, Et Al. Penetrating Keratoplasty For Keratoconus: Long-Term Results. *Cornea* 2005 Nov;24(8):959-61.
[115] Borderie Vm, Sandali O, Bullet J, Gaujoux T, Touzeau O, Laroche L. Long-Term Results Of Deep Anterior Lamellar Versus Penetrating Keratoplasty. *Ophthalmology* 2012 Feb;119(2):249-55.
[116] Guilbert E, Bullet J, Sandali O, Basli E, Laroche L, Borderie Vm. Long-Term Rejection Incidence And Reversibility After Penetrating And Lamellar Keratoplasty. *Am J Ophthalmol* 2012 Dec 6;(12):10.
[117] Kubaloglu A, Sari Es, Unal M, Koytak A, Kurnaz E, Cinar Y, Et Al. Long-Term Results Of Deep Anterior Lamellar Keratoplasty For The Treatment Of Keratoconus. *Am J Ophthalmol* 2011 May;151(5):760-7.
[118] Polack Fm. Lamellar Keratoplasty. Malbran's "Peeling Off" Technique. *Arch Ophthalmol* 1971 Sep;86(3):293-5.
[119] Barraquer Ji. Lamellar Keratoplasty. (Special Techniques). *Ann Ophthalmol* 1972 Jun;4(6):437-69.
[120] Anwar M. Dissection Technique In Lamellar Keratoplasty. Br J Ophthalmol 1972 Sep;56(9):711-3.
[121] Melles Gr, Lander F, Rietveld Fj, Remeijer L, Beekhuis Wh, Binder Ps. A New Surgical Technique For Deep Stromal, Anterior Lamellar Keratoplasty. *Br J Ophthalmol* 1999 Mar;83(3):327-33.
[122] Amayem Af, Anwar M. Fluid Lamellar Keratoplasty In Keratoconus. Ophthalmology 2000 Jan;107(1):76-9.
[123] Anwar M, Teichmann Kd. Big-Bubble Technique To Bare Descemet's Membrane In Anterior Lamellar Keratoplasty. *J Cataract Refract Surg* 2002 Mar;28(3):398-403.
[124] Parthasarathy A, Por Ym, Tan Dt. Using A "Small Bubble Technique" To Aid In Success In Anwar's "Big Bubble Technique" Of Deep Lamellar Keratoplasty With Complete Baring Of Descemet's Membrane. *Br J Ophthalmol* 2008 Mar;92(3):422.
[125] Fournie P, Malecaze F, Coullet J, Arne Jl. Variant Of The Big Bubble Technique In Deep Anterior Lamellar Keratoplasty. *J Cataract Refract Surg* 2007 Mar;33(3):371-5.
[126] Buzzonetti L, Laborante A, Petrocelli G. Standardized Big-Bubble Technique In Deep Anterior Lamellar Keratoplasty Assisted By The Femtosecond Laser. *J Cataract Refract Surg* 2010 Oct;36(10):1631-6.

[127] Anwar M, Teichmann Kd. Deep Lamellar Keratoplasty: Surgical Techniques For Anterior Lamellar Keratoplasty With And Without Baring Of Descemet's Membrane. *Cornea* 2002 May;21(4):374-83.
[128] Sugita J, Kondo J. Deep Lamellar Keratoplasty With Complete Removal Of Pathological Stroma For Vision Improvement. *Br J Ophthalmol* 1997 Mar;81(3):184-8.
[129] Suwan-Apichon O, Reyes Jm, Griffin Nb, Barker J, Gore P, Chuck Rs. Microkeratome Versus Femtosecond Laser Predissection Of Corneal Grafts For Anterior And Posterior Lamellar Keratoplasty. *Cornea* 2006 Sep;25(8):966-8.
[130] Rama P, Knutsson Ka, Razzoli G, Matuska S, Vigano M, Paganoni G. Deep Anterior Lamellar Keratoplasty Using An Original Manual Technique. *Br J Ophthalmol* 2013 Jan;97(1):23-7.
[131] Unal M, Bilgin B, Yucel I, Akar Y, Apaydin C. Conversion To Deep Anterior Lamellar Keratoplasty (Dalk): Learning Curve With Big-Bubble Technique. *Ophthalmic Surg Lasers Imaging* 2010 Nov;41(6):642-50.
[132] Hosny M. Common Complications Of Deep Lamellar Keratoplasty In The Early Phase Of The Learning Curve. *Clin Ophthalmol* 2011;5:791-5. Doi: 10.2147/Opth.S20943. Epub;%2011 Jun 10.:791-5.
[133] Jones Mn, Armitage Wj, Ayliffe W, Larkin Df, Kaye Sb. Penetrating And Deep Anterior Lamellar Keratoplasty For Keratoconus: A Comparison Of Graft Outcomes In The United Kingdom. *Invest Ophthalmol Vis Sci* 2009 Dec;50(12):5625-9.
[134] Sarayba Ma, Ignacio Ts, Binder Ps, Tran Db. Comparative Study Of Stromal Bed Quality By Using Mechanical, Intralase Femtosecond Laser 15- And 30-Khz Microkeratomes. *Cornea* 2007 May;26(4):446-51.
[135] Tan Dt, Anshu A, Parthasarathy A, Htoon Hm. Visual Acuity Outcomes After Deep Anterior Lamellar Keratoplasty: A Case-Control Study. *Br J Ophthalmol* 2010 Oct;94(10):1295-9.
[136] Busin M, Zambianchi L, Arffa Rc. Microkeratome-Assisted Lamellar Keratoplasty For The Surgical Treatment Of Keratoconus. *Ophthalmology* 2005 Jun;112(6):987-97.
[137] Bahar I, Kaiserman I, Srinivasan S, Ya-Ping J, Slomovic Ar, Rootman Ds. Comparison Of Three Different Techniques Of Corneal Transplantation For Keratoconus. *Am J Ophthalmol* 2008 Dec;146(6):905-12.
[138] Akdemir Mo, Kandemir B, Sayman Ib, Selvi C, Kamil Do. Comparison Of Contrast Sensitivity And Visual Acuity Between Deep Anterior Lamellar Keratoplasty And Penetrating Keratoplasty In Patients With Keratoconus. *Int J Ophthalmol* 2012;5(6):737-41.
[139] Sarnicola V, Toro P, Gentile D, Hannush Sb. Descemetic Dalk And Predescemetic Dalk: Outcomes In 236 Cases Of Keratoconus. *Cornea* 2010 Jan;29(1):53-9.
[140] Feizi S, Javadi Ma, Jamali H, Mirbabaee F. Deep Anterior Lamellar Keratoplasty In Patients With Keratoconus: Big-Bubble Technique. *Cornea* 2010 Feb;29(2):177-82.
[141] Watson Sl, Ramsay A, Dart Jk, Bunce C, Craig E. Comparison Of Deep Lamellar Keratoplasty And Penetrating Keratoplasty In Patients With Keratoconus. *Ophthalmology* 2004 Sep;111(9):1676-82.
[142] Sogutlu Se, Kubaloglu A, Unal M, Pinero Ld, Koytak A, Ofluoglu An, Et Al. Penetrating Keratoplasty Versus Deep Anterior Lamellar Keratoplasty: Comparison Of Optical And Visual Quality Outcomes. *Br J Ophthalmol* 2012 Aug;96(8):1063-7.

[143] Bohringer D, Reinhard T, Spelsberg H, Sundmacher R. Influencing Factors On Chronic Endothelial Cell Loss Characterised In A Homogeneous Group Of Patients. *Br J Ophthalmol* 2002 Jan;86(1):35-8.

[144] Patel Sv, Hodge Do, Bourne Wm. Corneal Endothelium And Postoperative Outcomes 15 Years After Penetrating Keratoplasty. *Trans Am Ophthalmol Soc* 2004;102:57-65; Discussion 65-6.:57-65.

[145] Kanellopoulos Aj. Comparison Of Sequential Vs Same-Day Simultaneous Collagen Cross-Linking And Topography-Guided Prk For Treatment Of Keratoconus. *J Refract Surg* 2009 Sep;25(9):S812-S818.

[146] Spadea L, Paroli M. Simultaneous Topography-Guided Prk Followed By Corneal Collagen Cross-Linking After Lamellar Keratoplasty For Keratoconus. *Clin Ophthalmol* 2012;6:1793-800. Doi: 10.2147/Opth.S37280. Epub;%2012 Nov 2.:1793-800.

In: Current Understanding and New Techniques …
Editor: Michael O'Keefe
ISBN: 978-1-62808-748-2

Chapter 16

Femtosecond Laser Cataract Surgery

Sheraz M. Daya and Marcela Espinosa-Lagana***
Centre for Sight, East Grinstead, UK

Abstract

Femtosecond lasers have been used successfully in corneal surgery for almost a decade. The benefits of the laser have been increased accuracy and reproducibility making surgery more safe and predictable [1 2]. The introduction of accurate anterior segment imaging techniques has now enabled safe use of femtosecond lasers in the anterior segment [3]. Procedures such as capsulotomy and lens fragmentation can now be carried out with confidence and these two areas in particular have facilitated the process of cataract surgery. Other corneal procedures including corneal incisions for entry into the eye [4], limbal relaxing incision and astigmatic keratotomy can also be accomplished at the same time [5]. All these highly reproducible processes have been demonstrated to improve the ease of lens removal with reduced ultrasound times, improved lens centration and refractive predictability [6, 7, 8]. Femtosecond laser cataract surgery is in its relative infancy and in time variations in technique as well as the developments of new implants that take advantage of laser accuracy promise to revolutionise cataract surgery.

Femtosecond lasers uses ultrashort near-infrared (1053nm) pulses to transect or cleave tissue with minimal collateral tissue damage. The short duration of the pulse of the laser (100 femtoseconds = 10^{-13} seconds) enables delivery of high power using low energy and in this way manages to accomplish tissue cleavage without dissipation of energy to the surrounding tissue. The highly focused pulse of energy results in a cavitation of plasma that expands and in doing so cleaves tissue.

The laser has been in use for flap creation since the early 2000s and is now common used in Lasik surgery. The laser is also used for accurate placement of intracorneal rings [9], lamellar [10] and penetrating corneal transplants [11] as well as astigmatic keratotomies [12].

* Address for Correspondence: Sheraz M. Daya, Centre for Sight, Hazelden Place, Turners Hill Road, East Grinstead RH19 4RH, UK, Tel: +44 1342 306028, Email: sdaya@centreforsight.com

More recently the femtosecond laser in combination with accurate anterior segment imaging techniques has been used to perform procedures within the anterior segment including anterior capsulotomy and lens fragmentation [6]. The addition of accurate anterior segment imaging to a femtosecond laser adds a new level of sophistication and complexity. Imaging has to be extremely accurate in terms of measurement and the lasers in turn need to be able to accurately deliver the laser pulses. The interface of the laser to the eye has a considerable impact in accomplishing accurate laser delivery. The ideal imaging system is one that is active and online in case of ocular movement, with automatic localization of anterior segment structures to accurately plan laser delivery. Femtosecond lasers are yet to accomplish this ideal, however in spite of some limitations are able to accomplish the goal of accurate capsulotomy and lens fragmentation. Unlike the creation of flaps, where corneal deformation can be tolerated, laser placement in the anterior segment is prone to error in the presence of corneal deformation. Avoidance of corneal deformation is achieved by either curved applanation with very light docking onto the corneal surface or through the use of a liquid interface between the cornea and the laser.

Conventional cataract surgery involves the following steps: 1) Incisions (typically corneal) 2) Capsulotomy 3) Lens removal 4) Irrigation and aspiration of cortex 5) Lens implantation. The femtosecond laser is able to address two components of the cataract procedure, corneal incisions and anterior capsulotomy as well as a portion of lens removal through lens fragmentation. Correction of astigmatism at the time of cataract surgery is becoming standard practice especially with the use of multifocal lenses and this can also be accomplished using the femtosecond laser which can use its capability of performing corneal incisions in the steep meridian of the cornea. Either astigmatic keratotomy or limbal relaxing incisions can be performed, however the latter is more commonly used for low levels (<2.00D) of astigmatism.

Femtosecond Laser Systems - 2013

Several manufacturers now have lasers in commercial use and they vary in terms of how the laser interfaces to the eye as well as how the anterior segment is imaged. Currently there are four femtosecond lasers commercially available for use in cataract and lens surgery.

Victus Femtosecond Laser (Bausch & Lomb – Technolas Perfect Vision)

The Victus laser (Figure 1) was developed and manufactured by Technolas Perfect Vision, Munich, Germany and acquired in 2013 by Bausch and Lomb. This platform is highly versatile in being able to perform lamellar flaps for Lasik, lamellar and penetrating corneal transplantation, tunnels for intracorneal rings and Intracor, a procedure to correct presbyopia. The laser performs cataract surgery at 80Khz (potentially can be increased to 320KHz) and uses high definition online real-time ocular coherence tomography for imaging the anterior segment (Figure 2). Interfacing the laser to the eye involves a curved applanation interface which is docked lightly on the cornea avoiding deformation.

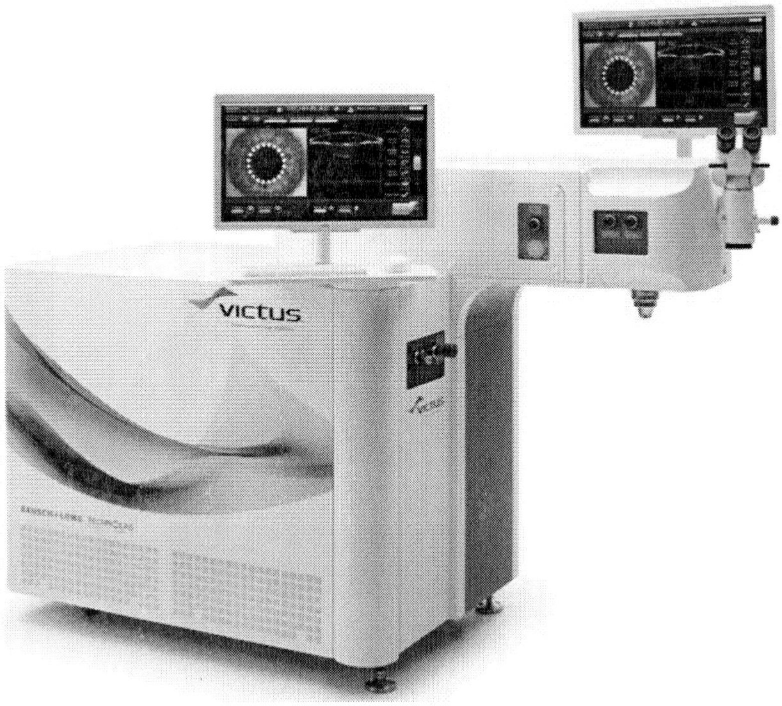

Figure 1. Victus Femtosecond Laser.

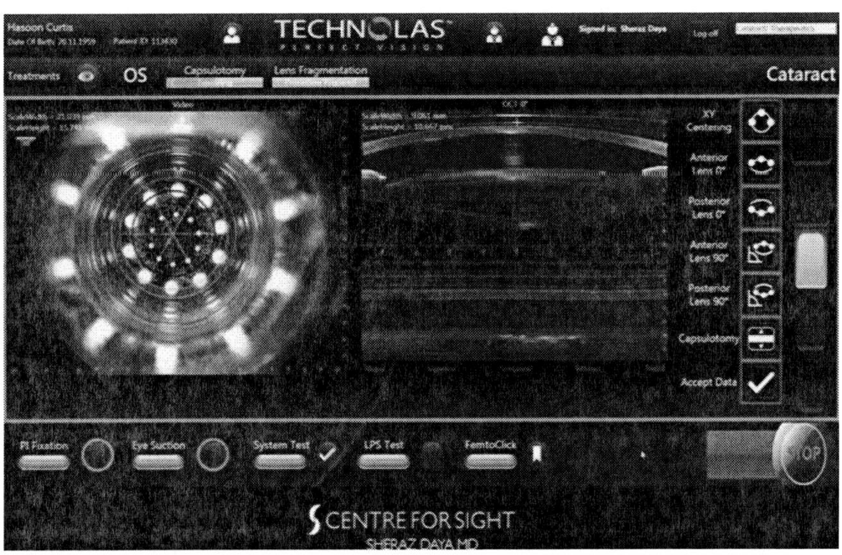

Figure 2. Online real time OCT imaging.

This is assisted by an intelligent pressure sensor mechanism that reduces and equalizes pressure on the corneal surface. With the more recently introduced 12.5mm interface, the laser is capable of performing limbal relaxing incisions, corneal incisions for entry of the phacoemulsification instrumentation. Anterior capsulotomy is performed prior to lens fragmentation. Patterns for fragmentation include rings and radial cuts or a combination. A unique pattern devised by KP Reddy in Hyderabad and called the "Quadrant pattern" (Figure 3) is well suited for hard lenses. A single quadrant has the additional partial ring fragmentation for easy dismantling of the first segment in turn facilitating removal of the remaining segments. While the laser ablation takes place, the OCT image online demonstrates the cross-section cleavage of the anterior capsule as well as lens fragmentation.

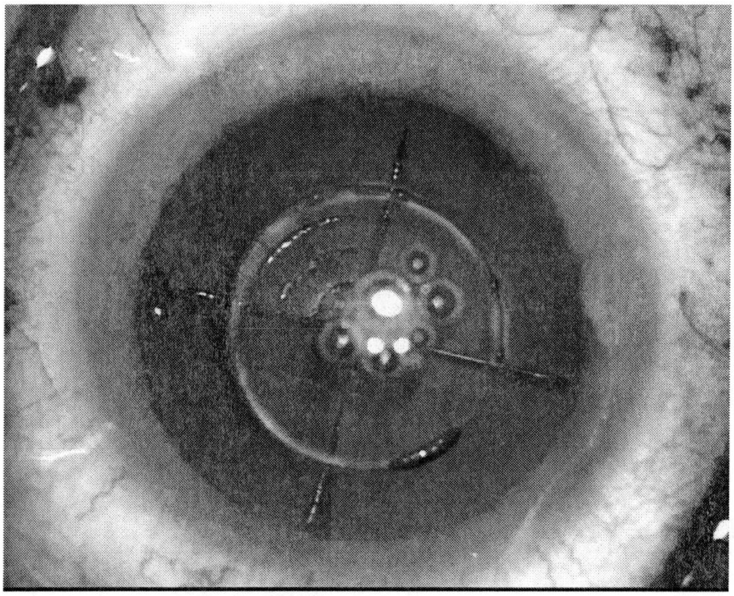

Figure 3. Lens fragmentation – radial and quadrant.

Catalys (Optimedica Corporation, CA, USA)

The Catalys femtosecond laser developed and manufactured by Optimedica Corporation, USA operates at 80KHz and is designed to perform corneal incisions for entry into the anterior chamber, limbal relaxing incision, anterior capsulotomy and lens fragmentation. To avoid corneal deformation, the system uses a proprietary liquid interface "Liquid Optics™". Imaging of the anterior segment is performed using a 3D Fourier-domain OCT imaging system. The software automatically identifies the relevant surfaces within the eye and plans laser delivery accordingly. Lens segmentation includes quadrants as well as grids segmenting the lens into cubes with sizing determined by the surgeon [13].

Lensx (Alcon Laboratories, TX, USA)

This laser was the first commercially available platform to perform femtosecond cataract surgery. The laser operating at 33KHz is able to perform corneal incisions, limbal relaxing incisions, anterior capsulotomy and lens fragmentation. The interface uses a curved applanation to minimise corneal deformation and imaging is by ocular coherence tomography. Like the Victus, the surgeon confirms the location of the anterior and posterior capsule prior to laser delivery.

LensAR (Lensar Inc, FL USA)

The LensAR femtosecond laser uses a proprietary imaging technology that provides a 3 dimensional view of the anterior segment. Called "Augmented Reality" this provides high contrast images that can be used for automated placement of landmarks for surgery. The image is a snapshot view and assumes there has been no movement between image capture and laser delivery. The interface is non-contact and like the Catalys uses liquid to interface between the laser and the eye to avoid corneal deformation. Like the other platforms the laser is able to perform corneal incisions for entry into the eye as well as correction of astigmatism.

Femtosecond Cataract / Lens Surgery

Incision Creation

Clear corneal cataract wound construction can be performed with the femtosecond laser. Masket et al. demonstrated the benefits of reproducible clear corneal stepped incisions in cadaver eyes, providing better strength and stability of the wound incision [4].

Capsulotomy

The precision of the capsulotomy in femtosecond laser cataract surgery changes the paradigm of cataract surgery. The appearance of a perfect circle and often absolutely well centered case after case provides confidence and assurance to the operating surgeon. Moving into an age where lens exchange surgery takes place for patients to avail themselves of the benefits of multifocal and accommodating lenses, the goal is emmetropia with minimal or no tilt to avoid inducement of astigmatism and high order aberrations such as coma. To accomplish this, precise effective lens position (ELP) is necessary with no change during the process of healing. Any procedure that helps accomplish this predictability is very welcome.

Nagy et al. in 2009 provided the first report of the use of the femtosecond laser in cataract surgery [6]. His group demonstrated improved accuracy of capsulotomy size for an intended 5.0mm capsulotomy in the laser group 5.020 (SD04) versus a manual curvilinear capsulorrhexis 5.880 (SD73). Later Nagy et al. and Friedman [14] demonstrated better circularity of a femtosecond laser capsulotomy. Perfectly smooth capsulotomy openings using scanning electron microscopy were described by Nagy et al. [6], Femtosecond laser capsulotomies are also stronger as demonstrated by Friedman who showed increased anterior capsulotomy strength at more than twice that of conventional manual capsulorrhexis [14]. The benefit of a predictable capsulotomy in terms of circularity, centration and size and in turn IOL overlap has been shown to improve lens centration with less decentrations using the femtosecond laser [15]. Sizing of a manual capsulotomy has been demonstrated not to be accurate and influenced by anterior chamber depth. This is possibly due to the effect of variable pupil size and also the influence of magnification where a manual capsulotomy was found to be often larger in myopic eyes [7]. .A larger than expected capsulotomy can lead to a lack of overlap and a reduction in lens stability [7]. Using the Crystalens, Szigeti et al. demonstrated less IOL tilt in cases where a 5.5 mm capsulotomy was performed compared with 6.0mm capsulotomy [16]. Minhaltz et al. demonstrated a significant reduction in internal ocular aberrations in eyes that underwent femtosecond laser cataract surgery in comparison to conventional cataract surgery [17]. They found that the femtosecond laser group had significantly lower values of intraocular vertical tilt (-0.05 +/- 0.36 vs 0.27 +/- 0.57) and coma (-0.003 +/- 0.11 vs 0.1 +/- 0.15). Strehl ratios (0.02 +/- 0.02 vs 0.01 +/- 0.01) and MTF values at all measured cycles per degree were significantly higher in the femtosecond laser group compared to the manual capsulorrhexis group [17]. This finding confirms the advantages of an accurate, well-centred and sized anterior capsulotomy over a manual and conventional approach.

Lens Fragmentation

Another major benefit of the femtosecond laser is its ability to accurately fragment the lens. A variety of patterns have been devised, from simple radial cuts, circular rings, grids and various combinations. Femtosecond laser fragmentation has resulted in a statistically significant reduction in phacoemulsification times with reports of a reduction of 43% reduction in power and 51% reduction in phacoemulsification time [6]. Abell et al. also demonstrated a significant reduction of effective phacoemulsification time (EPT) by 70% in the femtosecond laser group compared to a conventional cataract group ($P=<0.0001$) as well as 26 cases in requiring an EPT of 0 secs compared to only one in the conventional group ($p<0.0001$) [18]. The author using the Victus femtosecond laser compared the phacoemulsification parameters of 108 conventional cataract procedures prior to adoption of femtosecond cataract surgery to the first 108 cases using femtosecond technology and found a statistically significant reduction in ultrasound power, ultrasound time and EPT [19]. Prior fragmentation of the lens is akin to pre-chop described by Akahoshi [20] where the lens is chopped prior to phacoemulsification. Both Akahoshi and others have described reduced phacoemulsification times and rapid removal as a result of prior lens fragmentation [21]. The femtosecond laser provides a reproducible and accurate method of performing fragmentation.

Influence on the Retina

It has been postulated that use of the suction ring on the eye in the process of femtosecond laser cataract surgery might have an adverse influence on the retina and macula in particular [22]. The suction on the eye can theoretically lead to anterior displacement of the posterior segment and traction on the retina by the posterior hyaloid. Whether this has an effect on the retina and predisposes to retinal and macular oedema has been evaluated by Ecsedy and Nagy [22-23]. In a prospective study Ecsedy and co-workers compared the retinal thickness in laser cataract eyes compared with a control of conventional cataract surgery eyes. They found increased retinal thickness in both groups, however statistically significantly greater in the conventional group compared with the laser group [22]. A further study performed by the same group evaluated macular oedema and found that both laser and conventional cataract surgery groups developed early postoperative oedema located in the outer nuclear layer. The increase in thickness was worse in the conventional group. Nagy and colleagues also demonstrated that greater phacoemulsification times did not increase the amount of oedema, thus suggesting conventional cataract surgery disrupts the blood-retinal barrier (BRB) more than laser cataract surgery. This has relevance in those predisposed to disruption such as patients with diabetes as well as prior history of uveitis where use of a femtosecond laser may offer a significant advantage.

Deviations in Technique

The ability to perform a precise capsulotomy along with nuclear fragmentation has resulted in changes in the technique of phacoemulsification. Capsular block syndrome following conventional hydrodissection and loss of lens posteriorly into the vitreous has been described in two cases by Roberts et al. [24]. The cause of this problem was attributed to prior pneumo-dissection and collection of gas behind the lens and compounded by the accumulation of fluid in the capsular bag following conventional hydrodissection. The authors suggested technique changes to avoid this complication including reducing the amount of viscoelastic in the anterior chamber prior to removal of the anterior capsule; decompression of the anterior chamber before and during hydrodissection; decompressing the lens capsule during hydrodissection by elevating the anterior capsule with the cannula; slow hydrodissection gauged by the progression of a fluid wave; and dividing the lens with a chopper prior to hydrodissection. Other surgeons have advocated no hydrodissection and to concentrate on removal of the first fragment followed by shoe-horning each remaining fragment centripetally for removal by phaco-emulsification. Daya noticed when trying to hydrodissect conventionally difficulty in inserting the cannula immediately underneath the anterior capsule. The cortex immediately adjacent to the capsulotomy appeared to have coagulated and "mushroomed" on to the anterior capsule not permitting easy entry. Once entry was made forcefully and fluid injected, there was in effect a peripheral seal between the anterior capsule and cortex that did not permit easy egress of fluid as experienced in conventional cataract surgery. Capsular block with anterior displacement of the lens also occurred further arresting egress of fluid. Avoidance of capsular block can be achieved by the technique of "trans-lenticular hydrodissection" where a cannula is inserted into the fragmentation line of the nucleus and fluid injected. This allows fluid to hydrodissect the lens and for any excess fluid to egress at the point of entry of the cannula with less danger of entrapment [19]. Use of this technique assists in both lens mobilization and fragmentation with reduced phacoemulsification times.

While lens removal times are reduced using laser cataract surgery, cortical clean up is a little more challenging. Because of the remaining safety distance between the posterior extent of laser lens fragmentation and the posterior capsule, more cortex remains following lens removal. This is further affected in cases where the surgeon chooses not to hydrodissect. Additionally the anterior cortex adjacent to the capsulotomy is included during capsulotomy at the same position. Removal of the cortex therefore requires some caution to avoid capturing the anterior capsule in the aspiration port with potential zonular dehiscence. With experience removal of cortex becomes easier. The authors find the use of a bi-axial technique an advantage over a co-axial irrigation-aspiration handpiece.

Complications

Roberts et al. [25] in their first 200 cases reported a high incidence of complications in their initial 50 cases suggesting a steep learning curve. Of the first 200 cases, suction breaks (n=5), anterior capsule tags (10.5%), anterior radial tears (4%), posterior capsular ruptures (3.5%) and dropped nuclei (n=4 2%). These complications reduced considerably in a subsequent report of 1300 further cases by the same group [26]. The above reports illustrate the types of complications that can occur, however the frequency of complications by other femtosecond laser users, even in the early learning curve is not in any way similar and may be a result of better mentoring and caution based on the experiences and reports by early femtosecond laser cataract adopters.

Economics

Many would understandably argue that femtosecond lasers are not essential to providing good cataract surgery. This is possibly correct currently, however some of the advantages illustrated above are quite significant especially for obtaining consistently good visual outcomes. Refractive lens exchange has grown in popularity, mainly because of the advent of improved technology multifocal lenses. Trifocal lenses like the FINEvision (Physiol, Belgium) consistently provide patients with complete spectacle independence. However refractive outcomes are influenced by lens centration, effective lens positioning and the absence of tilt. Absence of cystoid macular oedema is also necessary in obtaining good visual outcomes. The laser has been shown in small studies to be better than conventional cataract / lens surgery.

The cost of the femotosecond laser currently is high and manufacturers are determined to charge a "per click" fee which further influences the cost of the procedure. The lack of a monopoly serves the interests of ophthalmologists and patients well and competition amongst the current four providers with more to follow will in the authors' opinion improve quality of lasers as well as reduce pricing. Meanwhile several economic models are being tested to assess the financial viability of femtosecond lasers.

For the moment the lasers are well positioned to take advantage of the refractive lens exchange market where patients are self paying and not reliant on reimbursement from a third party. As lasers develop and complications are seen to be significantly reduced compared to conventional surgery, a case may well be made for the adoption of lasers in the best interests of patients, like phacoemulsfication 25 years ago. Furthermore with rapid lasers, key use of surgical centre architectural layout and personnel, productivity will in the author's opinion improve and this will ultimately be the business case for acquisition of the laser in high volume cataract centres including the public health system. Finally patient demand is another factor that is likely to influence adoption.

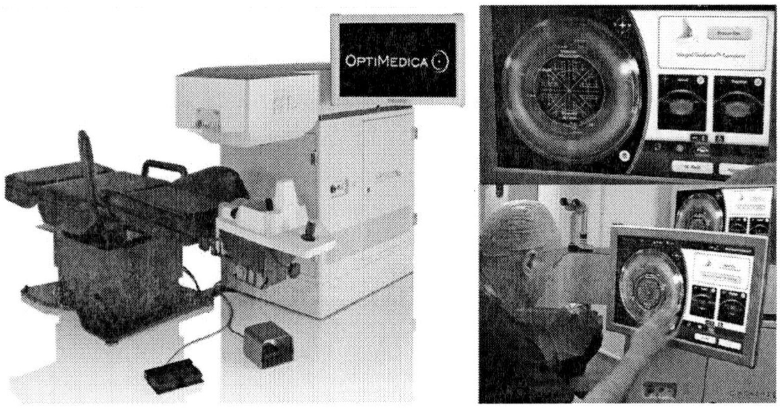

Figure 4. Optimedica Catalys Femtosecond Laser *(Courtesy Julian Stevens FRCOphth).*

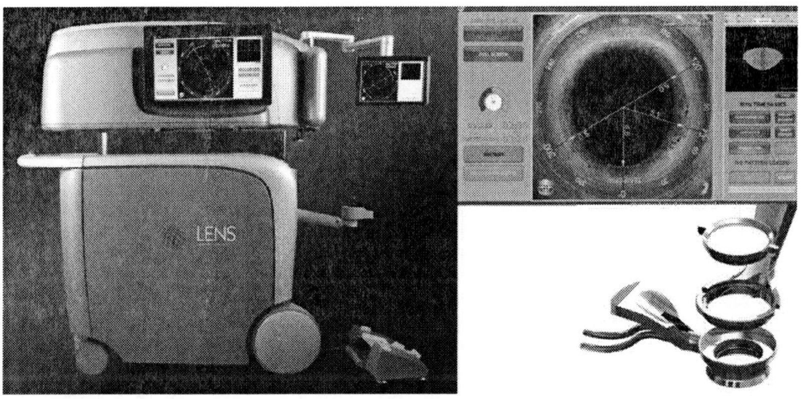

Figure 5. LensAR Femtosecond Laser *(Courtesy Frank Bucci, MD).*

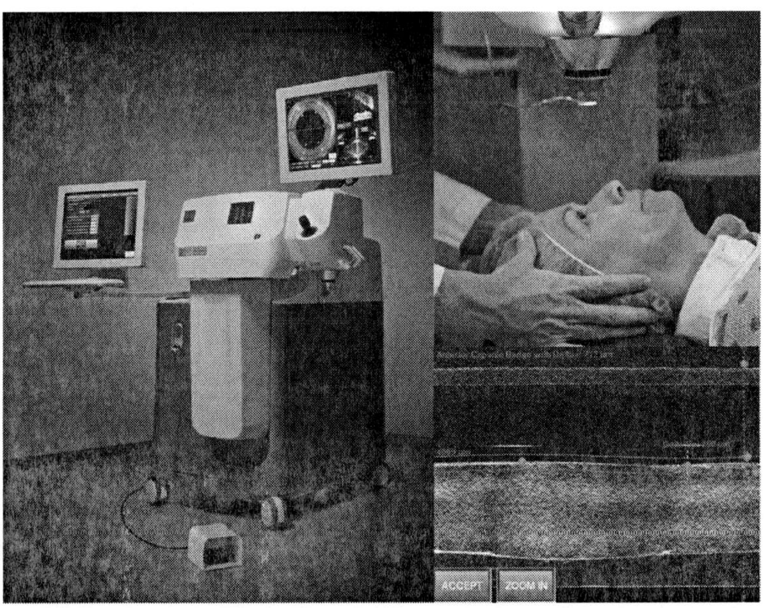

Figure 6. Lensx Femtosecond Laser.

Future

Femtosecond laser cataract surgery is still in its infancy. One has to only look at the evolution of excimer lasers over a two decades to see how technology has changed from what now appears to be very rudimentary to current state of the art technology with customized corrections, rapid delivery along with accurate and highly responsive trackers. Commensurate with the improvements has been an improvement in safety and visual outcomes. Similar evolutionary step changes are anticipated with femtosecond laser cataract surgery. Improvements in imaging with online real time imaging, integration with diagnostic devices to plan accurate astigmatic correction, accurate toric implantation as well as specifically designed intraocular lenses that benefit from the accuracy and reproducibility of the femtosecond laser will completely revolutionise cataract surgery as we know it today. The future looks very bright…

References

[1] Nordan, L. T.; Slade, S. G.; Baker, R. N.; Suarez, C.; Juhasz, T.; Kurtz, R., Femtosecond laser flap creation for laser in situ keratomileusis: six-month follow-up of initial U.S. clinical series. *J. Refract. Surg.* 2003, *19* (1), 8-14.

[2] Kezirian, G. M.; Stonecipher, K. G., Comparison of the IntraLase femtosecond laser and mechanical keratomes for laser in situ keratomileusis. *J. Cataract. Refract. Surg.* 2004, *30* (4), 804-11.

[3] Palanker, D. V.; Blumenkranz, M. S.; Andersen, D.; Wiltberger, M.; Marcellino, G.; Gooding, P.; Angeley, D.; Schuele, G.; Woodley, B.; Simoneau, M.; Friedman, N. J.; Seibel, B.; Batlle, J.; Feliz, R.; Talamo, J.; Culbertson, W., Femtosecond laser-assisted cataract surgery with integrated optical coherence tomography. *Science translational medicine* 2010, *2* (58), 58ra85.

[4] Masket, S.; Sarayba, M.; Ignacio, T.; Fram, N., Femtosecond laser-assisted cataract incisions: architectural stability and reproducibility. *J. Cataract. Refract. Surg.* 2010, *36* (6), 1048-9.

[5] Uy, H. S.; Edwards, K.; Curtis, N., Femtosecond phacoemulsification: the business and the medicine. *Current opinion in ophthalmology* 2012, *23* (1), 33-9.

[6] Nagy, Z.; Takacs, A.; Filkorn, T.; Sarayba, M., Initial clinical evaluation of an intraocular femtosecond laser in cataract surgery. *J. Refract. Surg.* 2009, *25* (12), 1053-60.

[7] Nagy, Z. Z.; Kranitz, K.; Takacs, A. I.; Mihaltz, K.; Kovacs, I.; Knorz, M. C., Comparison of intraocular lens decentration parameters after femtosecond and manual capsulotomies. *J. Refract. Surg.* 2011, *27* (8), 564-9.

[8] (a) Naranjo-Tackman, R., How a femtosecond laser increases safety and precision in cataract surgery? *Current opinion in ophthalmology* 2011, *22* (1), 53-7; (b) Lawless, M.; Bali, S. J.; Hodge, C.; Roberts, T. V.; Chan, C.; Sutton, G., Outcomes of femtosecond laser cataract surgery with a diffractive multifocal intraocular lens. *J. Refract. Surg.* 2012, *28* (12), 859-64.

[9] Ertan, A.; Bahadir, M., Intrastromal ring segment insertion using a femtosecond laser to correct pellucid marginal corneal degeneration. *J. Cataract. Refract. Surg* 2006, *32* (10), 1710-6.

[10] Farid, M.; Steinert, R. F., Deep anterior lamellar keratoplasty performed with the femtosecond laser zigzag incision for the treatment of stromal corneal pathology and ectatic disease. *J. Cataract. Refract. Surg.* 2009, *35* (5), 809-13.

[11] Farid, M.; Kim, M.; Steinert, R. F., Results of penetrating keratoplasty performed with a femtosecond laser zigzag incision initial report. *Ophthalmology* 2007, *114* (12), 2208-12.

[12] Kymionis, G. D.; Yoo, S. H.; Ide, T.; Culbertson, W. W., Femtosecond-assisted astigmatic keratotomy for post-keratoplasty irregular astigmatism. *J. Cataract. Refract. Surg.* 2009, *35* (1), 11-3.

[13] Conrad-Hengerer, I.; Hengerer, F. H.; Schultz, T.; Dick, H. B., Effect of femtosecond laser fragmentation of the nucleus with different softening grid sizes on effective phaco time in cataract surgery. *J. Cataract. Refract. Surg.* 2012, *38* (11), 1888-94.

[14] Friedman, N. J.; Palanker, D. V.; Schuele, G.; Andersen, D.; Marcellino, G.; Seibel, B. S.; Batlle, J.; Feliz, R.; Talamo, J. H.; Blumenkranz, M. S.; Culbertson, W. W., Femtosecond laser capsulotomy. *J. Cataract. Refract. Surg.* 2011, *37* (7), 1189-98.

[15] Kranitz, K.; Takacs, A.; Mihaltz, K.; Kovacs, I.; Knorz, M. C.; Nagy, Z. Z., Femtosecond laser capsulotomy and manual continuous curvilinear capsulorrhexis parameters and their effects on intraocular lens centration. *J. Refract. Surg.* 2011, *27* (8), 558-63.

[16] Szigeti, A.; Kranitz, K.; Takacs, A. I.; Mihaltz, K.; Knorz, M. C.; Nagy, Z. Z., Comparison of long-term visual outcome and IOL position with a single-optic accommodating IOL After 5.5- or 6.0-mm Femtosecond laser capsulotomy. *J. Refract. Surg.* 2012, *28* (9), 609-13.

[17] Mihaltz, K.; Knorz, M. C.; Alio, J. L.; Takacs, A. I.; Kranitz, K.; Kovacs, I.; Nagy, Z. Z., Internal aberrations and optical quality after femtosecond laser anterior capsulotomy in cataract surgery. *J. Refract. Surg.* 2011, *27* (10), 711-6.

[18] Abell, R. G.; Kerr, N. M.; Vote, B. J., Catalys femtosecond laser-assisted cataract surgery compared to conventional cataract surgery. *Clinical & experimental ophthalmology* 2012.

[19] Daya, S. M., Nanvaty M., Espinosa-Lagana, M., , Trans-lenticular hydrodissection, lens fragmentation and influence on ultrasound power in Femtosecond Laser Cataract Surgery. *J. Cataract. Refract. Surg.* 2013, *Submitted for Publication.*

[20] T, A., Phaco prechop: Manual nucleofracture prior to phacoemulsification. . *Op. Tech. Cataract. Ref. Surg.* 1998, *1*, 69-91.

[21] Pereira, A. C.; Porfirio, F., Jr.; Freitas, L. L.; Belfort, R., Jr., Ultrasound energy and endothelial cell loss with stop-and-chop and nuclear preslice phacoemulsification. *J. Cataract. Refract. Surg.* 2006, *32* (10), 1661-6.

[22] Ecsedy, M.; Mihaltz, K.; Kovacs, I.; Takacs, A.; Filkorn, T.; Nagy, Z. Z., Effect of femtosecond laser cataract surgery on the macula. *J. Refract. Surg.* 2011, *27* (10), 717-22.

[23] Nagy, Z. Z.; Ecsedy, M.; Kovacs, I.; Takacs, A.; Tatrai, E.; Somfai, G. M.; Cabrera DeBuc, D., Macular morphology assessed by optical coherence tomography image

segmentation after femtosecond laser-assisted and standard cataract surgery. *J. Cataract. Refract. Surg.* 2012, *38* (6), 941-6.

[24] Roberts, T. V.; Sutton, G.; Lawless, M. A.; Jindal-Bali, S.; Hodge, C., Capsular block syndrome associated with femtosecond laser-assisted cataract surgery. *J. Cataract. Refract. Surg.* 2011, *37* (11), 2068-70.

[25] Roberts, T. V.; Lawless, M.; Chan, C. C.; Jacobs, M.; Ng, D.; Bali, S. J.; Hodge, C.; Sutton, G., Femtosecond laser cataract surgery: technology and clinical practice. *Clinical & experimental ophthalmology* 2012.

[26] Roberts, T. V.; Lawless, M.; Bali, S. J.; Hodge, C.; Sutton, G., Surgical Outcomes and Safety of Femtosecond Laser Cataract Surgery: A Prospective Study of 1500 Consecutive Cases. *Ophthalmology* 2012.

In: Current Understanding and New Techniques …
Editor: Michael O'Keefe
ISBN: 978-1-62808-748-2

Chapter 17

Corneal Grafting

Tim Fulcher
Mater Misericordiae Hospital, Dublin, Ireland

Abstract

This chapter outlines the evolution of corneal graft surgery. It describes the currently used techniques and highlights the advantages and disadvantages of each. It also highlights specific management difficulties that can be encountered. It also outlines methods of dealing with the post-keratoplasty astigmatism.

Introduction

Corneal transplantation has been carried out now for over 100 years. The first human corneal allograft was performed by Zirm in 1905. Slow progress in evolving techniques was then made over the next 50 years. This included lamellar keratoplasties which then went out of favour following the development of a more standardised penetrating keratoplasty technique which allowed for improved quality of vision. Earlier lamellar techniques resulted in an interface scar that limited visual outcomes. Since then, with improved microscopes, instrumentation and materials, techniques have evolved resulting in changing indications and improved outcomes. Over recent years, there has been a significant change in techniques with a return to a variety of lamellar techniques. Newer techniques target only the diseased part of the cornea. The surgery is thus often less invasive and may result in more rapid visual rehabilitation.

The advent of eye banking has allowed corneas to be stored for longer periods before use. This allows for better utilisation of donor material and for planned surgery. Corneas can now be stored in tissue culture for up to six weeks. Prior to eye banking, eyes were harvested within 24 hours post-mortem, and kept in a moist chamber at 4 degrees Celsius for a further 24-48 hours before use. Eye banking also allows for quality assessment of donor material prior to use and more recently for pre-preparation of donor material for endothelial transplantation.

The establishment of corneal graft registries has been paramount in our understanding of graft indications and outcomes. In the United States, the Eye Bank Association of America (EBAA) demonstrates the rapidly changing indications for corneal transplantation and the move to endothelial transplantation. The number of grafts supplied for endothelial keratoplasties increased from 1,429 in 2005 to 18,221 in 2009. At the same time the number of grafts supplied for penetrating keratoplasties reduced from 45,821 in 2005 to 23,269 in 2009. Various graft registries also demonstrate the differing indications for surgery depending on the geographic location. In Australia, the main indication for a graft is keratoconus (31% in 2012) whereas in the US the main indication is Fuch's dystrophy (23.9% in 2009).

Indications for Corneal Grafting

There are many indications for performing corneal graft surgery. The vast majority of these are carried out to improve vision due to corneal pathology. The frequency of indication has changed significantly over the last number of decades. It also varies in different geographic areas.

The main groups of indications include:

- Keratoconus
- Bullous keratopathy
- Failed previous graft
- Corneal dystrophy
- Herpetic eye disease
- Corneal scars and opacities
- Corneal ulcers
- Trauma
- Non-herpetic infections

Less commonly corneal graft surgery is carried out for therapeutic reasons or cosmetic reasons. Therapeutic indications include performing tectonic grafting for corneal perforations or impending perforations. It also includes performing grafting to debride / debulk inflamed corneal tissue unresponsive to medical treatment (such as unresolving fungal keratitis). Corneal grafts can also rarely be performed for cosmetic reason for patients with a white cornea when no improved vision is expected due to either severe amblyopia or posterior segment disease.

Pre-Operative Evaluation

The most important aspect of corneal graft surgery is making the appropriate decision to proceed with surgery in the first place. This decision is based on both local ocular factors as well as general patient factors. This decision is aimed at selecting suitable patients that have a realistic chance of getting a significantly improved outcome. The outcome measure may vary from patient to patient depending on the indication for surgery and the patient's circumstances. Serious consideration should be given before deciding to graft a patient with mild to moderate unilateral corneal disease, when they have a normal fellow eye, especially if the eye is emmetropic. Will the patient really benefit, given the high probability that the patient will require a significant refractive correction in order to get good visual acuity?

Local Ocular Factors

- Diagnosis: The threshold for surgery is lower in patients with conditions with good outcomes. Keratoconus or Fuch's corneal dystrophy patients have excellent outcomes and so should be operated on at an earlier stage than a patient with a vascularised corneal scar secondary to herpetic eye disease.
- Associated ocular co-morbidity: Factors such as corneal vascularisation, glaucoma, uveitis, anterior synechiae, severe dry eyes, eyelid malposition, ocular surface cicatrising conditions all significantly increase the risk of corneal graft failure. The threshold for surgery in these patients should thus be significantly higher. These factors should be addressed as much as is possible before grafting. If risk factors still exist, consideration should be given to performing lamellar graft surgery or the use of immunosuppression.

General Patient Factors

- Patient motivation: It is important that the patient is motivated to undergo the surgery having been counselled about realistic outcome measures. It is important that the patient clearly understands the timeframe involved for visual rehabilitation. Following penetrating keratoplasty, it can be as long as 2 years before a stable refraction is achieved and the patient is fully visually rehabilitated.
- Patient reliability: Post-operative care is probably the most important factor in achieving a good outcome from corneal graft surgery. As a result serious consideration should be given before deciding to perform surgery on a patient who is unreliable. It is essential that patients use their post-operative drops as prescribed and that they attend all post-op outpatient appointments. All patients need to be advised about symptoms of potential complications and have direct telephone access to the clinic so that they can be seen at the earliest opportunity if these symptoms occur. Corneal graft rejection is treatable and reversible. Best outcomes are achieved with early and aggressive treatment. Similarly, loose corneal sutures need to be removed as they may become infected or stimulate corneal graft rejection.
- General medical history: Patients with general medical conditions should be reviewed in a pre-operative anaesthetic clinic to assess their suitability for a general anaesthetic. If the surgery is being carried out under local anaesthetic, the patient needs to be able to lie flat for the length of time needed for the surgery. Other medical issues are also important. Patients with rheumatoid arthritis may have

difficulty putting in eye drops. It is important to ensure that they have someone who can put them in for them. Patients with special needs have poorer outcomes from corneal graft surgery. This may be because putting in drops can be difficult and also because they may present late with complications. The threshold for surgery in these patients groups should thus be higher. However, they should not be excluded from surgery as they can often benefit greatly.

Timing of Surgery

The timing of surgery depends on many factors. It is variable depending on the diagnosis, and also within a group of patients with the same diagnosis. In general, surgery should be delayed for as long as is practically possible as graft survival reduces with time, and the younger the patient has the surgery, the longer it needs to survive. The success rate for repeat grafts reduces with each subsequent graft and so the number of grafts in any one patient needs to be minimised.

Patients with keratoconus should be managed with contact lens wear for as long as possible. Patients with early keratoconus showing signs of progression should undergo corneal cross linking treatment in an attempt to prevent progression and thus alleviate the need for graft surgery in the future. Surgery should be reserved for patients who become contact lens intolerant or who cannot get a good level of vision with contact lenses. In patients with bilateral progressive keratoconus, consideration may be given to earlier surgery in the worst eye, to allow time for visual rehabilitation in that eye before the better eye deteriorates.

The timing of surgery in patients with bullous keratopathy depends on many factors. Surgery for patients with Fuch's dystrophy largely depends on the patient's needs. A young patient who is working and finds driving in the mornings difficult will require surgery at an earlier stage than an elderly patient who is managing very well in their own home environment. This may be similar for patients with pseudophakic bullous keratopathy. These patients will often have a normally seeing fellow eye. The threshold for surgery is thus often higher. Often reserved in some patients for when they complain of pain.

However, the threshold for surgery for endothelial dysfunction has come down significantly since the advent of endothelial transplant surgery. This is because the surgery is less invasive and the visual rehabilitation is much faster.

Choice of Techniques

Penetrating keratoplasty has been the preferred technique for corneal transplantation since the 1950's. This is due to the better quality of vision achieved with it compared to earlier lamellar techniques and to a better understanding of corneal graft rejection and its prevention by the use of steroid eye drops. However, over the last 10 years there has been a significant shift back to lamellar corneal surgery. This is partly due to the limited very long term survival figures for penetrating keratoplasty and partly due to the improved technology and instrumentation allowing for better visual outcomes with lamellar surgery. Early lamellar techniques resulted in irregular surfaces and interface scars which limited visual outcome. Newer techniques can provide almost perfectly smooth interfaces with minimal or no interface scarring. As a result, excellent visual results are achievable.

Available Techniques

- Penetrating keratoplasty.
- Anterior lamellar keratoplasty.
- Posterior lamellar / endothelial keratoplasty.

Penetrating Keratoplasty

Penetrating keratoplasty is the full thickness excision of diseased corneal tissue and replacement with full thickness donor corneal tissue. The aims of surgery are to provide a clear central cornea and to take steps to minimise post-operative refractive errors.

Pre-operatively, ocular surface disease should be optimised. Patients with blepharitis should undergo rigorous eyelid hygiene and have pre-op antibiotic therapy. Patients with ocular surface inflammatory conditions (eg. allergic eye disease) should have this controlled with topical steroids.

The patient's pupil should be constricted pre-operatively with 2% pilocarpine to help protect the lens unless cataract surgery is planned to be performed at the same time. In which case, the pupil is dilated.

Patient preparation is as for all patients undergoing anterior segment surgery. Povidone iodine 5% should be instilled in the conjunctival sac and the eye draped to provide a sterile operating field. A steridrape is used to keep the eyelashes out of the operating field. A speculum is inserted taking care not to place any pressure on the globe.

The centre of the cornea is then marked and a decision is made about what sized graft is to be used. Some surgeons prefer to mark the centre of the pupil as this will centre the graft on the visual axis. However, decentration of a graft places the graft closer to the limbus and may increase the risk of graft rejection. Most grafts are between 7.5-8.5mm. This depends on the patient's corneal diameter, the extent of the corneal pathology and the indication for surgery. In general, patients who are high risk for graft rejection should have a smaller graft performed as a large graft introduces more antigenic material and places it closer to the limbus, thus increasing the risk of rejection. Patients with low risk for graft rejection can have larger grafts done as this probably reduces the amount of post-op astigmatism. A large graft may also be used in patients with endothelial dysfunction to introduce more endothelial cells and increase the chance of success.

The donor corneal is then prepared on a separate trolley. This is usually cut from the endothelial side. This results in a slightly smaller button than achieved when cut from the epithelial side and so the donor should be oversized by 0.25mm. The donor can be cut from the epithelial side with the aid of an artificial anterior chamber. In which case, the donor trephine can be the same size as the recipient trephine. In some patients with advanced keratoconus, the graft may be cut to the same size as the recipient bed, even when cut from the endothelial side, in an attempt to get a flatter corneal profile post-operatively and reduce the degree of myopia. However, care must be taken as this is more likely to result in a leaking corneal wound, and so additional sutures may be required.

The donor button is then covered with the preservation medium or with viscoelastic to protect the endothelium and covered until needed.

The recipient bed is then prepared. This is most commonly done with a disposable vacuum trephine. Care must be taken to ensure the initial placement of the trephine is well centred. This is achieved with the help of a crosswire which is centred on the corneal mark previously made. Centration should be confirmed as parallax errors can occur. Some trephines also have points which can be ink marked to mark the cornea and facilitate suture placement. The trephination is then carried out. Once the anterior chamber is entered, the suction is released to minimise the risk of damage to the iris or lens. The corneal excision is completed with curved corneal scissors. The scissors should be kept perpendicular to the wound to ensure a square edge for good wound apposition. This helps minimise post-operative astigmatism. Some surgeons leave a small rim at the posterior edge of the wound to facilitate wound closure and reduce the chances of a wound leak.

The anterior chamber is then filled with viscoelastic and the donor button placed into the wound taking care not to touch the endothelium. The graft is sutured in place using 10/0 or 11/0 nylon or polypropylene sutures. Four cardinal sutures are initially placed at the 12, 3, 6 and 9 o'clock positions. These sutures are the most important to ensure good placement of the graft. The graft and sutures should be inspected at this stage to ensure these sutures are well placed. Any poorly placed sutures should be removed and replaced. Suturing of the graft should then be completed with 12 further interrupted sutures or a continuous suture. Some surgeons use a combination of interrupted and continuous sutures. Interrupted sutures should be used in patients with any risk factors that may result in loosening of sutures at an early stage. Continuous sutures may be considered for patients with low risk graft failure. The benefit of a continuous suture is that it allows for post-operative suture adjustments. This may help reduce the amount of post-op astigmatism giving the patient better vision at an earlier stage. The main disadvantage is that the whole suture may need to be replaced if it becomes loose or breaks during a suture adjustment.

At the end of surgery, a keratometer may be used to facilitate intra-operative continuous suture adjustment or to identify any particularly tight or loose interrupted sutures that should then be replaced.

Anterior Lamellar Keratoplasty

Anterior lamellar keratoplasty should be considered in patients with stromal conditions in which there is a normally functioning endothelium. This includes anterior stromal scars following corneal infections, anterior stromal dystrophies and keratoconus.

The main advantage of anterior lamellar keratoplasty is the elimination of the risk of endothelial rejection, which remains the commonest cause for graft failure following penetrating keratoplasty. This is particularly important in vascularised corneal scars that would otherwise be at high risk for rejection. Other advantages include the fact that it is an extraocular procedure and consequently there is a lower risk of other complications occurring, including endophthalmitis and suprachoroidal haemorrhage. The eye is also tectonically stronger. This is important in young, active patients who may still engage in certain sporting activities. Lamellar grafting is also a good option for poorly compliant patients. It also allows the use of larger diameter grafts. This may help reduce the amount of post-operative astigmatism.

There are a number of methods used for anterior lamellar keratoplasty:

Manual lamellar keratoplasty. This is the originally described method, where a trephine is used to cut down to the desired depth, and then a lamellar dissection is performed manually. Care is taken to follow the natural lamellar planes. This is best achieved using a semi-sharp lamellar dissector. With better instrumentation and microscopes, a smoother bed can be achieved than by originally described methods many years ago. This results in less interface scarring, but some scarring will occur, resulting in poorer quality vision than can be achieved with penetrating keratoplasties. Further lamellar dissections can be performed on the bed if required until the desired depth is achieved. This can be facilitated by hydrating the bed with a balanced salt solution if required. This thickens the residual stromal bed and makes further dissection easier.

The donor graft is then prepared in the same way using an artificial anterior chamber and trephining down to the same depth as performed in the recipient bed.

Femtosecond lasers can now assist in cutting both the donor and recipient corneas. This is an emerging technology that can result in more precise lamellar dissections that should leave a smoother interface. This may result in better quality of vision due to reduced interface scarring.

Deep anterior lamellar keratoplasty (DALK). This describes removing all the corneal stroma down to Descemet's membrane. This results in a much smoother interface with no interface scar. Visual acuities similar to post penetrating keratoplasty can be achieved. This is performed by forcefully injecting air into the deep corneal stroma (Anwar's big bubble technique), or viscoelastic, to strip Descemet's membrane from the posterior corneal stroma. The resulting cleavage plane allows for an easier manual dissection of the corneal stroma leaving a bare Descemet's membrane. The main technical difficulty with this method is the risk of rupturing Descemet's membrane. This may occur at the time of the air injection or during the manual removal of the stroma. A significant sized perforation will result in the need to convert to a penetrating keratoplasty. A small perforation may be managed by injecting air into the anterior chamber and the patient posturing supine post-operatively to ensure attachment of Descemet's membrane. The technical difficulty associated with this technique, have limited its widespread use.

A full thickness donor button can then be sutured in place following removal of Descemet's membrane and the endothelium. This is easily performed with the help of a lint free sponge and fine forceps. The donor button should again be oversized by 0.25mm to allow for good wound apposition.

Microkeratome assisted anterior lamellar keratoplasty. Microkeratomes are used regularly to perform LASIK. They create a very smooth lamellar corneal plane which heals with negligible interface scarring. As a result, they have been used to assist anterior lamellar keratoplasties. They are limited by the size of heads available on the keratomes and so they can only be used for more superficial corneal pathology. The same head is then used to cut the donor using an artificial anterior chamber. The main disadvantage of this method is that the trephination may result in slightly different sized cuts, which causes a mismatch of the donor and host bed. This can result in delayed healing and epithelial ingrowth between the graft and host.

Posterior Lamellar / Endothelial Keratoplasty

Descemet's stripping (automated) endothelial keratoplasty (DS(A)EK) has rapidly become the procedure of choice for endothelial cell dysfunction. The advent of this procedure has resulted in a huge reduction in the number of penetrating keratoplasties performed in the US, from over 45,000 to less than 25,000 in just a 4 year period, between 2005 and 2009. At the same time, the number of endothelial keratoplasties increased from less than 1500 to over 18,000.

The main advantages of endothelial keratoplasty include the fact that it is performed through a small 4-5mm incision. This may be sutureless or may require minimal suturing. As a result, there is minimal induced astigmatism. The anterior corneal profile is also unchanged and so there is a minimal refractive change. This allows for rapid visual rehabilitation. A stable refractive outcome is usually achieved within 3 months. The eye is also tectonically stronger due to the small incision, allowing patient to return to work and physical activity at an earlier stage. There is also a suggestion that there may be a lower incidence of rejection due the presence of less transplanted tissue.

The main disadvantage of this procedure is the endothelial cell loss associated with inserting the donor graft which may result in primary graft failure. This has resulted in evolving techniques aimed at protecting the endothelium of the graft. The original technique described folding the graft in the so-called taco folding technique. The folding has been shown to damage the endothelium at the places where the inserting forceps grasp the donor. Techniques are evolving to develop methods to minimise iatrogenic endothelial cell loss. Many surgeons now use a pull through technique using a modified forceps to pull the graft into the anterior chamber from a glide or inserting device.

Technique

The corneal epithelium is marked with ink to define the size of graft to be used. A superior or temporal 4-5mm sclero-corneal tunnel is fashioned. An anterior chamber maintainer is inserted through a separate paracentesis. The endothelium can be stained with vision blue to facilitate visualisation. This is not always required, particularly in patients with Fuch's dystrophy when it is easily seen. The anterior chamber is then filled with viscoelastic or air. Descemet's membrane and the endothelium are then cut using a blunt tipped instrument at the marked diameter. This is then gently stripped and removed. The visco-elastic is then removed completely. If air is used, then an air-fluid exchange is performed.

The donor button is prepared using a keratome to cut to a depth of about 350 microns. The stroma is marked to aid orientation when the graft is in the eye. The posterior cornea is then trephined to the desired diameter. This may be pre-prepared in some eye banks.

The donor button is then inserted into the eye and filtered air in injected under the graft. The wounds are then made air tight. The graft is centred and then more air is injected into the anterior chamber with a 30G needle under the graft until a complete air fill and a firm pressure is achieved. Venting incisions may be performed in the mid peripheral cornea to aid drainage of interface fluid and to aid centration of the graft. Further interface fluid is removed with the aid of a LASIK roller. Most surgeons then wait for a period of between 5-20 minutes to ensure good adhesion of the graft. Some of the air is then released to lower the intraocular pressure to less than 20mmHg. The pupil is dilated with atropine 1% to prevent pupil block. The patient remains supine until the next morning.

Donor dislocation may occur the next morning in up to 50% of cases. With more experience and evolving techniques, this incidence has reduced. However, cases of graft dislocation will require reattachment with further injections of air with or without repositioning of the graft. This results in further endothelial cell loss and an increased incidence of primary graft failure.

Post-Operative Management

Good post-operative management following a corneal graft is essential to optimise the chances of long term graft survival. The general principles of management are the same for all methods of corneal graft. Certain differences will be highlighted below that are specific for different techniques.

Immediate Post-op Management

At the end of surgery, a subconjunctival injection of dexamethasone and an antibiotic are usually administered. A topical mydriatic may be applied in patients that there is a risk of pupil block. Topical or systemic analgesia should be given to facilitate pain relief. Systemic carbonic anhydrase should be considered for patients with pre-existing glaucoma or in whom intracameral viscoelastic material may have been left in. The eye should be covered with a pressure pad until the following morning. Patients who have had a DSEK procedure should be postured supine.

If the patient experiences severe pain, and/or nausea, during the first day after surgery, the dressing should be removed and the eye assessed. Particular attention should be paid to the intraocular pressure as this can become very high resulting in a fixed dilated pupil from iris ischaemia.

Early Post-op Management

The first routine post-operative check should be performed within the first 24 hours. At this stage, particular attention is paid to the wound integrity and intraocular pressure. A small wound leak may often be managed conservatively. This may be facilitated by replacing a pressure pad or a bandage contact lens. High intraocular pressure is usually managed with carbonic anhydrase inhibitors, alpha agonists and/or beta blockers. In patients having undergone a DSEK procedure, attachment of the graft is assessed. Non primary attachment requires further injection of filtered air into the anterior chamber below the graft, with or without repositioning of the graft. This is usually best done in the operating theatre, but partial non attachments may be managed at the slit lamp.

Patients should be commenced on steroid eye drops at least four times daily. Patients at high risk for rejection or patients with significant ocular inflammation should use them more frequently, up to one hourly. Systemic steroids may also be considered for high risk patients.

Patients should also be commenced on broad spectrum antibiotic eye drops four times daily. Systemic antiviral therapy should be commenced in patients undergoing surgery following herpes simplex keratitis.

Topical lubricants should be considered in some patients. Preservative free drops are preferable as this should facilitate epithelialisation.

Intermediate Post-op Management

Topical antibiotic therapy should be discontinued once the graft has fully epithelialized. Prolonged use may cause toxicity to the graft and may also encourage the development of resistant infections. Topical antibiotics should be re-introduced at any stage following suture manipulation or removal.

Topical steroid therapy should be continued in most patients for a minimum of six months. This is usually four times daily for the first three months, and then tapered down over the following three months. Patients who have undergone anterior lamellar grafting can stop steroids at a much earlier stage as they are not at risk of endothelial rejection. High risk patients for rejection may require longer term topical steroid therapy. Sometimes this may be lifelong.

Frequent post-operative outpatient visits are required. The minimum number of post-op reviews should be at one week, one month, three months and six months. Additional visits will often be required depending on many factors.

At each visit, the examination should include: visual acuity, refraction or keratometry, slit lamp examination to inspect the sutures and graft clarity and the intraocular pressure checked. The use of ultrasound pachymetry can be helpful to monitor clearing of the graft, particularly in endothelial grafts.

The patient's vision will often be quite poor at the earlier post-op visits due to lack of graft clarity or to astigmatism. Once the graft has cleared and an accurate measure of refraction and keratometry can be made, usually 2-4 weeks, suture adjustments can be made in an attempt to reduce the early astigmatism and improve vision. Caution should be taken about removing interrupted sutures at such an early stage as this may result in wound dehiscence. Certainly very loose sutures should be removed. Individual, very tight sutures can be removed, but these should probably be left until a later stage. Continuous sutures (single or double running) or combined interrupted and continuous suturing techniques allow for early suture adjustments. This is performed at the slit lamp under topical anaesthesia. Using a plain tying forceps, the suture is gathered from the flat axis and rotated to the steep axis. Care must be taken as it is possible to break the suture. The entire graft would then need to be re-sutured. A slit lamp keratometer is used to monitor the induced effect of the suture adjustment, and further adjustments are made until the graft appears regular. The patient can then be re-refracted and the change in refraction noted. Small adjustments in the early post-op period can result in big refractive changes. Topical antibiotics must be used for a week after the adjustment to prevent infections as the epithelium has been disrupted. The patient should then be review a few weeks later when further adjustments can be made if necessary.

The first six months following corneal graft surgery is the period that the graft is at the highest risk of rejection or infection. Consequently, patients must be aware of any symptoms and signs of these, and need to have a rapid access route to be seen in the event that they occur. Any patient presenting with symptoms of a red eye, a painful eye or reduced vision should be seen immediately. The key to managing corneal graft rejection is early recognition with prompt and aggressive treatment. Treatment should include using topical dexamethasone 0.1% hourly, subconjunctival dexamethasone injection and systemic steroids. Early treatment can result in reversal of the rejection episode and survival of the graft. Any precipitating factors, such as loose sutures, must be dealt with at the same time.

Late Post-op Management

Late post-operative management is mainly focused on visual rehabilitation. The main factor limiting post-op vision is the presence of significant amounts of astigmatism. The development of astigmatism is multifactorial and includes pre-op, intra-op and post-op factors.

The management of post-op astigmatism is initially based on suture management. Early suture adjustments can be performed as described above to reduce early astigmatism and attempt to give the patient better early visual acuity. However, significant changes in refraction can occur post suture removal, even when removed several years post-operatively.

When interrupted sutures are used, selective suture removal will flatten the steep axis. Care should be taken not to remove them too early, as early suture removal may weaken the wound integrity. Unless the sutures are very tight, it is usually better to wait for six months before selective suture removal. Similarly, the timing for complete suture removal or removal of a continuous suture should not be removed for a minimum of one year. Suture removal before this can result in wound dehiscence and ectasia with resultant high levels of astigmatism.

In patients who have good levels of visual acuity, sutures can be left in for longer. However, all sutures should ultimately be removed as the sutures will degrade and may become loose or break which may result in suture related infections or rejection of the graft.

Following suture removal, it is necessary to wait for a few months for the refraction to stabilise before further visual rehabilitation. Visual recovery is much more rapid following a DSEK procedure as there is less induced astigmatism. Usually the patient's refraction is stable after about three months.

Once the refraction is stable, most patients' require refractive correction. Small corrections can be corrected with glasses. Higher degrees of astigmatism will require contact lenses. Rigid gas permeable contact lenses are usually the preferred option, but toric soft lenses may be used. When the astigmatism is greater than six dioptres, it is difficult to fit contact lenses, and a refractive surgery procedure should be considered.

Refractive surgery procedures can be divided into compression techniques, relaxation techniques, excimer laser procedures or refractive lens procedures.

Compression techniques include the use of compression sutures or wedge resections. Compression sutures involve placing interrupted sutures on the flat axis with resultant corneal steepening. Wedge resections involve excising a crescentic wedge from either the donor or host interface and the resuturing the wound. This can be useful for very high degrees of astigmatism, but the results are often unpredictable.

Relaxing techniques usually involve the use of arcuate keratotomy (AK) incisions. These are placed on the steep axis at either the graft interface or just inside the interface. This will result in flattening of steep axis. The degree of correction can be variable and depends on the length of the incision, the depth of the incision, the distance from the visual axis and the number of cuts. Despite this, the effect can often be quite unpredictable. Relaxing incisions can be coupled with compression sutures in very high levels of astigmatism.

Excimer laser procedures can be used to reduce both the spherical and the astigmatic components of the refractive error. The effect on the spherical component is more predictable. PRK, LASEK and LASIK procedures have all been used. Surface ablations can be complicated by the development of significant haze. Intra-op application of mitomycin C has been shown to reduce this significantly. LASEK procedures are more likely to have flap related complications. The use of the femtosecond laser is more predictable and helps to minimise this. The effect of the cutting the flap may induce some refractive change, so some centres advocate preforming LASEK as a 2-step procedure.

Refractive lens procedures include the use of phakic intra-ocular lenses or refractive cataract surgery. Some patients will develop cataracts. This may be as a consequence of their surgery, their underlying condition, the use of prolonged steroid drops or simply age related. Removal of the cataract is an opportunity to accurately correct any refractive error. This will usually involve the use of toric intra-ocular lenses. In the absence of cataract, the use of phakic intra-ocular lenses can be used to correct any ametropia. This is particularly useful in pre-presbyopic patients in order to maintain their accommodation.

Conclusion

Despite many advances in surgical techniques for corneal graft surgery and a better understanding of the pathophysiology of wound healing and corneal graft rejection, the management of corneal graft patients still requires meticulous attention. With appropriate patient selection, appropriate selection of surgical technique and appropriate post-operative management the success rates for corneal grafting can be optimised.

References

Acar BT, Utine CA, Acar S, Ciftci F. Laser in situ keratomileusis to manage refractive errors after deep anterior lamellar keratoplasty. J Cataract Refract Surg. 2012 Jun;38(6):1020-7.

Al-Yousuf N, Mavrikakis I, Mavrikakis E, Daya SM. Penetrating keratoplasty: indications over a 10 year period. *Br. J. Ophthalmol.,* 2004 Aug;88(8):998-1001.

Anwar M, Teichmann KD. Big-bubble technique to bare Descemet's membrane in anterior lamellar keratoplasty. *J. Cataract. Refract. Surg.,* 2002 Mar;28(3):398-403.

Arenas E, Esquenazi S, Anwar M, Terry M. Lamellar corneal transplantation. *Surv. Ophthalmol.,* 2012 Nov;57(6):510-29.

Birnbaum F, Wiggermann A, Maier PC, Böhringer D, Reinhard T. Clinical results of 123 femtosecond laser-assisted penetrating keratoplasties. *Graefes Arch. Clin. Exp. Ophthalmol.,* 2013 Jan;251(1):95-103.

Buratto L, Böhm E. The use of the femtosecond laser in penetrating keratoplasty. *Am. J. Ophthalmol.,* 2007 May;143(5):737-742.

Busin M, Scorcia V, Zambianchi L, Ponzin D. Outcomes from a modified microkeratome-assisted lamellar keratoplasty for keratoconus. *Arch. Ophthalmol.,* 2012 Jun;130(6):776-82.

Ghaznawi N, Chen ES. Descemet's stripping automated endothelial keratoplasty: innovations in surgical technique. *Curr. Opin. Ophthalmol.,* 2010 Jul;21(4):283-7.

Ghosheh FR, Cremona FA, Rapuano CJ, Cohen EJ, Ayres BD, Hammersmith KM, Raber IM, Laibson PR. Trends in penetrating keratoplasty in the United States 1980-2005. *Int. Ophthalmol.,* 2008 Jun;28(3):147-53. Review.

Gorovoy MS. Descemet-stripping automated endothelial keratoplasty. *Cornea.* 2006 Sep;25(8):886-9.

Huang T, Zhang X, Wang Y, Zhang H, Huand A, Gao N. Outcomes of deep anterior lamellar keratoplasty using the big-bubble technique in various corneal diseases. *Am. J. Ophthalmol., 2012* Aug;154(2):282-289.

Jain S, Azar DT. New lamellar keratoplasty techniques: posterior keratoplasty and deep lamellar keratoplasty. *Curr. Opin. Ophthalmol.,* 2001 Aug;12(4):262-8.Review.

Jonas JB. Corneal endothelial transplantation using femtosecond laser technology. *Eye.* 2004 Jun;18(6):657-8.

Kang PC, Klintworth GK, Kim T, Carlson AN, Adelman R, Stinnett S, Afshari NA. Trends in the indications for penetrating keratoplasty, 1980-2001. *Cornea,* 2005 Oct;24(7):801-3.

Kaufman HE, Beuerman RW, Steinemann TL, Thompson TL, Varnell ED. Optisol corneal storage medium. *Arch. Ophthalmol.,* 1991;109,864-868.

Keenan TD, Jones MN, Rushton S, Carley FM; National Health Service Blood and Transplant Ocular Tissue Advisory Group and Contributing Ophthalmologists (Ocular Tissue Advisory Group Audit Study 8). Trends in the indications for corneal graft surgery in the United Kingdom: 1999 through 2009. *Arch. Ophthalmol.,* 2012 May 1;130(5):621-8.

Li JY, Terry MA, Goshe J, Davis-Boozer D, Shamie N. Three-year visual acuity outcomes after Descemet's stripping automated endothelial keratoplasty. *Ophthalmology,* 2012 Jun;119(6):1126-9.

Maeno A, Naor J, Lee HM, Hunter WS, Rootman DS. Three decades of corneal transplantation: indications and patient characteristics. *Cornea,* 2000 Jan;19(1):7-11.

McCarey BE, Kaufman HE. Improved corneal storage. Invest Ophthalmol. 1974;13,165-173.

Melles GR. Posterior lamellar keratoplasty: DLEK to DSEK to DMEK. *Cornea,* 2006 Sep;25(8):879-81.

Melles GR, Lander F, Nieuwendaal C. Sutureless, posterior lamellar keratoplasty: a case report of a modified technique. *Cornea,* 2002 Apr;21(3):325-7.

Melles GR, Lander F, Rietveld FJ. Transplantation of Descemet's membrane carrying viable endothelium through a small scleral incision. *Cornea,* 2002 May;21(4):415-8.

Melles GR, Lander F, Rietveld FJ, Remeijer L, Beekhuis WH, Binder PS. A new surgical technique for deep stromal, anterior lamellar keratoplasty. *Br. J. Ophthalmol.,* 1999 Mar;83(3):327-33.

Moorthy S, Graue E, Jhanji V, Constantinou M, Vajpayee RB. Microbial keratitis after penetrating keratoplasty: impact of sutures. Am J Ophthalmol. 2011 Aug;152(2):189-194.

Paufique L. Indications for the therapeutic lamellar corneal graft. *Am. J. Ophthalmol.,* 1950 Mar;33(3 Pt. 2):24.

Price FW Jr, Price MO. Descemet's stripping with endothelial keratoplasty in 50 eyes: a refractive neutral corneal transplant. *J. Refract. Surg.,* 2005 Jul-Aug;21(4):339-45.

Price MO, Price FW Jr. Descemet's stripping with endothelial keratoplasty: comparative outcomes with microkeratome-dissected and manually dissected donor tissue. *Ophthalmology,* 2006 Nov;113(11):1936-42.

Rahman I, Carley F, Hillarby C, Brahma A, Tullo AB. Penetrating keratoplasty: indications, outcomes, and complications. *Eye,* 2009 Jun;23(6):1288-94.

Sharif KW, Casey TA. Changing indications for penetrating keratoplasty, 1971-1990. *Eye,* 1993;7 (Pt 4):485-8.

Shimmura S, Tsubota K. Deep anterior lamellar keratoplasty. *Curr. Opin. Ophthalmol.,* 2006 Aug;17(4):349-55.

Szczotka LB, Lindsay RG. Contact lens fitting following corneal graft surgery. *Clin. Exp. Optom.,* 2003 Jul;86(4):244-9. Review.

Tan DT, Anshu A, Parthasarathy A, Htoon HM. Visual acuity outcomes after deep anterior lamellar keratoplasty: a case-control study. *Br. J. Ophthalmol.,* 2010 Oct;94(10):1295-9.

Tan DT, Anshu A. Anterior lamellar keratoplasty: 'Back to the Future'- a review. *Clin. Experiment. Ophthalmol.,* 2010 Mar;38(2):118-27.

Tan DT, Dart JK, Holland EJ, Kinoshita S. Corneal transplantation. *Lancet,* 2012 May 5;379(9827):1749-61.

Terry MA. Endothelial replacement: the limbal pocket approach. *Ophthalmol. Clin. North Am.,* 2003 Mar;16(1):103-12. Review.

Terry MA. A new approach for endothelial transplantation: deep lamellar endothelial keratoplasty. *Int. Ophthalmol. Clin.,* 2003 Summer;43(3):183-93. Review.

Thompson RW Jr, Price MO, Bowers PJ, Price FW Jr. Long-term graft survival after penetrating keratoplasty. *Ophthalmology,* 2003 Jul;110(7):1396-402.

Tourtas T, Laaser K, Bachmann BO, Cursiefen C, Kruse FE. Descemet membrane endothelial keratoplasty versus descemet stripping automated endothelial keratoplasty. *Am. J. Ophthalmol.,* 2012 Jun;153(6):1082-90.

Troutman RC. Corneal wedge resections and relaxing incisions for post-keratoplasty astigmatism. *Int. Ophthalmol. Clin.,* 1983;23,161-168.

Wietharn BE, Driebe WT Jr. Fitting contact lenses for visual rehabilitation after penetrating keratoplasty. *Eye Contact Lens,* 2004 Jan;30(1):31-3.

Wiley LA, Joseph MA, Springs CL. Tectonic lamellar keratoplasty utilizing a microkeratome and an artificial anterior chamber system. *Cornea,* 2002 Oct;21(7):661-3.

Zirm E. Eine erfolgreiche totale Keratoplastik. *Archiv. Ophthalmol.,* 1906;64:580-593.

About the Editor

Michael O Keefe first performed PRK twenty one years ago. Since then he has performed thousands of refractive procedures. He has been at the forefront of the newer techniques and is constantly pushing the boundaries. He has published many peer review papers and trained many ophthalmologist.

Professor O Keefe is also a paediatric ophthalmologist and has led the way on the use of refractive surgeries in paediatrics. He is actively involved in opening up new boundaries in presbyopia.

Index

A

acetylcholine, 207, 209
acid, 49
acne, 46
adaptation, 88, 228
adhesion, 28, 288
ADR, 153
adults, 89, 92, 93, 94, 96, 97, 99, 101, 103, 105, 106, 107, 179
advancements, 55, 92, 157, 162, 233
adverse effects, 213, 251
adverse event, 3, 152, 216, 239
aetiology, 82, 245, 246
age, 32, 38, 42, 45, 55, 56, 57, 58, 61, 63, 65, 75, 76, 80, 83, 93, 96, 97, 98, 99, 102, 105, 106, 108, 118, 129, 131, 140, 145, 156, 159, 169, 170, 173, 215, 229, 236, 240, 246, 248, 252, 255, 273, 292
aging population, 243
agonist, 48
albinism, 104, 111
alcohol exposure, 3, 18
algorithm, 69, 117, 198, 233
allergy, 5, 6, 7
amblyopia, 74, 75, 86, 89, 92, 94, 96, 98, 99, 101, 102, 103, 104, 108, 109, 112, 113, 149, 215, 251, 282
ametropia, 32, 92, 94, 103, 105, 109, 155, 157, 172, 175, 178, 201, 215, 229, 254, 292
amplitude, 79, 83, 85, 131
anatomy, 60
androgen, 38, 49
angulation, 99
anhydrase, 289
antibiotic, 7, 30, 285, 289, 290
antibiotic eye drops, 290
antidepressants, 50, 53, 76
anti-glaucoma, 8, 15
antihistamines, 38
anti-inflammatories, 212
anti-inflammatory agents, 4, 46, 49
anti-inflammatory drugs, 19
antimicrobial therapy, 7, 11
antispasmodics, 38
antiviral therapy, 290
apex, 32, 190, 196, 247
apoptosis, 40, 51, 64
argon, 21
arithmetic, 124, 191, 295
Artisan, 93, 101, 102, 109, 184, 203, 205, 206, 207, 212, 213, 216, 217, 218, 254, 263
Asia, 93
aspiration, 270, 275
assault, 146
assessment, 22, 32, 38, 40, 57, 62, 69, 74, 86, 88, 122, 133, 152, 221, 222, 228, 254, 281
asthma, 246
astigmatism, 15, 18, 22, 27, 32, 53, 55, 56, 58, 63, 65, 92, 104, 107, 112, 117, 128, 129, 143, 159, 160, 162, 171, 177, 179, 180, 182, 187, 191, 194, 197, 199, 205, 210, 212, 215, 218, 233, 236, 240, 245, 247, 248, 250, 253, 255, 256, 270, 273, 279, 281, 285, 286, 287, 288, 290, 291, 292, 294
asymmetry, 55, 56, 57, 61
asymptomatic, 29, 32, 74
atopy, 249
atrophy, 104, 203, 213
audits, 125, 150, 152, 153, 295
autism, 92, 94, 95, 96

B

bacteria, 30, 31
banking, 281
banks, 288
basal lamina, 41

base, 78, 79, 80, 81, 83, 85, 122
basement membrane, 1, 9, 17, 96, 112, 188
beams, 135, 137
behaviors, 30, 94
Beijing, 17
Belgium, 276
beneficial effect, 48, 49, 63, 131, 220
benefits, 84, 131, 138, 139, 142, 147, 151, 257, 269, 273
beta blocker, 289
bias, 157, 190
bicarbonate, 46, 47
bilateral, 107, 215, 261
biocompatibility, 231
biocompatible materials, 231, 232
biomechanics, 232
biopsy, 11
blepharitis, 30, 31, 37, 285
blood, 213, 275
bonds, 30
branching, 12
Brazil, 253
breakdown, 41, 213

C

cadaver, 273
CAM, 180
candidates, 5, 6, 10, 87
capsule, 138, 192, 209, 272, 273, 275, 276
carbon, 49, 234
carbonic anhydrase inhibitors, 289
carbonyl groups, 251
case law, 150
cataract, 8, 21, 45, 53, 56, 92, 93, 102, 107, 110, 111, 115, 116, 117, 119, 120, 121, 122, 125, 126, 137, 139, 140, 142, 148, 149, 153, 182, 187, 194, 197, 198, 205, 208, 209, 212, 213, 215, 216, 218, 255, 269, 270, 272, 273, 274, 275, 276, 278, 279, 280, 285, 292
cataract extraction, 45, 110, 111
categorization, 164
catheter, 95
cefazolin, 31
cell culture, 252
cell death, 40, 64
cell surface, 47
cerebral palsy, 92, 94, 95
challenges, 50, 91, 93, 94, 95, 116, 125, 232, 295
changing environment, 197
charge coupled device, 137
chemical bonds, 64
chemotaxis, 96
Chicago, 195
childhood, 94, 107, 110, 111, 113, 114, 129, 140
children, 88, 92, 93, 94, 95, 96, 97, 98, 99, 100, 101, 102, 103, 104, 105, 106, 107, 108, 109, 110, 111, 112, 113, 201, 215, 216
circulation, 232
civil law, 146
clarity, vii, 3, 97, 193, 248, 290
classification, 32, 40, 51, 86, 245, 246, 247
cleaning, 29, 32, 33
cleavage, 1, 96, 269, 272, 287
clinical application, 201, 215
clinical diagnosis, 35, 40, 50
clinical examination, 188, 254, 256
clinical trials, 49, 55
closure, 4, 5, 6, 7, 286
coherence, 116, 122, 124, 125, 201, 215, 217, 218, 270, 272, 278, 279
collagen, 10, 15, 21, 23, 30, 51, 58, 63, 64, 65, 69, 71, 72, 209, 245, 248, 251
Colombia, 232
color, 65, 188, 189, 190
coma, 127, 129, 131, 132, 133, 134, 135, 139, 247, 273, 274
combined effect, 106
commercial, 146, 189, 270
common sense, 152
communication, 92, 149, 153
compliance, 6, 30, 145
complications, vii, 1, 3, 5, 8, 12, 13, 17, 25, 26, 31, 34, 55, 56, 57, 68, 73, 92, 96, 97, 98, 99, 101, 102, 106, 113, 146, 176, 181, 201, 203, 208, 217, 226, 231, 232, 239, 240, 248, 249, 252, 253, 254, 255, 276, 283, 284, 286, 292, 294
compression, 291, 292
computer, 36, 94, 117, 152, 188, 189
conditioning, 36
configuration, 192
confocal microscopy, 2, 12, 22, 64, 71
conformity, 222
congenital cataract, 113
conjunctiva, 37
connective tissue, 5, 150, 246
conscious sedation, 95
consent, 36, 50, 146, 147, 149, 151, 153
construction, 45, 273
contamination, 29
contamination of the interface, 29
contour, 188
contrast sensitivity, 17, 129, 131, 134, 138, 139, 141, 142, 178, 227, 257
control group, 59
controlled studies, 255, 258

convergence, 74, 76, 79, 82, 83, 85
copolymer, 209, 236
cornea, 12, 16, 26, 27, 29, 30, 31, 32, 41, 42, 50, 55, 58, 59, 60, 61, 62, 63, 64, 68, 71, 92, 94, 96, 107, 116, 117, 119, 120, 122, 130, 131, 138, 140, 150, 170, 187, 188, 189, 190, 191, 192, 194, 195, 197, 220, 223, 227, 228, 229, 232, 233, 235, 237, 240, 241, 245, 246, 249, 250, 251, 252, 253, 257, 270, 281, 282, 285, 286, 288
corneal transplant, 65, 269, 270, 282, 284, 292, 293, 294
corneal ulcer, 30
correlation, 40, 121, 148, 170
cortex, 270, 275
corticosteroids, 11, 13, 20, 31
cosmetic, 74, 84, 86, 215, 282
cost, 125, 254, 276, 295
Court of Appeals, 146
covalent bond, 251
covering, 146, 190
crystalline, 40, 64, 131, 140, 192, 193, 201, 209, 213, 214, 215
culture, 281
cure, 6
cycles, 274
cyclosporine, 42, 49, 53
cyst, 2
cytochrome, 51
cytokines, 32, 96
cytology, 40, 45
cytotoxicity, 71

D

damages, 146
data collection, 155
database, 198
debridement, 2, 13, 14, 18, 252
defects, 29, 33, 40, 48, 73, 214, 254
deficiencies, 6
deficiency(ies), 30, 35, 36, 41, 51, 76
deficit, 30
deformation, 56, 99, 211, 270, 272, 273
degradation, 15, 40
dehiscence, 275
dehydration, 29, 36
delirium, 95
deposition, 232
deposits, 201, 212, 214, 254
depression, 190
deprivation, 75
depth, 12, 14, 26, 27, 31, 42, 74, 79, 80, 81, 84, 87, 93, 94, 106, 116, 118, 131, 138, 141, 142, 170, 175, 192, 202, 205, 207, 216, 218, 220, 229, 232, 234, 237, 238, 240, 254, 256, 274, 287, 288, 292
depth perception, 87, 94
desiccation, 28
destruction, 41, 106
detachment, 101, 217
detection, 69, 133, 137, 246
deviation, 74, 75, 76, 80, 82, 83, 84, 86, 88, 89, 127
diabetes, 150, 275
differential diagnosis, 30
diffuse lamellar keratitis, 1, 33, 34, 174
diffusion, 233
diffusivity, 233
digestion, 246, 251
dilation, 191, 194
diplopia, 73, 74, 76, 77, 78, 79, 80, 81, 83, 84, 85, 86, 87, 89, 138
discomfort, 3, 4, 8, 31, 35, 36, 41, 45, 49, 97, 212
disease progression, 251
diseases, 10, 35, 41, 51, 53, 140, 293
dislocation, 29, 102, 213, 214, 216, 289
disorder, 98
dispersion, 99, 209, 212, 214, 216
displacement, 28, 135, 205, 274, 275
disposition, 177
dissatisfaction, 14, 80, 87, 145, 148
distilled water, 30
distribution, 69, 70
divergence, 79
DNA, 12
doctors, 146, 148, 150, 197
dominance, 78, 82, 83, 236, 242
dosage, 5
Down syndrome, 246
drainage, 288
drug abuse, 5
drugs, 38, 49, 76, 95
dry eyes, 31, 44, 48, 50, 62, 197, 222, 283
dry-eye syndrome, 141
drying, 4

E

eczema, 246
edema, 27, 29, 64, 102
Ehlers-Danlos syndrome, 246
electron, 16, 112
electron microscopy, 16, 112
elongation, 156, 170
endothelial cells, 22, 285
endothelial dysfunction, 149, 284, 285
endothelium, 13, 22, 63, 64, 113, 205, 211, 212, 215, 251, 252, 257, 286, 287, 288, 293

energy, 26, 28, 45, 269, 279
England, 1, 146
entrapment, 211, 275
environment, 38, 59, 95, 96, 284
environmental factors, 36
environmental influences, 246
enzyme, 246
epidemiology, 51
epithelial cells, 6, 18, 27, 32, 33, 41, 47, 51
epithelial in-growth, 1
epithelium, 1, 2, 3, 4, 7, 9, 13, 25, 27, 28, 30, 31, 33, 41, 47, 49, 53, 63, 174, 184, 252, 288, 290
equilibrium, 233
equipment, 25, 91, 92, 95, 115, 122, 125, 151, 152, 157, 172, 295
erosion, 8, 9, 14, 20
esotropia, 74, 82, 83, 84, 85, 87, 88, 105, 107, 113
essential fatty acids, 49
estrogen, 49
ethanol, 17, 33, 96, 112
ethnic groups, 246
etiology, 17, 34, 75, 212
Europe, 31, 53, 93, 101, 199, 220
evacuation, 26
evaporation, 36
evidence, 13, 39, 42, 44, 45, 48, 58, 59, 60, 70, 86, 92, 119, 148, 149, 159, 222, 251
evolution, 142, 157, 278, 281
examinations, 190, 192
excimer lasers, 278
excision, 285, 286
excitation, 65
exotropia, 74, 83, 84, 85, 86
expertise, 107
exposure, 3, 17, 18, 27, 28, 29, 36, 252, 254
extracellular matrix, 233, 251
extraction, 35, 36, 44, 45, 53, 91, 111, 217
extrusion, 232
eye movement, 95
eye-tracking, 26

F

family history, 32
family members, 199
fatty acids, 49
FDA approval, 252
fears, 60, 64
fiber(s), 30, 63, 65, 71
fibroblasts, 12, 233
fibrosis, 96
field defect, 188
filters, 80, 81
financial, 145, 146, 228, 276
first generation, 118, 252
fixation, 74, 75, 78, 80, 81, 83, 84, 86, 87, 192, 210, 235, 237
flap melt, 1, 33
flap removal technique, 4
flexibility, 83, 232
fluid, 28, 47, 250, 275, 288
fluoroquinolones, 7, 31
Food and Drug Administration (FDA), 151, 152, 217, 252
force, 27, 189
formation, 4, 8, 9, 11, 13, 23, 96, 135, 136, 175, 176, 208, 209, 212, 213, 215, 216, 251
formula, 93, 115, 116, 117, 118, 119, 120, 121, 122, 123, 124, 125, 126, 295
Fourier analysis, 129
fovea, 81, 86
France, 104, 113
free radicals, 65, 251
fungi, 10
fusion, 73, 74, 75, 76, 78, 79, 83, 85, 86, 89, 96, 98, 100, 103, 105, 107, 112, 113

G

general anaesthesia, 91, 95, 97
geometry, 197
Germany, 91, 118, 125, 219, 220, 227, 240, 251, 270
gland, 36, 37, 41, 49, 50
glasses, 55, 73, 74, 75, 76, 77, 79, 80, 82, 83, 84, 85, 87, 92, 94, 105, 106, 129, 226, 236, 240, 242, 291
glaucoma, 20, 98, 99, 201, 208, 209, 212, 214, 283, 289
glucose, 232, 233
goblet cells, 31, 37, 41
governance, 152
grades, 76
grading, 39, 40, 194
grids, 272, 274
growth, 1, 30, 32, 33, 41, 47, 50, 56, 93, 105, 106, 107, 110
growth factor, 41, 50, 93
guidance, 147, 194
guidelines, 113, 116, 145, 150, 152, 195

H

halos, 97
hay fever, 246

haze, 1, 2, 4, 5, 8, 11, 12, 13, 16, 18, 20, 22, 23, 44, 62, 64, 75, 96, 97, 107, 163, 171, 175, 176, 177, 252, 292
head injury, 85
healing, 1, 2, 3, 5, 6, 8, 11, 19, 22, 48, 50, 64, 71, 96, 106, 175, 233, 237, 242, 273, 287
health, 12, 38, 46, 49, 94, 98
health care, 94
health problems, 98
hearing impairment, 94
height, 45, 69, 189, 191, 192, 198
hemorrhage, 97, 99, 109
herpes, 10, 21, 150, 290
herpes simplex, 10, 21, 290
herpes simplex keratitis, 10, 290
high risk patients, 290
histidine, 251
historical data, 125, 295
history, 5, 10, 36, 50, 56, 73, 74, 76, 84, 85, 86, 88, 115, 117, 119, 122, 123, 124, 126, 138, 150, 157, 187, 198, 205, 275, 295
HLA, 50
hormones, 49
host, 257, 287, 292
House, 147
human, 21, 51, 52, 68, 69, 70, 110, 113, 135, 140, 141, 145, 146, 198, 218, 220, 229, 251, 281
humidity, 28, 38
Hunter, 293
hybrid, 250
hydrogels, 231, 232
hydrops, 68, 245, 249, 257
hydroxyethyl methacrylate, 236
hygiene, 7, 30, 285
hyperemia, 30, 31
hyperopia, 12, 18, 19, 22, 45, 53, 75, 82, 83, 84, 85, 88, 105, 107, 112, 129, 149, 155, 157, 158, 159, 162, 163, 176, 178, 179, 180, 203, 205, 210, 215, 218, 229, 233, 235, 252, 256
hyperplasia, 96
hypersensitivity, 29, 31
hypertension, 8, 20
hypoplasia, 13, 104

I

iatrogenic, 1, 57, 71, 177, 201, 202, 256, 288
illumination, 63, 137, 191
image(s), 64, 76, 78, 79, 81, 83, 84, 86, 87, 92, 106, 127, 129, 131, 132, 134, 135, 138, 188, 189, 190, 191, 192, 193, 196, 197, 198, 272, 273, 279
immersion, 115, 116
immune reaction, 31
immunofluorescence, 96
immunosuppression, 283
impairments, 94
implants, 49, 56, 62, 93, 102, 108, 150, 177, 231, 232, 239, 253, 269
improvements, 13, 15, 49, 91, 92, 93, 96, 106, 108, 122, 139, 236, 251, 253, 278
impurities, 30
in vitro, 71
in vivo, 12, 71, 252
inadmissible, 150
incidence, 7, 10, 26, 29, 32, 42, 44, 45, 50, 56, 57, 60, 62, 65, 156, 176, 177, 187, 203, 211, 212, 213, 228, 246, 253, 276, 288, 289
indentation, 116
independence, 219, 228, 276
individuals, 3, 4, 131, 140, 242, 245, 246
induction, 1, 5, 14, 15, 64, 95, 131, 138, 139, 141, 143, 220, 227
infancy, 129, 138, 269, 278
infants, 110, 113
infection, 5, 6, 10, 30, 48, 56, 215, 291
inflammation, 3, 35, 36, 45, 49, 56, 96, 99, 201, 214, 290
inflammatory cells, 28, 29, 96
inflammatory mediators, 45, 213
informed consent, 16, 146, 147, 149, 151
inhibition, 8, 80
injections, 289
injury, 85, 146, 175
insertion, 15, 16, 32, 63, 215, 216, 219, 232, 242, 279
insulin, 41
integration, 33, 278
integrity, 41, 51, 60, 233, 289, 291
interface, 27, 28, 29, 30, 31, 32, 33, 37, 175, 187, 189, 257, 270, 271, 272, 273, 281, 285, 287, 288, 292
interference, 26, 51, 119
intervention, 30, 215
intra-lamellar flap complications, 1
intraocular, 8, 13, 20, 23, 35, 36, 70, 91, 92, 93, 95, 97, 100, 109, 110, 111, 112, 113, 114, 115, 116, 117, 120, 122, 125, 126, 127, 138, 142, 155, 163, 177, 184, 185, 201, 202, 212, 215, 217, 218, 219, 220, 228, 245, 274, 278, 279, 288, 289, 290
intraocular pressure, 8, 13, 20, 23, 70, 97, 202, 289, 290
iodine, 29, 285
ions, 47
ipsilateral, 23
Ireland, 55, 127, 147, 148, 150, 155, 222, 231, 237, 238, 245

iridotomy, 212
iris, 101, 102, 109, 112, 177, 178, 185, 201, 203, 205, 207, 208, 209, 211, 212, 213, 214, 215, 216, 217, 286, 289
irradiation, 64
irrigation, 29, 32, 276
Islam, 181, 261
isolation, 59, 60, 65, 104
issues, 57, 91, 92, 93, 94, 97, 98, 101, 105, 106, 116, 149, 188, 231, 242, 249, 283
Italy, 25, 253, 260

J

Japan, 48, 137
jurisdiction, 146

K

keratoplasty, 10, 11, 13, 15, 55, 57, 63, 71, 133, 140, 157, 245, 249, 250, 253, 254, 255, 256, 257, 258, 279, 281, 283, 284, 285, 286, 287, 288, 292, 293, 294

L

laser ablation, 2, 5, 7, 10, 11, 12, 13, 18, 28, 97, 133, 143, 149, 155, 177, 188, 194, 220, 272
lasers, 26, 93, 95, 107, 117, 157, 269, 270, 276, 287
later life, 156
lead, 36, 64, 65, 80, 138, 146, 211, 213, 214, 274
learning, 97, 153, 242, 257, 276
legislation, 150
lens dislocation, 201
lesions, 104
life expectancy, 216
light, 15, 26, 37, 63, 65, 70, 76, 77, 78, 79, 81, 108, 114, 127, 129, 131, 132, 135, 137, 143, 189, 192, 226, 227, 234, 235, 237, 242, 250, 270
light transmission, 234
linoleic acid, 49
liposomes, 49
litigation, 116, 145, 149, 152
localization, 270
low risk, 85, 254, 285, 286
lubricants, 5, 8, 9, 47, 48, 290
Luo, 51

M

magnitude, 75, 84, 87, 137, 155, 156, 158, 163, 164, 165, 174, 175
management, 3, 7, 10, 14, 17, 20, 34, 46, 49, 51, 74, 91, 95, 110, 149, 245, 246, 248, 249, 250, 253, 256, 258, 281, 289, 291, 292
manipulation, 32, 212, 290
manufacturing, 189
marketing, 145
masking, 76
materials, 40, 48, 228, 281
matrix metalloproteinase, 10, 20
measurement(s), 8, 11, 15, 59, 60, 61, 70, 111, 116, 117, 122, 123, 125, 126, 127, 135, 137, 141, 150, 188, 192, 196, 197, 199, 202, 204, 222, 251, 270, 295
medical, 9, 10, 92, 94, 103, 105, 107, 118, 145, 146, 147, 148, 150, 151, 152, 153, 192, 282, 283
medical history, 150, 283
medication, 6, 7, 8, 12, 13, 226, 237
medicine, 152, 278
melt(s), 1, 5, 8, 21
melting, 4, 10, 11, 12, 19, 22, 27, 29, 33
membranes, 47
memory, 198
mentoring, 276
meridian, 63, 76, 80, 189, 190, 198, 270
messages, 226
meta-analysis, 12, 18, 85, 171, 182
metalloproteinase, 8
methodology, 39
methyl methacrylate, 236
methylprednisolone, 49
Miami, 89
microscope, 235, 237
microscopy, 2, 12, 22, 64, 71, 150
miosis, 14
mitosis, 41
MMA, 236
MMP-9, 49
mobile phone, 226
modelling, 68
models, 33, 49, 123, 125, 204, 205, 208, 217, 276, 295
moderate myopia, 2, 17, 18, 19, 112, 156, 164, 172, 178, 181
molecules, 40, 232, 251
monocular clues, 80
monomers, 209
morbidity, 35, 36, 283
morphology, 255, 279
Moscow, 217

MR, 18, 22, 52, 142, 195, 199, 217
mucin, 31, 36, 37, 40, 41
mucous membrane, 46
mycobacteria, 30

N

National Health Service, 148, 293
nausea, 289
Nd, 137, 138, 140, 210
necrosis, 33, 47, 231, 232
negative outcomes, 74
Nepal, 18
nerve, 12, 31, 50, 84, 85, 104, 175
nerve fibers, 31
nerve growth factor, 50
Netherlands, 93, 101, 205, 206, 208, 233, 254
neurons, 41
neuropathic pain, 35, 41, 50
neuropathy, 50, 97
neurotransmitters, 41
neutral, 47, 294
NHS, 1, 148
nodules, 37
North America, 93
nuclei, 276
nucleus, 131, 275, 279
nutrient, 233, 236
nutrition, 231
nystagmus, 92, 104, 105, 107

O

occlusion, 46
oedema, 232, 254, 274, 276
oil, 36, 47
old age, 129
omega-3, 49
opacification, 99, 138
opacity, 30
operations, 25, 30
ophthalmologist, 58, 139, 146, 151, 188, 297
optic nerve, 92, 94, 104
orbit, 37
organ, 94
organism, 7
osmolality, 47
osteogenesis, 259
osteogenesis imperfecta, 246
outpatient, 9, 283, 290
oxygen, 48, 65, 95, 233, 251

P

pain, 1, 2, 3, 4, 5, 6, 11, 18, 19, 38, 96, 97, 147, 149, 252, 284, 289
pain management, 252
paracentesis, 288
parallel, 29, 129, 137
paresis, 76
pathogenesis, 26, 49
pathogens, 30
pathology, 91, 104, 107, 109, 129, 137, 188, 189, 203, 217, 235, 279, 282, 285, 287
pathophysiology, 18, 51, 292
perforation, 19, 254, 287
permanent wrinkling, 1
permeability, 213
personality disorder, 149
pH, 47
pharmaceutical, 48
pharmacotherapy, 20
Philadelphia, 90
photodetectors, 137
photographs, 192
photophobia, 26, 30
photorefractive keratectomy (PRK), 1, 2, 3, 4, 5, 7, 8, 10, 11, 12, 13, 15, 16, 17, 18, 19, 20, 21, 22, 23, 26, 27, 28, 30, 32, 35, 36, 41, 44, 50, 52, 56, 59, 60, 61, 62, 68, 70, 74, 80, 89, 91, 93, 96, 97, 98, 109, 111, 112, 113, 120, 121, 126, 141, 153, 156, 160, 179, 180, 181, 182, 183, 184, 188, 192, 199, 235, 255, 256, 258, 292, 297
physical activity, 288
physical properties, 239, 240
physiology, 47, 60, 141, 232, 233
pilot study, 237, 238, 239
placebo, 49
plaque, 33
plasticity, 86
platform, 17, 98, 180, 229, 270, 272
plexus, 31, 175
PMMA, 101, 204, 205, 253
point spread function, 131, 133, 134
pollen, 37
poly(methyl methacrylate), 253
polymer, 209, 232
polymer chains, 232
polypropylene, 286
polyvinylidene fluoride, 234
population, 37, 38, 45, 70, 73, 91, 92, 111, 138, 156, 159, 178, 182, 216, 217, 245, 251
postoperative outcome, 110
postoperative pain, 4, 19, 96
potassium, 46, 47

predictability, 2, 21, 82, 116, 120, 125, 157, 158, 159, 163, 164, 171, 176, 177, 178, 182, 201, 202, 204, 205, 216, 224, 227, 255, 258, 269, 273
pregnancy, 248
prematurity, 95, 216
presbyopia, vii, 44, 45, 52, 53, 85, 86, 87, 89, 140, 159, 219, 220, 222, 227, 228, 229, 231, 233, 242, 270, 297
preservation, 19, 201, 216, 286
preservative, 5, 6, 7, 8, 10, 13, 46
prevention, 17, 29, 51, 88, 284
probe, 116
profit, 148
prognosis, 69, 151, 184, 199
pro-inflammatory, 32
proliferation, 32
prophylactic, 7, 10, 175
proteinase, 246
proteins, 29, 232
proteoglycans, 251
pseudophakia, 110, 111
pterygium, 12, 22
ptosis, 104
public health, 276

Q

quality of life, vii, 15, 38, 108

R

race, 145
radial keratotomy, 13, 121, 125, 141, 188
radiation, 260
radius, 117, 189, 190, 197
reactive oxygen, 64
reactivity, 93
reading, 36, 83, 85, 94, 116, 119, 194, 195, 196, 222, 226, 227, 236, 240, 242, 247
reality, 37
reasoning, 146
recall, 38, 149
recalling, 157
recession, 148
recognition, 34, 150, 157, 291
recommendations, 46, 53, 124, 295
reconstruction, 192
recovery, 1, 2, 4, 5, 6, 7, 8, 18, 41, 47, 75, 78, 79, 95, 175, 201, 202, 216, 291
recurrence, 33, 175, 256
refractive index, 131, 140
regeneration, 6, 50
registries, 256, 282
regression, 11, 13, 15, 22, 42, 52, 62, 75, 82, 93, 96, 106, 117, 121, 123, 126, 155, 156, 157, 158, 159, 162, 163, 164, 165, 167, 169, 170, 171, 172, 173, 174, 175, 176, 178, 183, 184, 201, 202, 231
regression analysis, 117
regression equation, 123
rehabilitation, 2, 15, 55, 56, 57, 70, 201, 202, 245, 249, 254, 256, 258, 281, 283, 284, 288, 291, 294
rejection, 92, 256, 257, 283, 284, 285, 286, 288, 290, 291, 292
relative size, 241
relaxation, 30, 291
relevance, 149, 197, 275
relief, 5, 84, 99, 289
repair, 29, 63, 147
replication, 12
requirements, 123, 151
resection, 31, 70
residual error, 162
resistance, 251
resolution, 5, 9, 14, 59, 86, 92, 93, 98, 153
response, 8, 11, 31, 39, 49, 77, 78, 83, 106, 108, 155, 248
restoration, 97, 99
restrictions, 84, 222
retina, 92, 94, 129, 137, 227, 242, 251, 252, 274
retinal detachment, 101, 202, 205
retinopathy, 216
rheumatoid arthritis, 150, 283
riboflavin, 21, 23, 63, 64, 65, 70, 71, 251, 252
rings, 32, 33, 44, 63, 188, 190, 269, 270, 271, 274
risk(s), 1, 5, 8, 9, 11, 12, 15, 16, 32, 33, 36, 48, 50, 52, 55, 56, 58, 59, 60, 61, 62, 63, 65, 70, 73, 75, 81, 82, 83, 84, 85, 86, 87, 88, 89, 98, 101, 137, 147, 148, 149, 151, 153, 163, 172, 175, 176, 177, 182, 183, 184, 188, 195, 202, 209, 211, 215, 216, 220, 248, 249, 252, 254, 255, 283, 285, 286, 287, 289, 290, 291
risk factors, 50, 52, 60, 61, 63, 65, 70, 148, 149, 153, 177, 182, 183, 184, 283, 286
RNA, 12
root, 127, 211, 247
rosacea, 46
rules, 30

S

safety, 2, 22, 32, 55, 58, 91, 93, 96, 150, 163, 183, 201, 204, 205, 208, 215, 227, 243, 252, 254, 255, 258, 275, 278
salivary gland, 46
scanning electron microscopy, 273

sclera, 12
sclerosis, 156
scotoma, 74, 77, 80, 81, 83, 84, 86
secretion, 20, 41, 50
sensation, 3, 30, 31, 36, 40, 41, 42, 44, 50, 51, 52, 53
sensitivity, 39, 52, 64, 139, 226
sensors, 135
sequencing, 40
serum, 32, 48, 53
sex, 38, 248
shape, 41, 47, 58, 127, 131, 133, 138, 140, 188, 189, 190, 194, 197, 201, 215, 232, 245, 246, 247, 253, 255, 258
showing, 12, 42, 43, 66, 87, 97, 133, 190, 225, 253, 284
signs, 5, 7, 9, 10, 11, 39, 40, 41, 51, 57, 66, 96, 150, 226, 256, 284, 291
silicon, 205
SLA, 18
slit lamp, 9, 13, 28, 30, 33, 40, 150, 191, 289, 290
slit lamp examination, 9, 40, 290
smoothness, 49
social interactions, 94
society, 88, 148
sodium, 47, 48
software, 116, 123, 124, 125, 190, 272, 295
solution, 1, 3, 19, 22, 48, 49, 63, 116, 120, 126, 155, 158, 242, 287
South Africa, 148
species, 7, 10, 64
sponge, 9, 29, 30, 287
stability, 2, 11, 16, 22, 62, 63, 64, 99, 150, 155, 156, 157, 158, 159, 162, 163, 164, 165, 169, 171, 172, 173, 175, 176, 177, 178, 180, 181, 184, 185, 210, 251, 252, 254, 255, 258, 273, 274, 278
stabilization, 15, 63, 163, 174
standard deviation, 123, 160, 161, 222, 227
standard error, 256
state(s), 35, 36, 41, 92, 114, 129, 131, 150, 253, 278
stem cells, 63
sterile, 6, 20, 30, 31, 238, 252, 285
steroids, 8, 13, 21, 26, 252, 285, 290, 291
stimulant, 48
stimulus, 248
strabismus, 73, 74, 75, 76, 77, 82, 83, 84, 85, 86, 87, 88, 89, 92, 94, 105, 112, 113, 147
stress, 40, 51, 60, 73, 74, 82, 83, 84, 85, 251
stress test, 82, 83, 84, 85
stretching, 28, 147
striae, 29, 30, 174, 249
stroma, 1, 9, 29, 30, 33, 60, 64, 65, 96, 175, 205, 232, 233, 251, 252, 255, 287, 288
stromal flaps, 1
structural changes, 51, 64
structure, 37, 58, 65, 191, 233
subepithelial fibrosis, 183
success rate, 284, 292
Sun, 52, 125
suppression, 74, 76, 77, 78, 80, 81, 82, 83, 84, 86, 87, 89
Supreme Court, 147, 153
surface tension, 28
surface treatment, 32, 61, 63, 65, 151
surgical intervention, 10, 13, 155, 249
surgical technique, 25, 26, 93, 94, 98, 101, 105, 188, 201, 203, 211, 292, 293
survival, 256, 284, 289, 291, 294
suture, 207, 254, 286, 290, 291
swelling, 6, 27, 30
Switzerland, 233, 237, 240, 254
symptoms, 5, 8, 9, 10, 11, 14, 26, 35, 36, 38, 40, 41, 42, 44, 45, 46, 48, 49, 50, 51, 53, 76, 80, 83, 127, 146, 162, 226, 283, 291
syndrome, 8, 9, 14, 20, 41, 42, 45, 48, 51, 53, 107, 108, 109, 237, 275, 280
systemic lupus erythematosus, 10

T

target, 73, 75, 76, 79, 80, 81, 82, 85, 116, 124, 158, 162, 163, 176, 220, 221, 223, 224, 225, 227, 281, 295
Task Force, 46, 89
task performance, 236
techniques, vii, 2, 18, 35, 36, 64, 92, 94, 95, 98, 111, 116, 117, 125, 152, 155, 157, 159, 162, 171, 183, 193, 202, 220, 227, 252, 256, 257, 258, 269, 270, 281, 284, 288, 289, 290, 291, 292, 293, 295, 297
technological advancement, 155
technological advances, 127, 129
technological change, 107
technology(ies), vii, 14, 57, 61, 98, 106, 107, 108, 115, 116, 123, 124, 125, 137, 142, 157, 175, 188, 191, 193, 201, 202, 216, 231, 232, 233, 242, 273, 274, 276, 278, 280, 284, 287, 293, 295
teens, 92, 245
telephone, 151, 283
temperature, 28
tensile strength, 60, 61, 70
tension, 232
testing, 40, 88, 108
testosterone, 49
tetracyclines, 7, 8
therapeutic use, 187, 194
therapy, 9, 10, 28, 49, 53, 71, 74, 92, 100, 103, 215, 285, 290

thinning, 32, 58, 60, 64, 232, 245, 248, 254
threshold level, 252
time frame, 55, 63
tissue, 2, 26, 29, 58, 60, 62, 64, 93, 107, 177, 205, 207, 213, 232, 233, 249, 251, 253, 255, 269, 281, 282, 285, 288, 294
topical anesthetic, 19
topical antibiotics, 5, 252
torsion, 74, 76
toxicity, 5, 6, 7, 29, 45, 47, 63, 64, 251, 290
trajectory, 108
transforming growth factor, 49, 53
transparency, 11, 13, 22, 233, 248
transplant, 31, 32, 284
transplantation, 46, 65, 281, 282, 293, 294
transport, 47, 232, 233
trauma, 28, 76, 99, 212, 213, 214
treatment methods, 65, 94
trial, 2, 17, 18, 19, 21, 22, 38, 48, 49, 60, 77, 83, 86, 87, 108, 112, 142, 148, 151, 179, 183, 217, 221, 256
trigeminal nerve, 44

U

ultrasonography, 116
ultrasound, 65, 115, 125, 188, 192, 269, 274, 279, 290, 295
United Kingdom, (UK), 39, 88, 89, 93, 99, 113, 131, 147, 148, 150, 152, 217, 237, 257, 266, 269, 293
unmasking, 159
USA, 31, 40, 93, 98, 137, 232, 233, 252, 253, 272, 273, 282, 293
UV, 15, 65
UV irradiation, 65
UVA irradiation, 64, 252
uveitis, 98, 203, 208, 216, 275, 283

V

vacuum, 44, 240, 286
variables, 118, 156, 163
variations, 69, 74, 155, 157, 162, 171, 257, 269
vascular diseases, 10
vascularization, 48
VDF, 234
vector, 255
velocity, 38, 116
vertebrates, 49
vessels, 213
viscosity, 47, 49
visual acuity, 6, 7, 16, 26, 30, 31, 32, 40, 48, 64, 80, 83, 86, 90, 94, 96, 98, 103, 104, 110, 131, 138, 160, 161, 174, 175, 176, 177, 193, 202, 212, 214, 219, 221, 222, 233, 235, 236, 248, 249, 251, 253, 283, 290, 291, 293
visual field, 80
visual recovery, 1, 2, 4, 6, 7, 8, 18, 216
vomiting, 95

W

Wales, 146
water, 30, 47, 209, 232, 233
wear, 3, 38, 44, 48, 63, 85, 94, 105, 249, 284
workers, 94, 101, 102, 103, 274
wound dehiscence, 290, 291
wound healing, 11, 12, 21, 47, 155, 159, 175, 292

Y

young adults, 105